HEALTHCARE TECHNOLOGIES SERIES 54

Medical Equipment Engineering

Other volumes in this series:

Volume 1	**Nanobiosensors for Personalized and Onsite Biomedical Diagnosis** P. Chandra (Editor)
Volume 2	**Machine Learning for Healthcare Technologies** D.A. Clifton (Editor)
Volume 3	**Portable Biosensors and Point-of-Care Systems** S.E. Kintzios (Editor)
Volume 4	**Biomedical Nanomaterials: From design to implementation** T.J. Webster and H. Yazici (Editors)
Volume 6	**Active and Assisted Living: Technologies and applications** F. Florez-Revuelta and A.A. Chaaraoui (Editors)
Volume 7	**Semiconductor Lasers and Diode-based Light Sources for Biophotonics** P.E. Andersen and P.M. Petersen (Editors)
Volume 9	**Human Monitoring, Smart Health and Assisted Living: Techniques and technologies** S. Longhi, A. Monteriù and A. Freddi (Editors)
Volume 13	**Handbook of Speckle Filtering and Tracking in Cardiovascular Ultrasound Imaging and Video** C.P. Loizou, C.S. Pattichis and J. D'hooge (Editors)
Volume 14	**Soft Robots for Healthcare Applications: Design, modelling, and control** S. Xie, M. Zhang and W. Meng
Volume 16	**EEG Signal Processing: Feature extraction, selection and classification methods** W. Leong
Volume 17	**Patient-Centered Digital Healthcare Technology: Novel applications for next generation healthcare systems** L. Goldschmidt and R.M. Relova (Editors)
Volume 19	**Neurotechnology: Methods, advances and applications** V. de Albuquerque, A. Athanasiou and S. Ribeiro (Editors)
Volume 20	**Security and Privacy of Electronic Healthcare Records: Concepts, paradigms and solutions** S. Tanwar, S. Tyagi and N. Kumar (Editors)
Volume 23	**Advances in Telemedicine for Health Monitoring: Technologies, design and applications** T.A. Rashid, C. Chakraborty and K. Fraser
Volume 24	**Mobile Technologies for Delivering Healthcare in Remote, Rural or Developing Regions** P. Ray, N. Nakashima, A. Ahmed, S. Ro and Y. Soshino (Editors)
Volume 26	**Wireless Medical Sensor Networks for IoT-Based eHealth** F. Al-Turjman (Editor)
Volume 29	**Blockchain and Machine Learning for e-Healthcare Systems** B. Balusamy, N. Chilamkurti, L.A. Beena and P. Thangamuthu (Editors)
Volume 31	**Technologies and Techniques in Gait Analysis: Past, present and future** Nachiappan Chockalingam (Editor)
Volume 33	**Electromagnetic Waves and Antennas for Biomedical Applications** L. Wang
Volume 34	**The Internet of Medical Things: Enabling technologies and emerging applications** S.K. Pani, P. Patra, G. Ferrari, R. Kraleva and H. Wang (Editors)
Volume 36	**Applications of Machine Learning in Digital Healthcare** M.H. Silveira and S.-S. Ang (Editors)
Volume 37	**Technology-Enabled Motion Sensing and Activity Tracking for Rehabilitation** W. Zhoa
Volume 38	**Healthcare Monitoring and Data Analysis Using IoT: Technologies and applications** V. Jain, J. M. Chatterjee, P. Kumar and U. Kose (Editors)
Volume 39	**Digital Tools and Methods to Support Healthy Ageing** P.K. Ray, S.-T. Liaw and J.A. Serano (Editors)
Volume 40	**Applications of Artificial Intelligence in E-Healthcare Systems** Munish Sabharwal, B. Balamurugan Baluswamy, S. Rakesh Kumar, N. Gayathri, and Shakhzod Suvanov (Editors)
Volume 41	**Innovations in Healthcare Informatics: From interoperability to data analysis** M. Abouhawwash, S. Tanwar, A. Nayyar and M. Naved (Editors)
Volume 42	**Smart Health Technologies for the COVID-19 Pandemic: Internet of Medical Things perspectives** C. Chakraborty and J.J.P.C. Rodrigues (Editors)
Volume 44	**Medical Information Processing and Security: Techniques and applications** A. Kumar Singh and H. Zhou (Editors)
Volume 46	**Digital Twin Technologies for Healthcare 4.0** R.K. Dhanaraj, S. Murugesan, B. Balusamy, and V.E. Balas
Volume 50	**Explainable Artificial Intelligence in Medical Decision Support Systems** Agbotiname Lucky Imoize, Jude Hemanth, Dinh-Thuan Do and Samarendra Nath Sur (Editors)

Medical Equipment Engineering

Design, manufacture and applications

Edited by
Wai Yie Leong

The Institution of Engineering and Technology

Published by The Institution of Engineering and Technology, London, United Kingdom

The Institution of Engineering and Technology is registered as a Charity in England & Wales (no. 211014) and Scotland (no. SC038698).

First published 2023

The Institution of Engineering and Technology
Futures Place
Kings Way, Stevenage
Hertfordshire SG1 2UA, United Kingdom

www.theiet.org

British Library Cataloguing in Publication Data
A catalogue record for this product is available from the British Library

ISBN 978-1-83953-706-6 (hardback)
ISBN 978-1-83953-707-3 (PDF)

Typeset in India by MPS Ltd

Cover Image: Martin Barraud / OJO Images via Getty Images

Contents

About the editors

Wai Yie Leong is a senior professor at INTI International University, Malaysia, and is the chairperson of The Institution of Engineering and Technology Industry Revolution 4.0 Technical Network. She is involved with numerous professional engineering societies including a position as the vice president of the International Network of Women Engineers and Scientists (INWES), and chairman of The Institution of Engineering and Technology (Malaysia Local Network) and committee member of World Federation of Engineering Organisation (Women in Engineering Committee). Her specialisms include Industry 4.0, wireless sensor networks, ultra-wideband and wireless communications, and brain signal processing for signal conditioning and classification.

Preface

The future of Medical Equipment Engineering is shaping up in front of our very eyes with advances in digital healthcare technologies, such as artificial intelligence, VR/AR, 3D-printing, robotics or nanotechnology. We have to familiarize with the latest developments in Medical Equipment Engineering in order to be able to control technology and not the other way around. The future of Medical Equipment Engineering lies in working hand-in-hand with technology and healthcare workers have to embrace emerging healthcare technologies in order to stay relevant in the coming years.

A holistic Medical Equipment Engineering will affect many areas, most notably:

- Equipment services and engineering business models
- Equipment reliability and continuous productivity
- IT security
- Machine safety, standard and maintenance
- Equipment product lifecycles
- Industry value chain
- Technicians and workers' education and skills
- Healthcare and socio-economic factors
- Industry demonstration

In this book, we will discuss on Medical Equipment Engineering Revolution and technology requirements that bring robots closer to humans in smart equipment manufacturing environments where computer-integrated equipment manufacturing, high levels of adaptability and rapid equipment design changes, digital information technology, and more flexible technical working training are required. Medical Equipment Engineering can also assist in surveying workplace inefficiencies and worker safety. Efficiency optimization is a huge focus for adopters of "smart" systems, which is done through data research and intelligent learning automation. We will discuss the benefits of the integration of lean manufacturing, smart sensors, 5G technology, IoTs, virtual reality, 3D printing, robotics and automation.

Medical Equipment industry requires Human–Machine Interface (HMI) technologies to reduce complexity and processes and adding value to Medical Equipment Engineering. However, while business processes are changing rapidly, industries and manufacturers are struggling to exploit the full potential of digitization. This book will present the roadmap, from both a strategic and technological perspectives, to visualize each step on the route towards smart Medical Equipment manufacturing.

The importance of the human factor will be studied through the implementation of the "Sand Cone Model." A new framework will be proposed in order to explain the quality measures to the quality skills, and how it will improve efficiency and effectiveness of an industrial process.

Medical equipment engineers design tools, methods, and medical equipment to treat, cure, or otherwise benefit from medical disorders. While the precise tasks a biomedical engineer completes on a daily basis vary depending on the project, some of the most typical ones include:

- Create medical equipment like pacemakers or prosthetic limbs
- Repairing and setting up medical equipment
- Conduct novel analysis of biological systems and current biomedical devices
- Teach medical personnel how to use modern instruments

To explore engineering and medical care, you need to build a special set of abilities and knowledge if you want to join the ranks of professional medical equipment engineers who are applying cutting-edge science and technology to some of the most challenging issues in healthcare.

Medical equipment engineers have the chance to develop medical devices and other technology that enhances and saves lives as a medical equipment engineer and biomedical engineer. The inventions could improve healthcare and provide patients with improved chances of recovery. A medical equipment engineer applies knowledge and abilities to improve the lives of others.

Wai Yie Leong

Chapter 1

Medical equipment engineering revolution

Wai Yie Leong[1]

The application of engineering principles, technology, and design principles to medicine and biology for healthcare reasons is known as medical equipment engineering (BEE) or biomedical system engineering (BSE) (e.g., diagnostic or therapeutic). BEE is a traditional logical science used to promote therapy, monitoring, and diagnosis in the field of medicine (Figure 1.1). The management of modern medical equipment in hospitals and the healthcare sector while complying with pertinent industry standards falls under the purview of a biomedical engineer. This is a job that also goes by the name of clinical engineering or biomedical equipment technician (BMET), and it entails purchasing, routine testing, preventive maintenance, and providing equipment recommendations.

In contrast to many other engineering disciplines, medical equipment engineering has just lately been a separate field of study. A new subject frequently undergoes this transformation as it transitions from being an interdisciplinary specialty among already-established topics to being regarded as a field in and of itself. Research and development are a large portion of the job in medical equipment engineering and biomedical engineering, which encompasses a wide range of subfields (bioinformatics, biomechanics, biomaterials, tissue engineering, genetic engineering, pharmaceutical technology, medical imaging, implants technology, hospital, and medical devices) (Figure 1.2). Development of biocompatible prostheses, different diagnostic and therapeutic medical devices ranging from clinical equipment to microimplants, common imaging equipment such as magnetic resonance imaging (MRI) and EKG/ECG, regenerative tissue growth, pharmaceutical drugs, and therapeutic biologicals are a few notable applications of biomedical engineering [1].

1.1 Medical devices

This is a very broad category that essentially includes all medical goods that do not produce their desired effects primarily through chemical (e.g., pharmaceuticals) or biological (e.g., vaccines) means and do not involve metabolism.

[1]The Institution of Engineering and Technology, Malaysia

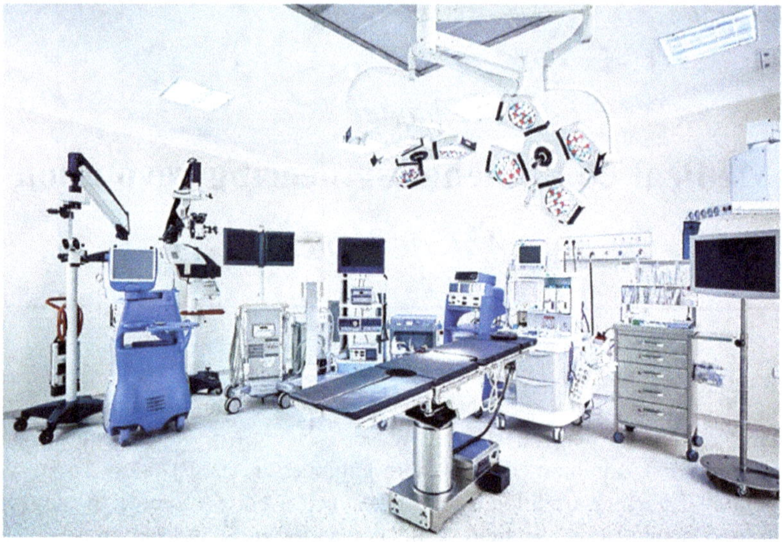

Figure 1.1 Medical equipment devices [2]

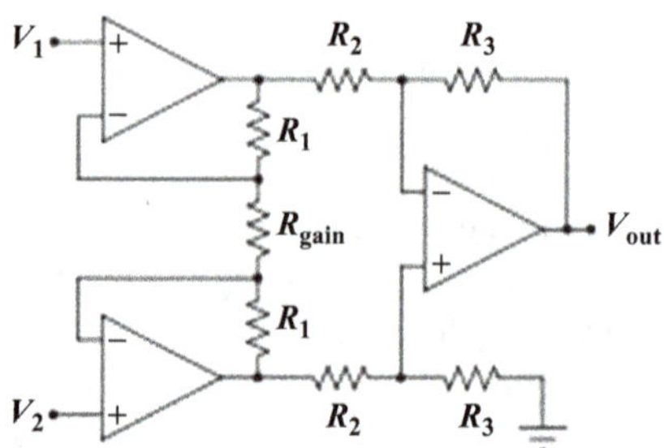

Figure 1.2 An illustration of a biomedical engineering application of electronic engineering to electrophysiology is a biomedical instrumentation amplifier schematic used in detecting low-voltage biological signals [3]

An intended purpose for a medical gadget is as follows:

- The diagnosis of sickness or other disorders
- In the treatment, mitigation, prevention, or cure of disease

Pacemakers, infusion pumps, heart–lung machine, dialysis units, artificial organs, implants, and artificial limbs are a few examples. Other examples include corrective lenses, cochlear implants, ocular prosthetics, face prosthetics, somato-prosthetics, and dental implants.

A real-world illustration of medical modeling is applied to the production of actual items is stereolithography. Emerging engineering techniques are now applied in the study and development of new devices for cutting-edge therapies, treatments, patient monitoring, and complex diseases, in addition to modeling organs and the human body.

In the United States, medical devices are categorized and subject to the following regulations:

Class I devices often have simpler designs than Class II or Class III devices and pose the least risk to the user of injury. Tongue depressors, bedpans, elastic bandages, exam gloves, handheld surgical instruments, and other items of comparable common equipment fall under this category.

Special controls in addition to the standard controls for Class I devices apply to Class II devices. Unique controls may include post market monitoring, mandated performance standards, and special labeling requirements. This category of equipment includes powered wheelchairs, infusion pumps, picture archiving and communication systems (PACS), X-ray machines, and surgical drapes. These devices are normally noninvasive.

In addition to the usual regulations of Class I, Class III devices typically need premarket approval (PMA) or premarket notification (510k), a scientific study to assure the device's safety and effectiveness. Examples include implanted brain stimulators, hip and knee replacement joints, endosseous (inside-the-bone) implants, silicone gel-filled breast implants, and replacement heart valves.

1.2 Medical imaging

A significant subset of medical equipment is biomedical and medical imaging. This topic focuses on giving physicians the ability to "see" things that are not immediately obvious (e.g., because of their size or position). Utilizing ultrasound, magnetic, UV, radiography, and other techniques may be necessary for this.

Imaging technologies, which include fluoroscopy, MRI, nuclear medicine, positron emission tomography (PET), PET-CT scans, projection radiography, including X-rays and CT scans, tomography, ultrasound, optical microscopy, and electron microscopy, are frequently crucial to medical diagnosis (Figure 1.3). They are also typically the most complex equipment found in a hospital.

1.3 Implants

A type of medical implant is a device designed to replace and function as a missing biological structure (as compared with a transplant, which indicates transplanted biomedical tissue). Depending on what is most functional, the surface of implants that come into contact with the body may be made of a biomedical substance such as titanium, silicone, or apatite. Electronic components may be found in some implants such as cochlear implants and artificial pacemakers (Figures 1.4 and 1.5). Some implants are bioactive, such as stents that distribute drugs subcutaneously or implantable pills that do the same.

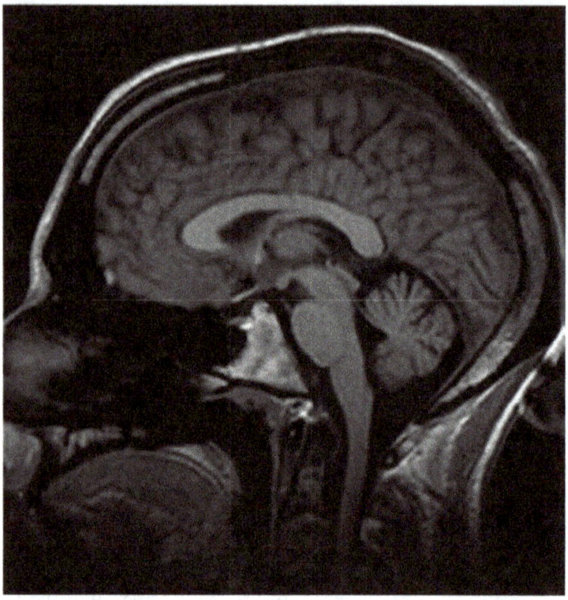

Figure 1.3 An illustration of a biomedical engineering application of electrical engineering to diagnostic imaging is an MRI scan of a human head [3]

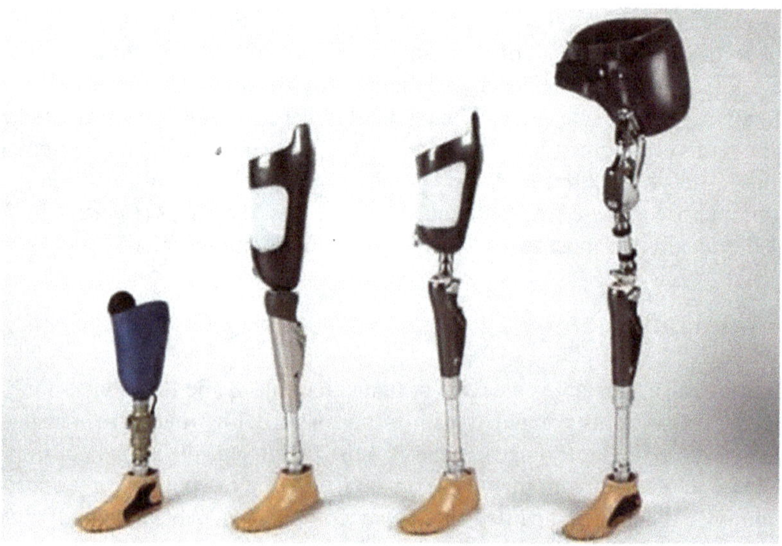

Figure 1.4 The prosthetic limb, popularly known as Jaipur Foot [4]

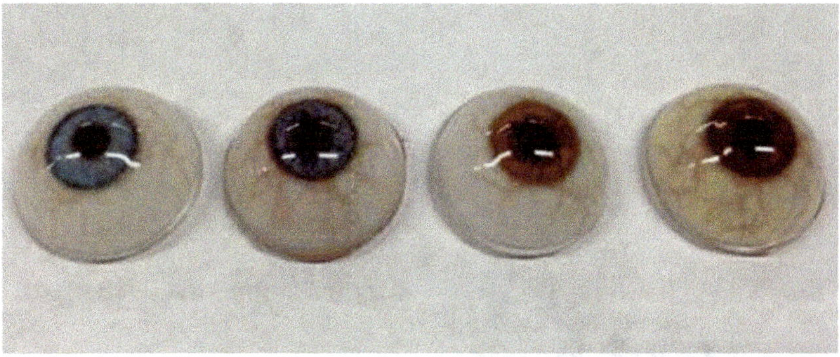

Figure 1.5 A prosthetic eye is an illustration of how mechanical engineering and biocompatible materials are used in biomedical engineering to advance ophthalmology [5]

1.4 Bionics

Replacement of artificial bodily parts is just one of the many uses for bionics. Bionics is a branch of engineering that deals with the deep and extensive research of the characteristics and operation of human body systems. Improvements to cameras, television, radio transmitters, and receivers, among other tools, were made possible by careful research of the various processes and functions of the eyes, ears, and other organs.

1.5 Biomedical sensors

Microwave-based biological sensors have drawn increased interest in recent years. For example, microwave sensors can be used as a supplemental method to X-ray to monitor lower extremity trauma. Different sensors can be developed for specific usage in both diagnosing and monitoring illness states. When measuring at various points during the healing process, the sensor's response will change as the trauma heals since the sensor monitors the dielectric properties and may thus detect changes in tissue (bone, muscle, fat, etc.) under the skin (Figure 1.6).

Medical equipment engineer may use their engineering skills to flourish in healthcare because engineering is the only industry that uniquely connects engineering and healthcare. If you are interested in medicine but are unable to pursue an engineering career, there is a bonus field for you. Mechanical engineers can easily specialize in biomedical engineering. It includes studying several types of engineering such as electronics, computer, mechanical, biochemical, and nanotechnology.

If you have ever wanted to work alongside a doctor, this is a wonderful field to pursue because medical equipment engineers collaborate closely with medical professionals including doctors and scientists. Not to mention the rewarding earnings in this industry, which inspire students to major in medical equipment engineering all over the world.

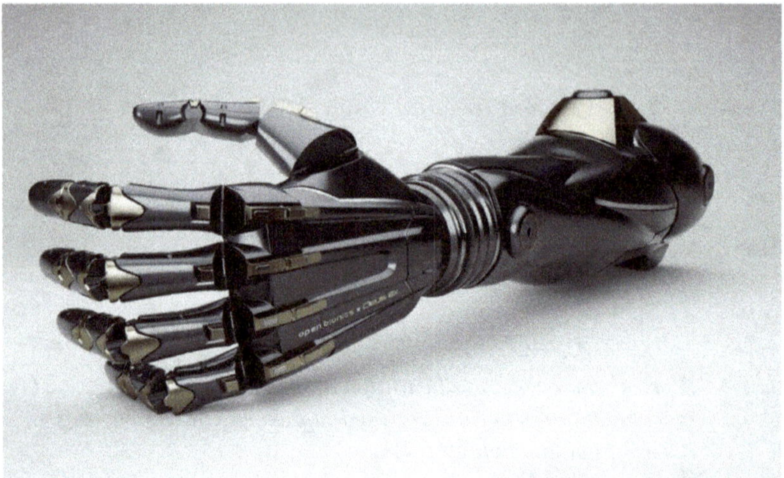

Figure 1.6 Open bionics bionic arm [6]

1.6 Industry perspectives

The market for smart medical devices was valued at USD 3.58 billion in 2016 and is projected to grow at a compound annual growth rate (CAGR) of 24.0% to USD 24.46 billion by 2025 (Figure 1.7). The market has been examined based on the product type, end user, distribution channel, and geographic location.

The healthcare sector is significantly impacted by smartphones. Global smartphone adoption increase, escalating need for wireless and smartphone compatible medical devices, rising public awareness of and interest in health and fitness, and rising home healthcare demand are all projected to drive market expansion.

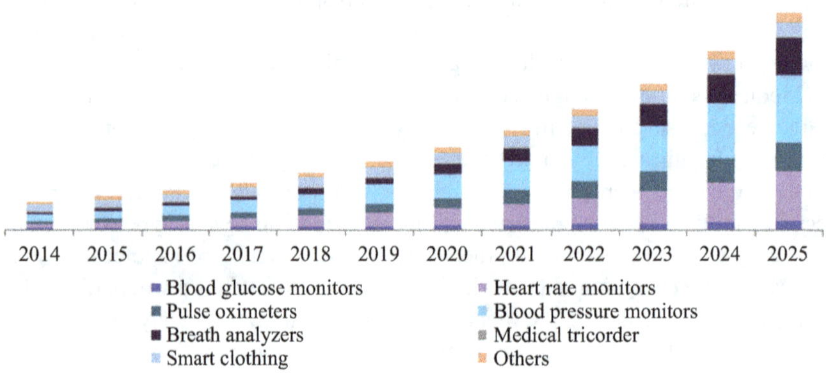

Figure 1.7 US smart medical devices market by product, 2014–2025 [7]

Global health concerns, the prevalence of chronic diseases, rising healthcare costs, and a rise in wearable gadget demand are all predicted to have a positive impact on the industry. Innovative products have been released by businesses such as Apple, Inc., Fitbit, Inc., and Medtronic, which is also anticipated to support market growth. Over the projection period, smart blood pressure monitors and smart apparel are anticipated to capture a sizable market share.

1.7 Regional perspectives

Asia Pacific accounted for more than 19.0% of the market's overall revenue in 2016 and was noted as the region with the fastest growing smart medical device market (Table 1.1). The state of emerging economies has been improving, including China and Japan. Population growth, higher living standards brought on by rising disposable income, and consumer demand for innovative, and cutting-edge products have all boosted the market for smart medical devices in the area [7].

Due to the high acceptance of cutting-edge technology and the presence of a highly developed healthcare industry, which is projected to foster the expansion of smart medical devices in the area, North America held the greatest market share in 2016. The region's healthcare system has benefited significantly from the positive economic climate, increased per capita income, and enhanced living standards.

Over the projection period, Europe is anticipated to increase its market share. The Reflection and Orientation Paper states that in 2016, the European Union contributed USD 43.5 million to innovative and team projects for wearable medical devices.

Table 1.1 Revenue growth at global, regional, and country levels and an analysis of the industry trends in each of the subsegments from 2014 to 2025

Attribute	Details
Base year for estimation	2016
Actual estimates/historical data	2014–2016
Forecast period	2017–2025
Market representation	Revenue in USD million and CAGR from 2017 to 2025
Regional scope	North America, Europe, Asia Pacific, Latin America, and Middle East Asia
Country scope	United States, Canada, United Kingdom, Germany, China, Japan, Mexico, Brazil, and South Africa
Report coverage	Revenue forecast, company share, competitive landscape, growth factors and trends
15% free customization scope (equivalent to five analyst working days)	If you need specific market information, which is not currently within the scope of the report, we will provide it to you as a part of customization

1.8 Market share insights for smart medical devices

Abbott, Apple, Fitbit, Dexcom, F. Hoffmann-La Roche Ltd., Zephyr, Sonova, NeuroMetrix, Inc., Medtronic, and Johnson & Johnson are a few of the major competitors in the market [7].

Industry participants engage in a variety of methods including mergers and acquisitions and the introduction of new products. For instance, in January 2015, Medtronic purchased Covidien Plc. With this acquisition, the business hopes to cut production costs and broaden its product offering in order to gain more market share. The same goes for Philips, which in 2016 unveiled five new smart medical products including a health watch, an ear thermometer, a body analysis scale, an upper arm blood pressure monitor, and a wrist blood pressure monitor.

References

[1] Leong, W.Y. *EEG Signal Processing: Feature Extraction, Selection and Classification Methods (Healthcare Technologies)*, 1st edn., The Institution of Engineering and Technology, Stevenage, 2019. ISBN: 101785613707.

[2] Scott Reedy, A. Pulse on Quality 4.0 for medical device manufacturing, *Quality Magazine*, https://www.qualitymag.com/articles/95844-a-pulse-on-quality-40-for-medical-device-manufacturing. Accessed December 10, 2019.

[3] Rasmeni, M. Hundreds of people set to benefit from prosthetic limb camp, *Namibia Economist*, https://economist.com.na/46991/health/hundreds-of-people-set-to-benefit-from-prosthetic-limb-camp/. Accessed September 4, 2019.

[4] Leong, W.Y. *Human Machine Collaboration and Interaction for Smart Manufacturing: Automation, Robotics, Sensing, Artificial Intelligence, 5G, IoTs and Blockchain*, Institution of Engineering and Technology, Stevenage, 2022. ISBN: 101839534141.

[5] Owano, N. British project uses 3D printing for prosthetic eyes, *Hi Tech & Innovation*. https://phys.org/news/2013-11-british-3d-prosthetic-eyes.html. Accessed November 30, 2013.

[6] Smart Medical Devices Market Size, Share & Trends Analysis Report By Product (Diagnostic & Monitoring and Therapeutic Device). *By Distribution Channel (Pharmacies, Online Channel), By End User, And Segment Forecasts,* 2018–2025, Grand View Research, Report ID: GVR-1-68038-495-6. https://www.grandviewresearch.com/industry-analysis/smart-medical-devices-market.

[7] Dahl, B. *Open Bionics Bionic Arm, Cool Material*. https://coolmaterial.com/tech/open-bionics-bionic-arm/.

Chapter 2
Medical device manufacturing

Wai Yie Leong[1]

The fourth industrial revolution, often known as Industry 4.0, is the source of Quality 4.0. The first revolution began with the development of machine manufacture, steam power and the emigration of farmers to urban areas before the fourth revolution [1,2]. Production was mechanised during the second industrial revolution, and the cost of consumer and industrial goods was reduced through mass production. The third industrial revolution includes the introduction of electronics and control systems, which helped reduce prices while increasing product complexity and lowering expenses. New quality paradigms, methods and technologies are being driven by the fourth industrial revolution of today (Figure 2.1).

There are many obstacles to designing and manufacturing safer products, particularly in the medical device manufacturing industry. Regulatory requirements are only one factor; if device companies want to stay competitive and use cutting-edge technologies, including the Internet of Things (IoT), artificial intelligence (AI), machine learning, augmented reality and even robotics, they must step up their game and incorporate emerging and constantly evolving technologies (Figure 2.2). These modern manufacturing technologies have come together to form Quality 4.0.

2.1 Restructuring the market and industry with technology

The third revolution, which connected the natural and physical worlds, marked the beginning of the digital transformation, and version 4.0 is where it is now. This fourth industrial revolution is powered by the influence of digital data, analytics, connectivity, scalability and collaboration, which also inform Quality 4.0 plans. The democratisation of technologies is bringing transformative capabilities in analytics, material science and networking as we discover new ways to connect people, devices and data. Such solutions enable a high-quality change of culture, leadership, collaboration and standards for the medical device business.

[1]The Institution of Engineering and Technology, Malaysia

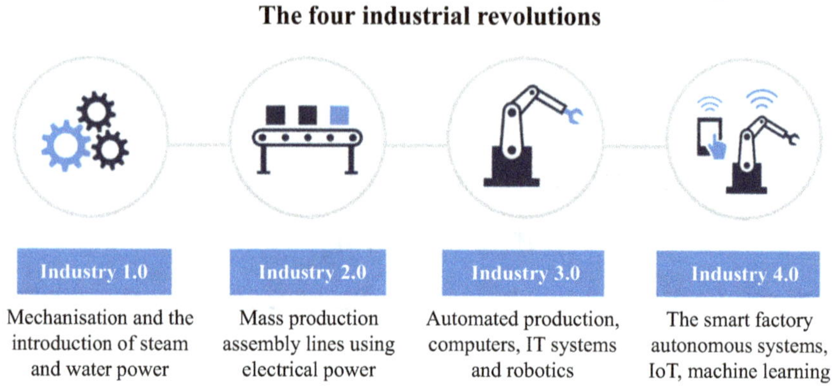

Figure 2.1 The industry evolvement has changed the competitive landscape of many industrial processes [1]

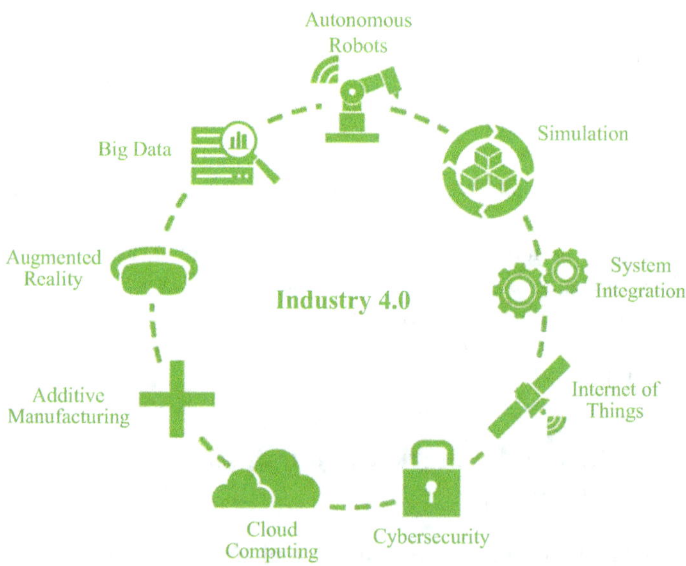

Figure 2.2 Modern manufacturing technologies have come together to form Quality 4.0

Device designs, functionality, manufacturing procedures, supply chain management, customer service and ways to keep quality systems compatible with regulatory bodies such as the FDA and ISO are all being changed by Quality 4.0. Intelligent and linked technologies are being used more and more frequently as businesses look for a competitive edge to offer innovative items before their rivals [3,4].

2.2 Digitalisation

By 2030, the medical device market is expected to reach $850 billion, according to [5]. The global medical devices market was valued at US$550 billion in 2021 and is expected to reach US$850 billion by 2030, poised to grow at a compound annual growth rate (CAGR) of 5.5% during the forecast period 2022–2030 (Figure 2.3). The state of healthcare is being improved through the development of smarter, more automated, linked technology that enables remote procedures with medical professionals from across the world. The success of medical device companies on the market in the coming years will depend on their ability to utilise Quality 4.0 technologies. Quality 4.0, the use of Industry 4.0 technology to quality initiatives, is seen by LNS Research as following in the footsteps of IoT. In fact, according to industry experts, a quarter of medical device manufacturers use digital transformation technology to boost quality. The design and delivery of items are both done using the same technologies. What does this signify for companies that make medical devices?

To begin with, Quality 4.0 plans were developed with the aid of digital transformation trends to do away with the need for various paper-based quality management systems (QMSs) and procedures [5]. Eliminating manual systems lowers errors, silos, hurdles to collaboration and traceability problems. Additionally, small and international businesses may swiftly grow their design and supply chain processes thanks to the digitisation and automation of production and design processes (Figure 2.4). RefleXion Medical, a pioneer in biology-guided radiation systems for the treatment of cancer, is one such business that was aware of the need to build a fully linked QMS that could grow to support its route to digital transformation and greater compliance. They needed a platform that was

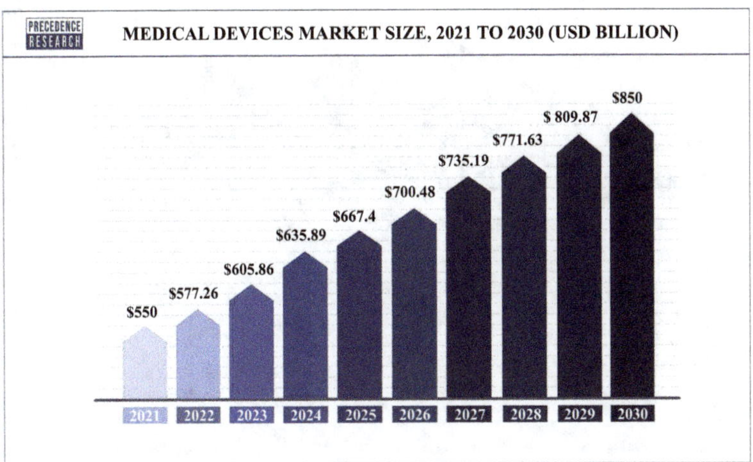

Figure 2.3 Global medical devices market was valued at US$550 billion in 2021 and is expected to reach US$850 billion by 2030 [5]

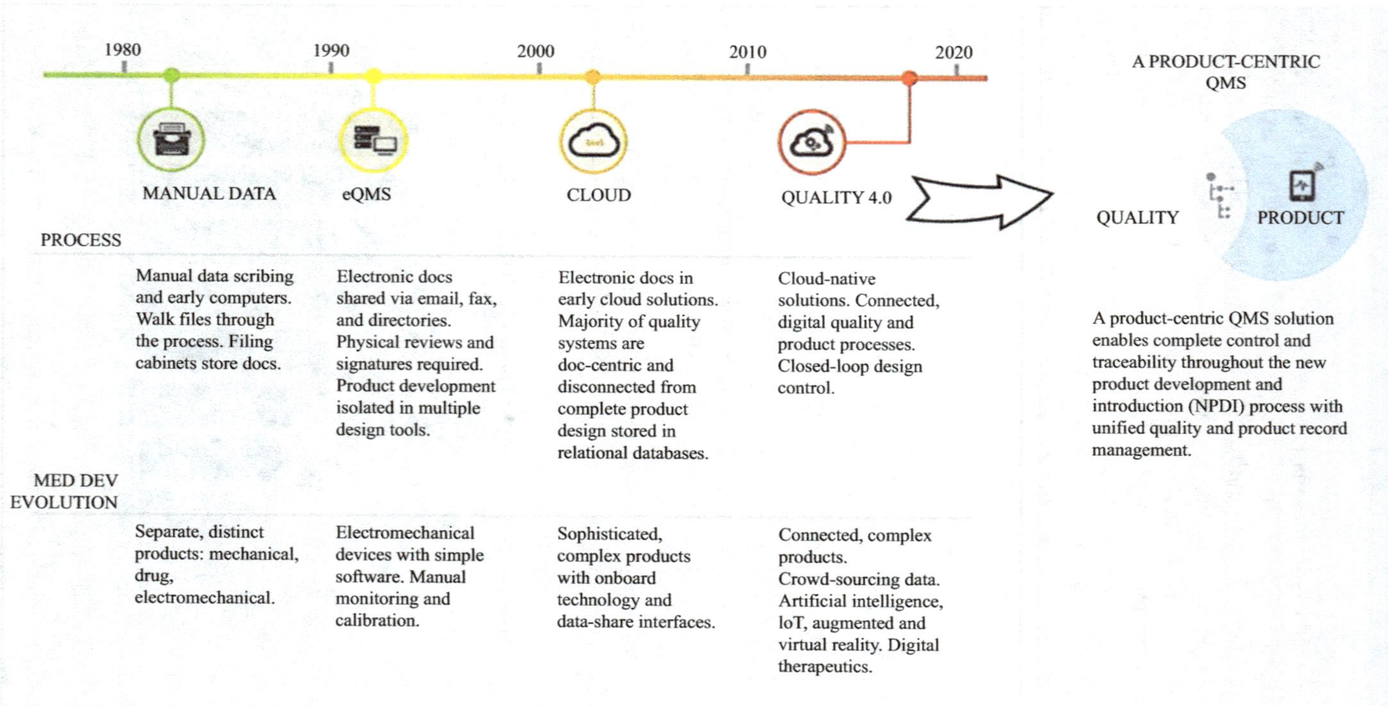

Figure 2.4 Quality 4.0 for medical equipment manufacturing [6]

adaptable and could expand along with their workforce, their goods and their road towards quality compliance.

2.3 Supply chain quality standards

Today's medical device makers rely on distributed teams and supply chains, including contract manufacturers, design partners and tier-based component suppliers, to speed products to market. The particular advantages that digital transformation technologies may bring to a device manufacturer's product requirements, product capabilities and regulatory compliance objectives are understood by businesses that have embraced new technology and cloud-based systems.

Digital treatments, medical diagnostic tools, implantable devices and disposable devices are just a few examples of the large range of devices used in the life sciences industry that aim to be error-free while delivering higher throughput and preserving compliance.

2.4 Linking to connected teams

To satisfy the needs brought on by Quality 4.0 trends, a networked or more product-centric QMS can be used. Quality teams need a unified system to spot problems, handle audits and address quality incidents as product complexity rises due to AI, IoT, robotics and associated 4.0 technologies. This makes sure that a single system contains the entire, intricate product design, which consists of electrical, mechanical and software components.

As teams communicate through each stage of new product development and introduction, this foundation makes it possible to keep complete, integrated quality and corrective action records. It also increases visibility and transparency.

More intelligence-driven product and quality process insights will provide medical device companies a competitive edge. Better data-driven decisions and cross-functional visibility with the supply chain, engineering and quality teams will follow from this. Meeting stringent criteria for medical device compliance is made more difficult by these Quality 4.0 transformative technologies:

- ISO quality system standards
    - (a) FDA 21 CFR Part 11
    - (b) Complaint Management and Corrective and Preventive Action (CAPA)
    - (c) ISO 13485
    - (d) FDA 21 CFR Part 820
- A product-centric QMS solution makes it possible to:
    - (a) Establish quality production processes to avoid audit issues
    - (b) Ensure traceable design and change controls
    - (c) Manage product bills of materials linked directly to quality records
    - (d) Encourage closed-loop quality and CAPA processes to accelerate resolution
    - (e) Boost quality compliance and supplier management processes

The final aspect of supplier management is crucial because the correct QMS solution can integrate quality and product record management to provide total control and traceability, streamline audits and lower risks.

2.5 Use cases by device manufacturers

Swan Valley Medical is a producer of surgical tools and add-ons used in the discipline of urology. They had to deal with ineffective paper-based manual processes that exposed them to significant compliance risks since they lost important documents. When missing or incorrect information was discovered during audits, recovery was challenging and could require hundreds of hours or even many months.

Accelerated root cause analysis and risk management observation processes were developed using a cloud-based product-centric QMS technology. Through linked product and quality records, this made it possible for various processes to communicate with one another, supporting audits with cross-linked evidence chains.

Quality teams can identify, examine and fix problems with quality more quickly with the aid of closed-loop CAPA processes. As an illustration, Pulse Biosciences implemented a closed-loop quality system throughout their business. With a product-centric QMS, all team members were able to collaborate on the most recent product definition and quality records. Pulse Biosciences was able to resolve important corrective actions quickly and with stronger audit trails because to streamlined CAPA processes.

The first doctor-recommended and FDA-cleared smart thermometers are available from Kinsa. To aid in the creation of the first-ever linked gadget for the company, they established a product-centric QMS. Kinsa has revolutionised how healthcare may be reimagined in an IoT world through connected technology to speed up product development, enhance quality control and reduce the amount of time it takes to resolve customer complaints.

2.6 Maintaining Quality 4.0

More intelligent devices are being delivered at a rapid clip. Newer technologies such as IoT, AR and robotics are being used by both large, established medical device businesses and smaller innovators in a race to enhance healthcare by linking people and data and providing better outcomes to patients around the world.

Industry 4.0 innovations have influenced Quality 4.0 technologies and approaches to enhance quality compliance. In order to compete in the modern global economy, it is essential to be able to synchronise complicated product development and quality processes. We can now execute surgeries and do healing when patients and doctors are separated by various time zones thanks to clever robotics and augmented reality technology. We can build products virtually with remote teams.

So, think about your objectives and constraints for developing and delivering complicated products that adhere to standards set by the FDA and ISO. To safeguard your patients' health as well as your revenue and long-term viability, be sure you can provide a completely traceable, low-risk environment.

Smarter, linked tactics are needed to keep up with Quality 4.0 developments and prevent your business from falling behind.

References

[1] Spectral Engines. *Industry 4.0 and how smart sensors make the difference.* https://www.spectralengines.com/articles/industry-4-0-and-how-smart-sensors-make-the-difference#:~:text=This%20shows%20how%20Spectral%20Engines,the%20smartness%20to%20spectral%20sensors [Accessed 26 Feb 2018].

[2] Leong W.Y., Chuah J.H., and Tuan T.B. (eds.). *The Nine Pillars of Technologies for Industry 4.0.* London: Institution of Engineering and Technology, 2020.

[3] Leong W.Y. *EEG Signal Processing: Feature Extraction, Selection and Classification Methods (Healthcare Technologies)*, 1st edn. Edison, NJ: The Institution of Engineering and Technology, 2019.

[4] Leong W.Y. *Human Machine Collaboration and Interaction for Smart Manufacturing: Automation, Robotics, Sensing, Artificial Intelligence, 5G, IoTs and Blockchain*. Stevenage: Institution of Engineering and Technology, 2022.

[5] Precedence Research. *Medical Devices Market (By Type: Cardiovascular Devices, Orthopedic Devices, Diagnostic Imaging, MIS, IVD, Diabetes Care, Wound Management, Dental, Nephrology, Ophthalmic Devices, and Others; By End User: Clinics, Hospitals & Ambulatory Surgical Centers, and Others) – Global Market Size, Trends Analysis, Segment Forecasts, Regional Outlook 2022–2030*. Report Code: 1129, 2021. https://www.precedenceresearch.com/medical-devices-market.

[6] Scott Reedy A. Pulse on Quality 4.0 for Medical Device Manufacturing. *Quality Magazine*. https://www.qualitymag.com/articles/95844-a-pulse-on-quality-40-for-medical-device-manufacturing [Accessed 10 Dec 2019].

Chapter 3

Challenges and impact of medical equipment engineering

Alex Looi Tink Huey[1,2]

The COVID-19 pandemic has shown how vulnerabilities in global healthcare systems can have profound implications for physical and mental health, economic recovery, confidence and trust in government, and social cohesion [1]. Organisation for Economic Co-operation and Development (OECD) reported that since 2020, COVID-19 cases had totaled around 500 million across the world, with over 6 million deaths registered [2]. These numbers are underrated as many COVID-19 cases were not reported, especially in lower- and middle-income countries. This public health crisis has also led to cascading health and economic crises from which most countries are only now beginning to emerge (Figure 3.1).

It is of utmost importance to strengthen health system preparedness and broader resilience to manage and contain emerging infectious pathogens or other potential shocks [2]. Resilient health systems are required to build stronger and fast recovering economies further contributing to greater health and social and economic productivity.

The World Health Organization (WHO) plays a central role in facilitating the sharing of knowledge across countries on health policies and practices, as well as providing a broad range of global public goods (GPGs). GPGs in this context denote protecting and promoting global public health. Three categories of GPGs were highlighted to strengthen the global health systems: research and assessment, normative functions, and managing externalities [3]. Figure 3.2 illustrates the relationship between spending on resilience and pandemic preparedness, at the national and international levels [2] where the research and assessment portfolio is subcategorized into health technology research and development, marketing approval, health technology assessment, product quality assessment, treatment guidelines, delivery, and health systems research; normative functions portfolio is subcategorized into standard setting, regulations, and policies; and managing externalities is subcategorized into infectious disease surveillance, strategic stockpiles of drugs and vaccines, and early warning systems.

[1]Malim Consulting Engineers Sdn Bhd, Malaysia
[2]IEC Young Professional, International Electrotechnical Commission (IEC), Malaysia

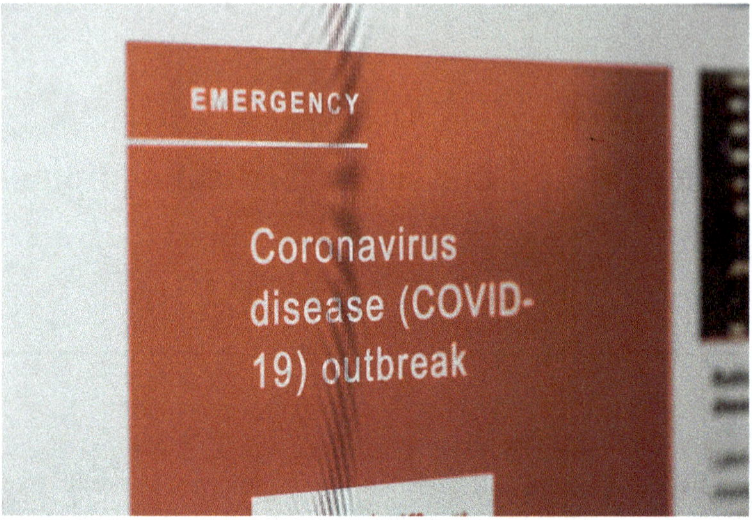

Figure 3.1 What are the effects of COVID-19 pandemic outbreak?

3.1 Challenges and impact

Medical equipment engineering is a field of engineering and a highly regulated industry that comprises designing, developing, manufacturing, testing, and maintaining medical devices and equipment used in healthcare. Medical devices and equipment range from simple heating blankets, electrical hospital beds, or electronic fever thermometers, to complex programmable electronic equipment such as medical lasers, incubators, electroencephalogram (EEG) monitors, cardiac monitors, imaging systems such as X-ray and magnetic resonance imaging (MRI) scan, and life-support devices; as well as wearable devices that include telemedicine, biometrics, big data, artificial intelligence (AI), etc. [4]. The advancement in sensor technologies and Internet of Things (IoT), improved network connections, wide adoption of smartphones and connected devices for the management of critical illnesses, increasing focus on patient-centric healthcare delivery, and increasing demand for home healthcare services are driving digital and mobile health technologies.

According to Ernst and Young, the pandemic continues to offer significant challenges and disruptions to global supply chains [5]. As a result, it becomes difficult for manufacturers to procure raw materials that are the supply of components for medical devices and equipment. The factors affecting the disruption of supply chains are due to extraordinary levels of global demand, temporary trade restrictions, and the disruptions in logistics and transportation industries from the pandemic outbreak. This translates to manufacturers being unable to accelerate production. Aside from labor shortages and losses due to closures, the pandemic has also accelerated and amplified problems that already existed in the supply chain prepandemic period.

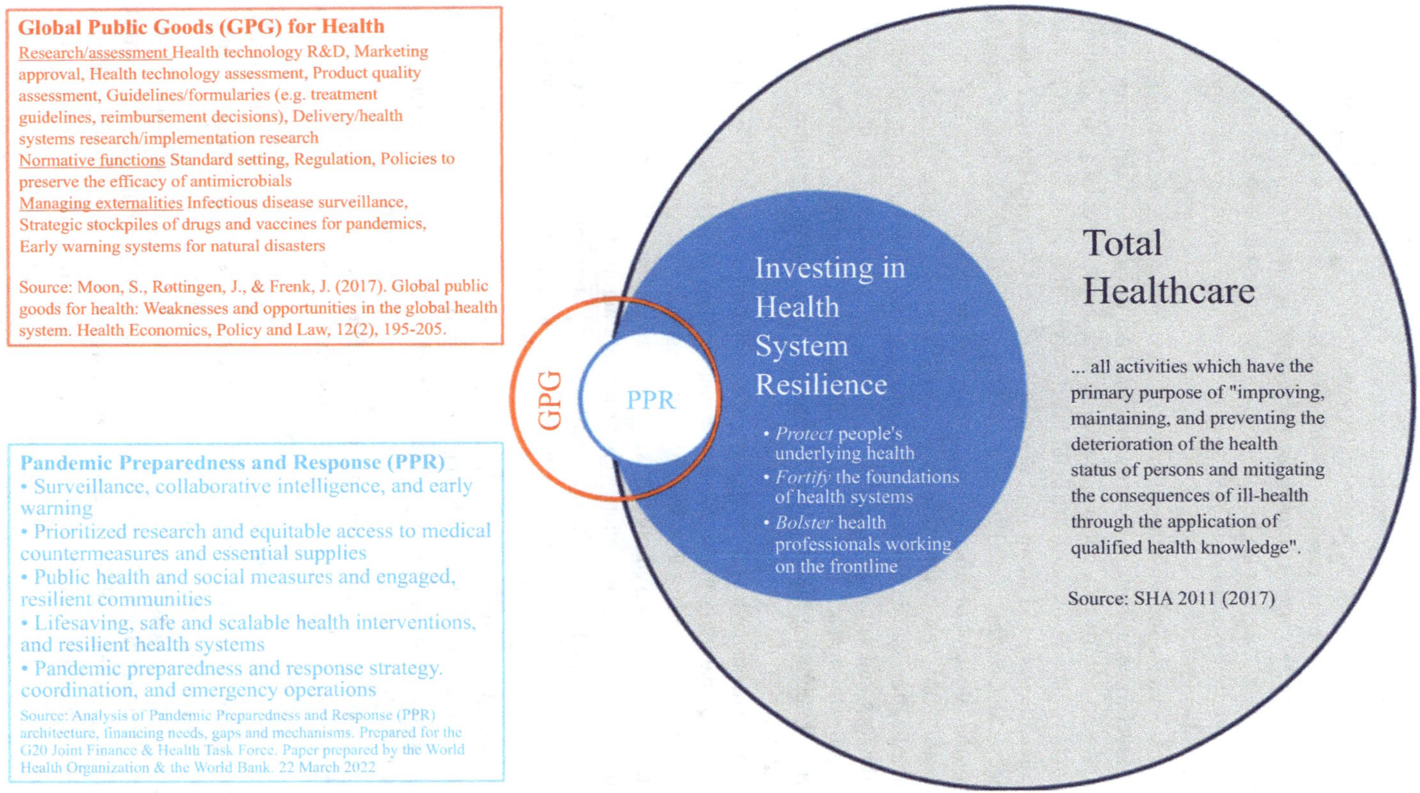

Figure 3.2 Relationship between spending on resilience and pandemic preparedness, at the national and international levels [2]

During the peak of the pandemic, there is a global shortage of many essential medical devices and equipment as well as critical medical supplies, from personal protective gear to ventilators and test kits [6]. The lack of medical devices and equipment to respond to the COVID-19 crisis had put healthcare systems and hospitals under tremendous stress. This situation is further aggravated by measures taken in higher-income countries to ban exports of essential and critical medical supplies in response to their own shortage of supplies in times of pandemics.

Medical devices and equipment must be designed and tested properly with very high level of certification. Poor quality medical devices and equipment could lead to end-user injuries or death-threatening situations, especially for high-risk devices such as pacemakers and artificial heart valves. It is challenging to produce novel medical devices and equipment at speed. In accordance with the International Electrotechnical Commission (IEC), all medical devices and equipment need to meet a complicated set of safety requirements, where regulation, standardization, and verification are closely interrelated [4]. Compliance with respect to regulations and standardization can heavily affect the design and manufacturing process of medical devices and equipment. Aside from that, it is important to have harmonized and globally agreed standards to enable system compatibility and avoid difficulty when integrating different technologies or using equipment from different manufacturers.

Modern medical devices and equipment often incorporate critical components or sophisticated materials that require a specialized set of technological skills to produce [7]. It is arduous for a single entity to possess the breadth of technological capabilities to produce everything by itself. Take an example, the growing number of electronic components in modern vehicles where automotive manufacturers are not equipped to create touchscreen displays in the entertainment and navigation systems or the countless microprocessors required to control the engine, steering wheel, and other functions [7].

The outbreak has also caused a high market demand for personal protection and medical products. Interpol announced a significant rise in counterfeit or defective medicines and medical products related to COVID-19 under Operation Pangea, a collective action between police, customs, and health regulatory authorities from 90 countries against illicit sales of counterfeit and unauthorized medicines and medical products [8]. Counterfeit medical devices pose a serious risk to patients and healthcare providers' safety as these devices may not perform as intended, fail to carry out necessary diagnosis or treatment, or cause harm. Counterfeit medical devices do not undergo rigorous testing and quality control measures to ensure their safety, quality, and performance.

The pandemic has accelerated the paradigm shift toward digitization and servitization of the global economy today, which is quickly becoming the main driving force of economic growth. The accelerating pace of the digital economy requires businesses and organizations to embrace digital transformation. Businesses and organizations that embrace digital solutions have greater resiliency in the face of economic uncertainty, a sudden drop-off in demand, and faster recovery [9].

As healthcare systems are focused and occupied on preventing and treating COVID-19, population drastically alter their behaviors to limit the possibilities of infections because of lockdown policies; consequently, social interaction activities and many essential in-person healthcare services were either postponed or cancelled [10]. These changes include a large reduction in healthcare utilization services and population who have missed out on much required care for vaccination, disruptions in treatments, or life-extending interventions for critical illnesses. A WHO survey detailed that the disruption to healthcare services was greatest among lower-income countries [11].

Aside from the pandemic, businesses and organizations will also need to anticipate multiple disruptions from geopolitical risks, cyber threats, and economic instability that will continue to put pressure on the global supply chains [5].

The IEC indicated a massive 45% increase in cyber-attacks on healthcare organizations globally in the last 2 months of 2020 [12]. Hospitals make easy targets for cyber-criminals due to obsolete information and communication technology (ICT) systems, and medical devices and equipment with weak or no protection. The increasing implementation of connected medical devices has only aggravated the situation. In hospitals, life-saving and life-support medical equipment must continue to run permanently to ensure patient safety. Unfortunately, cyber-attacks could stop these critical medical devices from functioning, and a hacked-connected medical device could provide a gateway for cyber-criminals into the hospital network to steal sensitive patient data and health records.

Apart from that, medical devices and equipment manufacturing and engineering require huge investments in research and development, clinical studies, and testing which translates to challenges to develop affordable medical devices and equipment.

3.2 The way forward

Implementing digitalization in healthcare systems requires a clear understanding and a well-designed digital strategy road map, digital literacy trainings, a shared and common vision of digital transformation and its potential, building an agile and competent digital talent pool, and a policy and education environment that encourages its implementation.

United Nations (UN) Sustainable Development Goal (SDG) target 3.8 states that "all people have access to needed health services (including prevention, promotion, treatment, rehabilitation and palliation) of sufficient quality to be effective while also ensuring that the use of these services does not expose the user the financial hardship" [13]. In other words, to achieve universal health coverage, access to quality essential healthcare services and affordable essential medicines and vaccines made available to all is an important element of a strong healthcare system.

Business sectors such as healthcare, manufacturing, real estate, retail, and financial services can leverage digital business models and digital technologies to

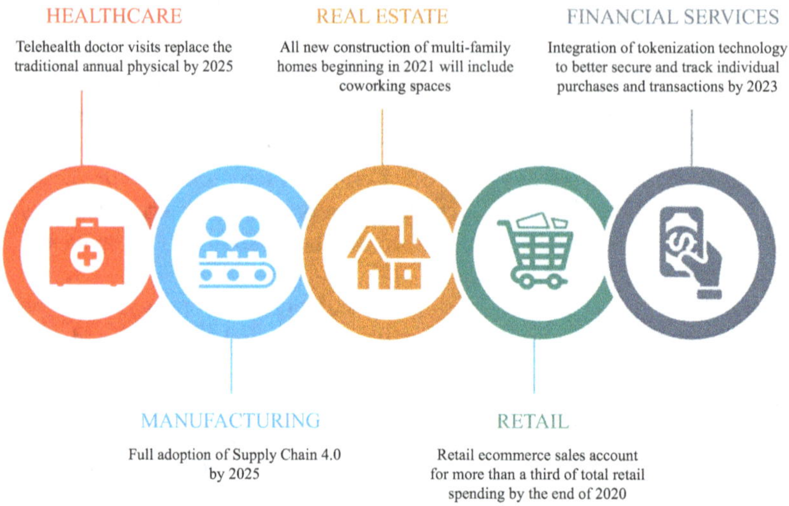

Figure 3.3 New reliance on digital solutions during COVID-19 [8]

enable a conducive and sustainable doing-business environment (Figure 3.3). Digital business models and digital technologies such as the IoT, big data, AI, and additive manufacturing are driving the change of current business models and shifting global economics and market structures.

Businesses and organizations are shifting from linear supply chains to more integrated networks connecting many stakeholders. Technology enablers such as IoT devices that provide valuable data on where goods are in the chain, cloud-based platforms for collaboration among suppliers, and supply chain orchestration have helped accelerate the adoption of integrated supply chain networks. The manufacturing industry needs to diversify its sources and stockpile key materials or items by mapping the process of its full supply chain [7].

The healthcare systems today must adopt a digital approach to alleviate the strain imposed by the pandemic. Telemedicine and remote diagnostics or consultations services have scaled up during the pandemic which caused a massive shift in healthcare system performance [10] (Figure 3.4). With telemedicine, patients can receive medical care from the comfort of their own homes or from a remote location, without the need to travel or physically visit a doctor's office or the hospital. Doctors can perform diagnosis and treatment, routine check-ups, provide mental health counseling, and monitor patients' condition via videoconferencing, phone consultations, and other forms of virtual communication platforms.

The cost of implementing automation into the manufacturing line will continue to decline, and people will see that robots can operate safely alongside humans as the technology continues to evolve with more kinds of tasks or work being automated. Robotics are currently being used in surgery to enhance precision and

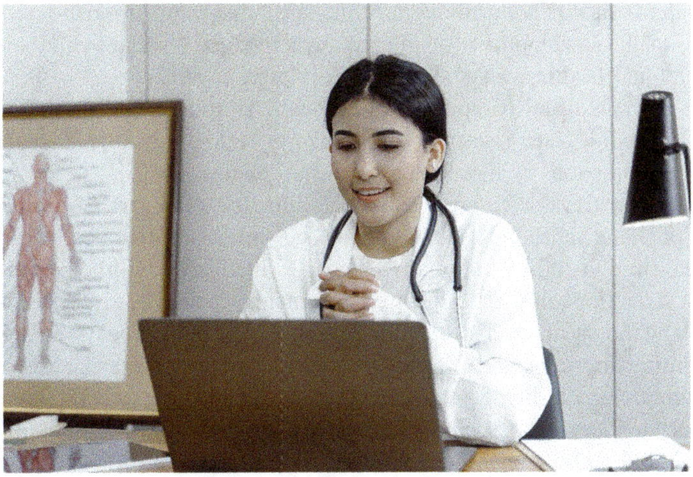

Figure 3.4 Telemedicine is the interconnected future of healthcare

accuracy (better outcomes and fewer complications), reduce surgical scarring and trauma (minimally invasive), speed up recovery times, increased dexterity (robotic arms can move in ways which human hands cannot), and improved visualization (3D visualization of the surgical site). 3D printing is also known as the production method of additive manufacturing, which can significantly reduce the number of steps or processes required to make complex shapes and reduce the dependence on suppliers of the machinery and tools needed [7]. Rapid advancement in 3D printing is allowing manufacturers to economically produce materials in much higher quantities.

Health data are critical and should not remain "data rich but information poor". AI technologies have been progressively integrated into medical equipment and are used to manage big data and a myriad of applications for data gathering, data integration, data governance, and advanced analytics. AI helps to improve the accuracy and efficiency of diagnosis, treatment, and patient care by identifying patterns and anomalies.

Standardized medical technologies that are tested and certified for safety, quality, and performance contribute to overall risk management. Standards ensure medical devices and equipment are safe for patients, and medical professionals, and practitioners to use and provide the basis for greater regulatory convergence [4]. The trade in medical devices and equipment is global; hence, it is important for medical equipment manufacturers to adopt an international approach to comply with standards and regulations. The use of harmonized and globally agreed technical rules helps increase the availability of safe, affordable, and quality medical devices and equipment. In return, this translates to broader access to better healthcare. Clear, harmonized regulatory medical guidelines also help in fostering investment in research and development and innovations. Key stakeholders such as manufacturers, healthcare providers, clinicians, and regulators are required to contribute to the development of international medical standards and ensure that the international healthcare standards fit seamlessly together.

Ernst and Young also reported that industrial products and high-tech manufacturing companies are investing massively in technology to reduce employee exposure to infection in more labor-intensive industries [5]. In the past, cost reduction was achievable through lean operations (business strategy driven by the principle of doing more with less), longer lead times, and low-cost labor. Today, agility, real-time visibility, automation, and upskilled labor will be key to not only drive cost reductions in the business environment but improved decision-making, process standardization, and streamlining supply chains and ecosystem partners.

According to Ernst and Young, 45% of supply chains are expected to be mostly autonomous utilizing robots in warehouses and stores, driverless forklifts and trucks, delivery drones, and fully automated planning by 2035 [5]. Simply utilizing digital technologies does not equate to creating a digitized and autonomous supply chain; an integrated digitized supply chain network requires supply chain technologies across planning, procurement, manufacturing, and logistics ecosystem taken into consideration beyond the organization's boundary.

The circular economy approach ensures that there is minimal to no waste in the manufacturing process to provide a competitive advantage with business sustainability by maximizing resource efficiency. Businesses and organizations must explore ways to redesign and engineer medical devices and equipment to achieve this circular economy with business sustainability by redesigning products and processes to minimize wastages, and promoting collaboration.

Equipped with real-time visibility and transparency through digital supply chain, businesses can make fast and efficient decision-making that drives agility and opportunities for growth across planning, procurement, manufacturing, and logistics.

Protecting, retraining, and reskilling the workforce should be the main priority, along with investing to make the digital and autonomous global supply chain to be a reality. There is a growing need for multidisciplinary skills; in addition to medical professionals, the manufacturing industry needs to use professionals with technical–mechanical and electrical and electronics engineering background, software engineering, material science, and data analysis.

Cyber security standards define the roles, responsibilities, and activities that are essential for risk management of ICT networks that integrate with medical devices and equipment. These standards manage the safety and effectiveness, as well as data and system security of medical devices and equipment, and serve as guidelines for medical equipment manufacturers and engineers. To strengthen trust in digital health solutions, there is a need to ensure personal data protection and enable privacy, digital security, and governance of health data.

Not only do digital technologies have the potential to create huge value in healthcare systems, but it also helps to drive down costs (Figure 3.5). McKinsey Global Institute provided an indication between \$1.5 trillion and \$3 trillion in cost savings per year by 2030 with the influx of automation, AI, and remote monitoring [14].

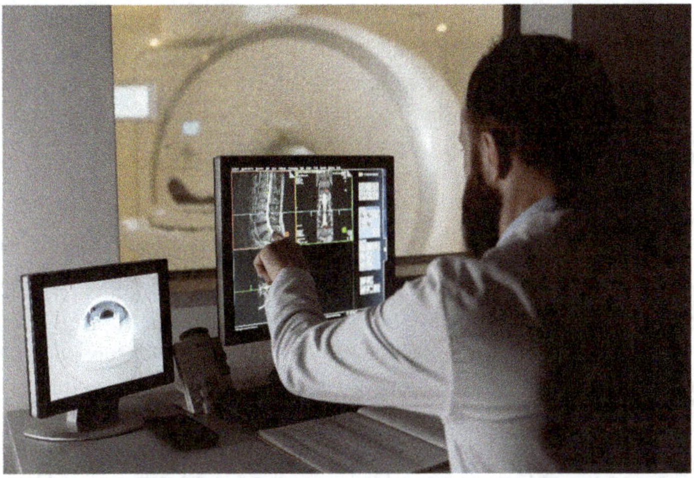

Figure 3.5 Digital technologies create huge value in healthcare systems

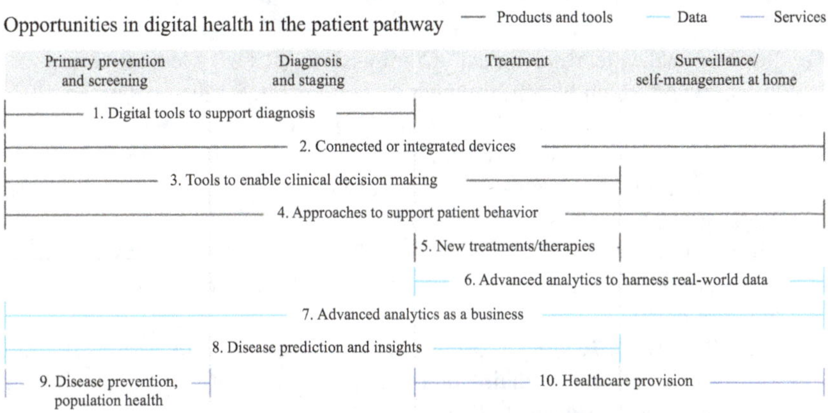

Figure 3.6 Opportunities in digital health in patient pathway [14]

Digital technology enablers open up new opportunities for medical equipment manufacturers along the entire patient pathway from primary prevention and screening through diagnosis and staging to treatment [14]. Figure 3.6 depicts how digital-centric tools devices and products can be used to address different pain points (specific problems faced by users) along the patient journey by becoming more precise and personalized with improved performance. One example of this is a modern pacemaker. Early designs of pacemakers can only be monitored via near-field or wireless technology. Today, pacemakers can focus on patients' needs which allows them to check the battery life of their devices, log and track their symptoms, and monitor physical activities, all through their smartphones.

Digital transformation allows medical devices and equipment engineering to take a more holistic approach to find responses to enhancing the capabilities and performance of medical devices and equipment, process innovation, greater user-centric strategy, smart data-gathering, user-specific adaptation, reducing manufacturing cost, shortened lead time, and efficient use of resources.

References

[1] Organisation for Economic Co-operation and Development (OECD). The Impact of COVID-19 on Health and Health Systems. https://www.oecd.org/health/covid-19.htm#:~:text=The%20COVID%2D19%20pandemic%20has,virus%20continue%20to%20be%20essential. AccessedNovember 2022.

[2] Morgan, D. and James, C. *Investing in Health Systems to Protect Society and Boost the Economy: Priority Investments and Order-of-Magnitude Cost Estimates*. Paris: Organisation for Economic Co-operation and Development (OECD), 2022.

[3] Moon, S., Røttingen, J., and Frenk, J. Global public goods for health: weaknesses and opportunities in the global health system. *Health Economics, Policy and Law*, 2017;12(2):195–205.

[4] International Electrotechnical Commission (IEC). Medical Equipment. https://www.iec.ch/healthcare/medical-equipment. Accessed January 2023.

[5] Harapko, S. *How COVID-19 Impacted Supply Chains and What Comes Next*. https://www.ey.com/en_my/supply-chain/how-covid-19-impacted-supply-chains-and-what-comes-next. Ernst & Young Global Limited. Accessed January 2023.

[6] Millar, A. *COVID-19: The Med Tech Bottlenecks*. https://www.medicaldevice-network.com/features/covid-19-the-med-tech-bottlenecks/. Accessed November 2022.

[7] Shih, WC. *Global Supply Chains in a Post-Pandemic World*. https://hbr.org/2020/09/global-supply-chains-in-a-post-pandemic-world. Harvard Business Review. Accessed August 2022.

[8] Interpol. *Global Operation Sees a Rise in Fake Medical Products Related to COVID-19*. https://www.interpol.int/en/News-and-Events/News/2020/Global-operation-sees-a-rise-in-fake-medical-products-related-to-COVID-19. Accessed August 2022.

[9] BDO International. *COVID-19 is Accelerating the Rise of the Digital Economy*. https://www.bdo.com/insights/business-financial-advisory/strategy,-technology-transformation/covid-19-is-accelerating-the-rise-of-the-digital-e. Accessed August 2021.

[10] Organisation for Economic Co-operation and Development (OECD). *The Future of Telemedicine after COVID-19*. https://www.oecd.org/coronavirus/policy-responses/the-future-of-telemedicine-after-covid-19-d46e9a02/. Accessed January 2023.

[11] Moynihan, R., Sanders, S., Michaleff, Z. A., *et al.* Impact of COVID-19 pandemic on utilisation of healthcare services: a systematic review. *BMJ Open*. 2021;11:e045343.

[12] International Electrotechnical Commission (IEC). *Cyber Security for Connected Medical Devices*. https://www.iec.ch/blog/cyber-security-connected-medical-devices. Accessed November 2022.

[13] Organisation for Economic Co-operation and Development (OECD). *Strengthening Health Systems During a Pandemic: The Role of Development Finance*. https://read.oecd-ilibrary.org/view/?ref=134_134620-xueji119ph&title=Strengthening-health-systems-during-a%20pandemic-The-role-of-development-finance. Accessed November 2022.

[14] Bartlett, R., Somauroo, A., and Zerbi, C. *How the Medtech Industry Can Capture Value from Digital Health*. https://www.mckinsey.com/industries/life-sciences/our-insights/how-the-medtech-industry-can-capture-value-from-digital-health. McKinsey & Company. Accessed November 2022.

Chapter 4

Physiotherapy on e-health platforms

Surya Vishnuram[1], Vinodhkumar Ramalingam[1] and Kumaresan Abathsagayam[1]

In recent years, e-health, or the use of technology to deliver healthcare services, has grown in popularity [1]. Physiotherapy is a branch of healthcare that deals with the treatment of physical conditions and injuries through various therapeutic techniques such as exercise, manual therapy, and education. With the rise of technology, physiotherapy has evolved, and now e-health platforms have emerged as a new way of delivering physiotherapy services [2].

Physiotherapy is one industry where e-health has had a substantial impact. Physical therapy, usually referred to as physiotherapy, is a discipline of medicine that focuses on the rehabilitate the problems from musculoskeletal, neurological, cardiopulmonary, sports, and various specialties. Exercise prescriptions, electrical modalities, manual therapy, and other hands-on therapy methods are used to assist patients in healing from dysfunctions or problems and enhancing their general physical function [3].

E-health platforms are online platforms that allow patients to access physiotherapy services from the comfort of their homes. These platforms provide a range of services such as teleconsultation, online appointment booking, and access to physiotherapy exercise programs.

This chapter will explore the application of e-health platforms in physiotherapy. The advantages and challenges of using these platforms will be discussed, along with the numerous e-health tools and technologies that are currently accessible for physiotherapy globally.

4.1 Need of e-platforms in physiotherapy

The usage of e-platforms to deliver patient care has increased in the field of physiotherapy in recent years. Physiotherapists and patients can collaborate and communicate more easily by using a variety of digital tools and technologies known as “e-platforms,” or electronic platforms. This covers everything from

[1]Saveetha College of Physiotherapy, SIMATS, Tamil Nadu, India

online workout regimens and patient portals to video conferencing and telerehabilitation.

There are a number of reasons why physiotherapy needs e-platforms. The rising need for remote care is one of the primary causes. It is getting harder and harder for physiotherapists to see every patient in person due to an ageing population and an increase in patients living in rural places. E-platforms enable physiotherapists to treat patients remotely and reach more people, which can be especially beneficial for those who have difficulty getting around or who live in remote areas [4].

The increasing emphasis on patient-centered care is another factor driving the need for e-platforms in physiotherapy. E-platforms give patients access to information and resources, such as exercise plans and educational materials, enabling them to play a more active role in their own care and treatment. This can improve results and patient satisfaction with care by assisting people in better understanding their diseases and how to manage them [5].

Both physiotherapists and patients benefit from saving money by using e-platforms. They can lessen the need for extra staff and equipment, as well as the requirement for patients to travel to clinics or hospitals for care. This can contribute to a reduction in overall healthcare costs, which is crucial for individuals with limited financial resources.

To address the demand for remote care and the emphasis on patient-centered care, e-platforms are becoming more and more important in the field of physiotherapy. They also provide financial advantages to physiotherapists and patients.

4.2 Types of e-health platforms for physiotherapy

There are a variety of e-health platforms currently available for physiotherapy. Some of the most common types include the following.

4.2.1 Video conferencing

Patients can schedule virtual appointments with their physiotherapist using this type of e-health platform. Real-time communication between patients and their physiotherapists allows them to ask questions and get advice on their workout regimen.

The practice of physiotherapy has advanced significantly in recent years, with technological advancements having a big impact on how patients are treated. The use of video conferencing for physiotherapy consultations is one of the most remarkable advancements in this area. As a result, patients who may not be able to visit them in person, such as those who reside in distant places or have mobility challenges, can receive remote therapy from physiotherapists.

In physiotherapy, video conferencing has numerous advantages (Figure 4.1). It eliminates the need for patients to travel to a clinic or hospital and lets them receive care in the convenience of their own homes. Patients who struggle to move around, such as those with mobility issues, and those who live in remote areas may particularly benefit from this.

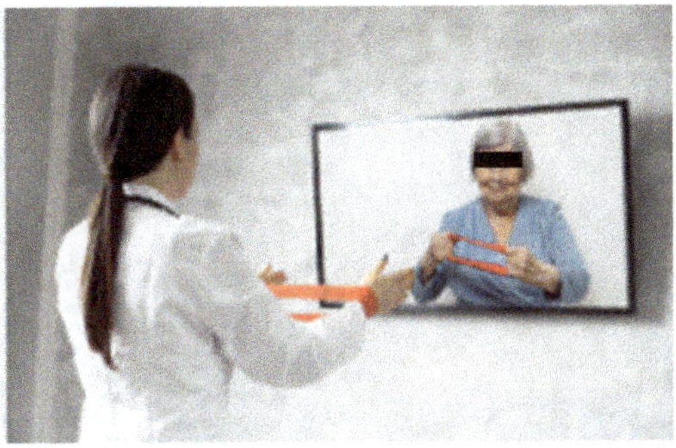

Figure 4.1 Physiotherapy on video call

Additionally, physiotherapists can treat patients with injuries or chronic conditions that necessitate ongoing care thanks to video conferencing. Physiotherapists can monitor their patients' progress and make necessary adjustments to their treatment plans by doing this on a regular basis.

Video conferencing in physiotherapy is a way to provide remote care to patients, which can be especially beneficial for those living in remote areas or who have mobility issues. It also allows physiotherapists to provide ongoing care to patients with chronic conditions [6].

There are also cost-saving benefits to using video conferencing in physiotherapy. This can be especially important for patients who may not have access to physiotherapy services in their area, or for those who have limited financial resources.

4.2.2 Telerehabilitation

Remote monitoring technology is used in this kind of e-health platform to monitor a patient's progress and provide feedback on their exercise program.

The field of telerehabilitation, which makes use of technology to deliver healthcare services from a distance, is expanding rapidly. One of the fields in which telerehabilitation has shown great promise is physiotherapy. It enables physiotherapists to treat patients who are unable to visit them in person, such as those with mobility issues or who live in remote areas.

In physiotherapy, telerehabilitation can take many forms, including interactive exercises, remote monitoring, and video conferencing as shown in Figure 4.2. Physiotherapists can treat a wide range of injuries and conditions, including musculoskeletal, neurological, and chronic pain, with the help of these techniques.

The fact that patients can receive treatment in the privacy of their own homes is one of the main advantages of telerehabilitation in physiotherapy. Patients who struggle to move around, such as those with mobility issues, and those who live in remote areas may particularly benefit from this.

Physiotherapists can also treat patients with chronic conditions or injuries that need to be treated on an ongoing basis, thanks to telerehabilitation. Physiotherapists

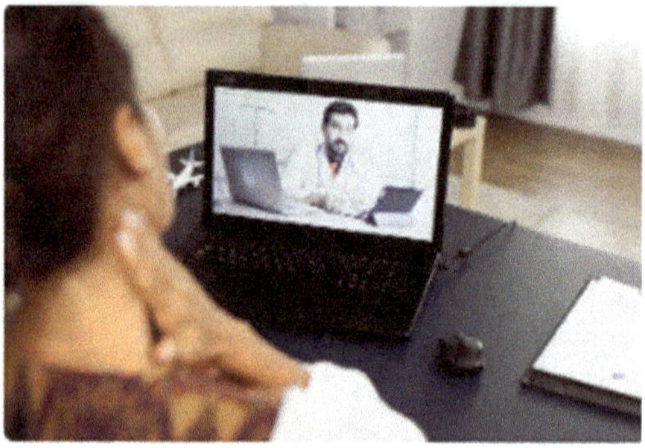

Figure 4.2 Video consultation

can monitor their patients' progress and make necessary adjustments to their treatment plans by doing this on a regular basis. Furthermore, telerehabilitation may be less expensive than in-person traditional physiotherapy. Patients no longer have to travel to a clinic or hospital, and staff and additional equipment may be required less frequently.

Telerehabilitation in physiotherapy is a way to provide remote care to patients, which can be especially beneficial for those living in remote areas or who have mobility issues. It also allows physiotherapists to provide ongoing care to patients with chronic conditions [7].

It is an effective and valuable tool for providing care to patients. With the right technology and support, it can help physiotherapists reach more patients and improve the quality of care that they provide.

4.2.3 Wearable technology

This kind of e-health platform keeps track of a patient's activity levels and gives them feedback on their exercise plan with smartwatches or fitness trackers.

In the field of physiotherapy, wearable technology is becoming an increasingly popular tool. The ability to track and monitor various aspects of physical activity, including movement, muscle activity, and heart rate, is provided by these wearable devices (Figure 4.3). Physiotherapists can use this information to help their patients recover from injuries, manage chronic conditions, and improve their physical health as a whole.

Physiotherapists can now monitor their patients' progress in real time, which is one of the main advantages of the practice. Patients who suffer from injuries or chronic conditions that necessitate ongoing care may find this particularly beneficial. Physiotherapists can use wearable technology to monitor patients' progress over time and make necessary adjustments to treatment plans [8].

Additionally, wearable technology can assist patients in increasing their level of physical activity, which is an essential component of physiotherapy. Fitness trackers are one type of device that can keep track of your physical activity and

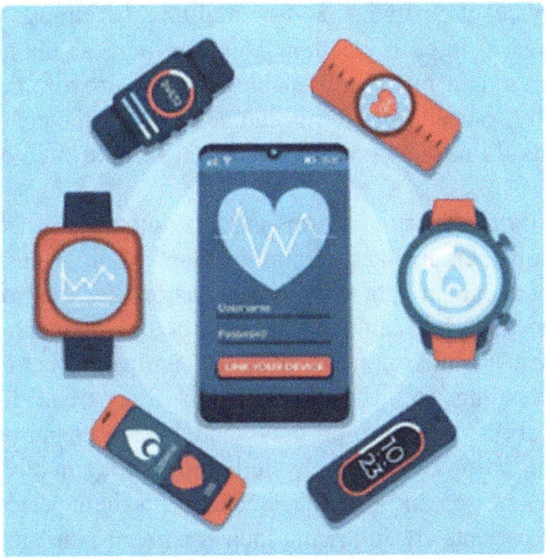

Figure 4.3 Wearable devices

offer suggestions for how to get better. Patients can use this to set goals and keep track of their progress, which can be a big incentive to stay active. Patients can now receive treatment in the convenience of their own homes thanks to wearable technology in physiotherapy. Wearable technology in physiotherapy is a way to monitor patients' progress in real time and provide them with feedback on how to improve. It can also help patients become more active, which is an important aspect of physiotherapy.

4.3 Benefits of e-health platforms in physiotherapy

E-health platforms offer a number of benefits for physiotherapy. One of the biggest advantages is that they allow patients to access physiotherapy services remotely. This is particularly useful for patients who live in remote areas or who have mobility issues that make it difficult for them to attend in-person appointments. One of the main benefits of e-health platforms for physiotherapy is that they enable patients to access care from anywhere, at any time. Patients can receive physiotherapy services remotely, without the need to travel to a physical clinic. This is particularly beneficial for individuals who live in remote or rural areas, have mobility issues, or are unable to leave their homes due to illness or disability.

E-health platforms can also provide patients with greater convenience and flexibility in accessing physiotherapy services. They can book appointments at a time that suits them, without having to take time off work or rearrange their schedule. This can lead to greater patient satisfaction and adherence to treatment plans [3].

In addition to these benefits, e-health platforms can also provide physiotherapists with greater flexibility in the delivery of services. They can deliver physiotherapy services to patients across multiple locations, without the need to be physically present in each location. This can increase the number of patients that a physiotherapist can reach and enable them to provide services more efficiently. Additionally, e-health platforms can also reduce the cost of physiotherapy services, as patients do not need to pay for travel or take time off work to attend appointments [9].

Primary benefit of e-health platforms in physiotherapy is that they can provide patients with a more personalized treatment plan. Many e-health platforms use algorithms to analyze patient data and create a customized treatment plan based on their individual needs. This can help to ensure that patients receive the most appropriate treatment for their condition, which can lead to better outcomes.

The major advantage of using e-platforms for patient follow-up in physiotherapy is the ability to track progress and outcomes more effectively. For example, telerehabilitation can allow physiotherapists to remotely monitor patients' progress through exercises and provide feedback on their performance. This can help to ensure that patients are following their treatment plan and making progress towards their goals.

Many of the e-health platforms provide patients with access to educational resources and support groups, which can help to empower them to take an active role in their own care. For example, patients can use a patient portal to access exercise videos, educational materials, and communicate with their physiotherapists (Figure 4.4).

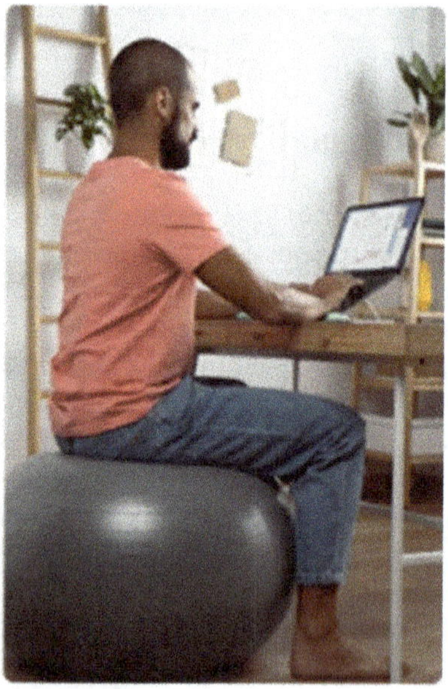

Figure 4.4 Online exercise guidance

Overall, e-health platforms have the potential to revolutionize the delivery of physiotherapy services, providing patients with greater access to care and physiotherapists with greater flexibility in the delivery of services. However, careful consideration must be given to the potential challenges associated with these platforms, to ensure that they are implemented in a safe and effective way [10–12].

4.3.1 Application of e-platforms in physiotherapy clinic management

The application of e-platforms in physiotherapy clinic management is driven by several factors. One of the main reasons is the increasing demand for efficiency and productivity in clinics. E-platforms allow physiotherapists and clinic staff to manage patient records (Figure 4.5), appointments, and billing more efficiently, which can help to reduce wait times and improve overall clinic flow.

Another reason for the use of e-platforms in physiotherapy clinic management is the growing focus on patient-centered care. E-platforms can provide patients with access to their own health records, appointment scheduling, and telerehabilitation services, which can help to improve communication and collaboration between patients and their physiotherapists [13].

E-platforms also offer cost-saving benefits to clinic management. They can reduce the need for paper records, reduce administrative staff, and improve billing and reimbursement process. This can help to lower the overall cost of clinic operations, which is especially important for clinics that have limited financial resources.

4.3.2 Role of e-platforms in rehabilitation

E-platforms, such as telerehabilitation and virtual reality, can play a significant role in physiotherapy rehabilitation by providing patients with increased access to therapy services, particularly in remote or underserved areas. These platforms can also be used to provide patients with personalized and interactive exercises, tracking their progress and providing feedback to both patients and therapists.

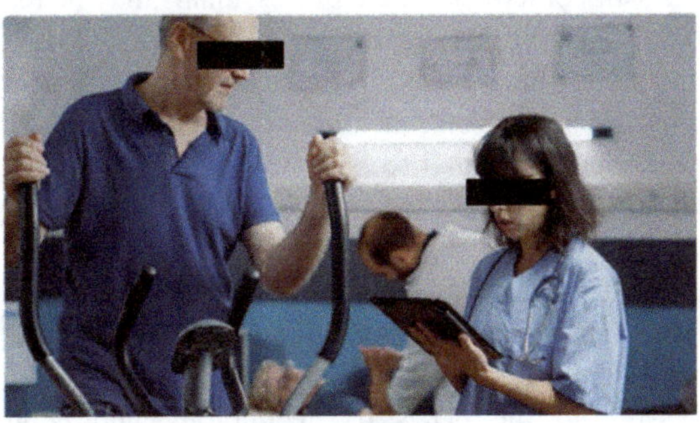

Figure 4.5 Patient record and progress

Additionally, e-platforms can help to reduce costs and increase the efficiency of physiotherapy rehabilitation [14].

Online platforms have been increasingly used in physiotherapy rehabilitation in recent years, due to the benefits they provide such as access to therapy services, personalized and interactive exercises, tracking of progress, and cost-effectiveness.

One example of an e-platform used in physiotherapy rehabilitation is tele-rehabilitation, which involves the use of video conferencing technology to provide therapy services remotely. This can be particularly beneficial for patients in remote or underserved areas, or for those who have difficulty accessing in-person therapy due to mobility issues.

Another example is the use of virtual reality (VR) in physiotherapy rehabilitation. VR can be used to provide patients with immersive and interactive exercises, as well as to track their progress and provide feedback to both patients and therapists [15].

This can help to increase the effectiveness of physiotherapy rehabilitation and also make it more engaging and motivating for patients. It is important to mention that e-platforms should be used under the supervision of a physiotherapist, and it should be taken into account that not all patients are suitable for this kind of rehabilitation, it will depend on the patient's condition and the stage of the rehabilitation.

4.4 Challenges of e-health platforms in physiotherapy

While e-health platforms have many benefits, there are also some challenges that need to be addressed. One of the biggest challenges is that e-health platforms may not be accessible to all patients. For example, some patients may not have access to the internet or may not be able to afford the technology needed to use e-health platforms. Additionally, e-health platforms may not be able to provide the same level of hands-on care as in-person physiotherapy appointments [7]. The following were some of the significant challenges of E-platforms:

1. Making sure that patients are familiar with the technology and can use it effectively for follow-up care.
2. Physiotherapists and other healthcare professionals may be required to provide training and assistance in this regard.
3. Ensuring that students have access to the necessary equipment and technology for e-platforms. Examples of this include a reliable internet connection, a computer or mobile device, and so on.
4. Ensuring that students are proficient users of the technology. Training and assistance may be required for this from teachers and other support staff.
5. Training patients to be familiar with the technology and can use it effectively. Training and assistance in this area may be required from physiotherapists and other healthcare professionals.
6. Patients accessing to the necessary technology and equipment for tele-rehabilitation. Examples of this include a reliable Internet connection, a computer or mobile device, and so on.

4.5 Conclusion

E-health platforms have the potential to revolutionize the field of physiotherapy. They can provide patients with access to physiotherapy services remotely, as well as a more personalized treatment plan. However, there are also challenges that need to be addressed, such as accessibility and the lack of hands-on care [16].

Nonetheless, the future of physiotherapy looks bright with the integration of e-health technologies. It is also important to note that more research is needed to fully understand the potential of e-platforms in physiotherapy rehabilitation and to optimize their use in clinical practice.

There are several areas where further research is needed in order to fully understand the potential of e-platforms in physiotherapy rehabilitation and to optimize their use in clinical practice.

Effectiveness: More research is needed to determine the effectiveness of e-platforms, such as telerehabilitation and virtual reality, in comparison to traditional in-person physiotherapy.

Patient satisfaction: Research is needed to understand patient satisfaction with e-platforms, and to identify any barriers or facilitators to their use.

Cost-effectiveness: Research is needed to determine the cost-effectiveness of e-platforms in physiotherapy rehabilitation, compared to traditional in-person therapy.

Implementation and adoption: Research is needed to understand the barriers and facilitators to the implementation and adoption of e-platforms in physiotherapy rehabilitation, both from the perspective of patients and healthcare providers.

Tailoring the treatment: Research is needed to understand how to tailor the treatment to each patient, to achieve the best results, taking into account the patient's condition, stage of rehabilitation, and individual needs.

Keeping the security and privacy: Research is needed to understand how to keep the security and privacy of patient's information and data when using e-platforms in physiotherapy rehabilitation.

Long-term follow-up: Research is needed to understand the long-term effects of e-platforms in physiotherapy rehabilitation, and to evaluate whether the benefits are maintained over time. Overall, the potential of e-platforms in physiotherapy and rehabilitation needs more research in order to optimize their use in clinical practice.

References

[1] Madanian S. The use of e-health technology in healthcare environment: The role of RFID technology. In: *2016 10th International Conference on e-Commerce in Developing Countries: With Focus on e-Tourism (ECDC)*, 2016 April 15 (pp. 1–5). New York, NY: IEEE.

[2] Cottrell MA and Russell TG. Telehealth for musculoskeletal physiotherapy. *Musculoskeletal Science and Practice*. 2020;48:102193.

[3] Martínez de la Cal J, Fernández-Sánchez M, Matarán-Peñarrocha GA, *et al.* Physical therapists' opinion of E-health treatment of chronic low back pain. *International Journal of Environmental Research and Public Health.* 2021;18(4):1889.

[4] Robinson A, Oksuz U, Slight R, Slight S, and Husband A. Digital and mobile technologies to promote physical health behavior change and provide psychological support for patients undergoing elective surgery: meta-ethnography and systematic review. *JMIR mHealth and uHealth.* 2020; 8(12):e19237.

[5] Liu R, Menhas R, Dai J, Saqib ZA, and Peng X. Fitness apps, live streaming workout classes, and virtual reality fitness for physical activity during the COVID-19 lockdown: an empirical study. *Frontiers in Public Health.* 2022;10: 852311.

[6] Aggarwal D, Ploderer B, Vetere F, Bradford M, and Hoang T. Doctor, can you see my squats? Understanding bodily communication in video consultations for physiotherapy. In: *Proceedings of the 2016 ACM Conference on Designing Interactive Systems*, 2016 Jun 4 (pp. 1197–1208).

[7] Albahrouh SI and Buabbas AJ. Physiotherapists' perceptions of and willingness to use telerehabilitation in Kuwait during the COVID-19 pandemic. *BMC Medical Informatics and Decision Making.* 2021;21(1):1–2.

[8] Blumenthal J, Wilkinson A, and Chignell M. Physiotherapists' and physiotherapy students' perspectives on the use of mobile or wearable technology in their practice. *Physiotherapy Canada.* 2018;70(3):251–261.

[9] Pathak N, Misra S, Mukherjee A, and Kumar N. HeDI: healthcare device interoperability for IoT-based e-health platforms. *IEEE Internet of Things Journal.* 2021;8(23):16845–16852.

[10] Du S, Liu W, Cai S, Hu Y, and Dong J. The efficacy of e-health in the self-management of chronic low back pain: a meta-analysis. *International Journal of Nursing Studies.* 2020;106:103507.

[11] Kim J, Kim S, Kim H, Kim K, Yang S, and Shin Y. Development of implementation strategies for u-health services based on the healthcare professionals' experiences. *Telemedicine and e-Health.* 2011;17(2):80–87.

[12] Martínez-Ballesté A, Gimeno P, Mariné A, Batista E, and Solanas A. e-PEMICU: an e-health platform to support early mobilisation in intensive care units. In: *2019 10th International Conference on Information, Intelligence, Systems and Applications (IISA), 2019 Jul 15* (pp. 1–6). New York, NY: IEEE.

[13] Jain S. Telemedicine: an innovation growing indispensable. In: *Digital Marketing Outreach* 2023 (pp. 157–169). India: Routledge.

[14] Valdés BA, Glegg SM, Lambert-Shirzad N, *et al.* Application of commercial games for home-based rehabilitation for people with hemiparesis: challenges and lessons learned. *Games for Health Journal.* 2018;7(3):197–207.

[15] Brepohl PC and Leite H. Virtual reality applied to physiotherapy: a review of current knowledge. *Virtual Reality*. 2022;3:1–25.

[16] van der Meer HA, Doomen A, Visscher CM, Engelbert RH, Nijhuis-van der Sanden MW, and Speksnijder CM. The additional value of e-Health for patients with a temporomandibular disorder: a mixed methods study on the perspectives of orofacial physical therapists and patients. *Disability and Rehabilitation: Assistive Technology*. 2022;12:1–3, doi: 10.1080/17483107.2022.2094000.

Chapter 5

Adoption of Building Information Modelling in Malaysia medical facilities building construction

Chee Fui Wong[1] *and Chun Chieh Yip*[1]

Abstract

The Malaysia government acknowledged the importance of BIM technology for the medical facilities building, and the first pilot project that adopted BIM in Malaysia was the medical facilities building known as the National Cancer Institute (NCI) in the 2010. Building Information Modelling (BIM) is a new innovative technology for the construction industry stakeholders. BIM is a modelling technology and processes to communicate, produce and utilise the digital data information for the integration of the construction data and information throughout the project life cycle, with the purpose to enhance the efficiency, increase the productivity as well as enhance the collaboration among the project stakeholders. The government of Malaysia acknowledges the paramount importance of BIM technology for the transformation toward a more sustainable construction environment particularly in the construction of the medical facilities building construction. This study focused on the adoption of BIM technology in the construction of medical facilities building in Malaysia. The benefits of BIM for facilities management and the benefits of the implementation of NCI as the pilot medical facilities building are discussed.

5.1 Fourth Industrial Revolution and BIM in Construction 4.0

Globally, the term "Fourth Industrial Revolution" refers to the emerging trends in the technologies such as artificial intelligence (AI), Internet of Things (IoT), cloud computing, augmented and virtual reality (AR/VR), automation, autonomous robot; additive manufacturing, big data analysis, cyber security, and system integration. However, in the Malaysia context, we have redefined the main technology for Construction 4.0 under "CIDB Construction 4.0 – Strategic Plan" to encompass also "Building Information Modelling (BIM)," "Prefabrication & Modular Construction" and "Advance Building Material." The concept of Construction 4.0

[1]Universiti Tunku Abdul Rahman, UTAR Sungai Long Campus, Malaysia

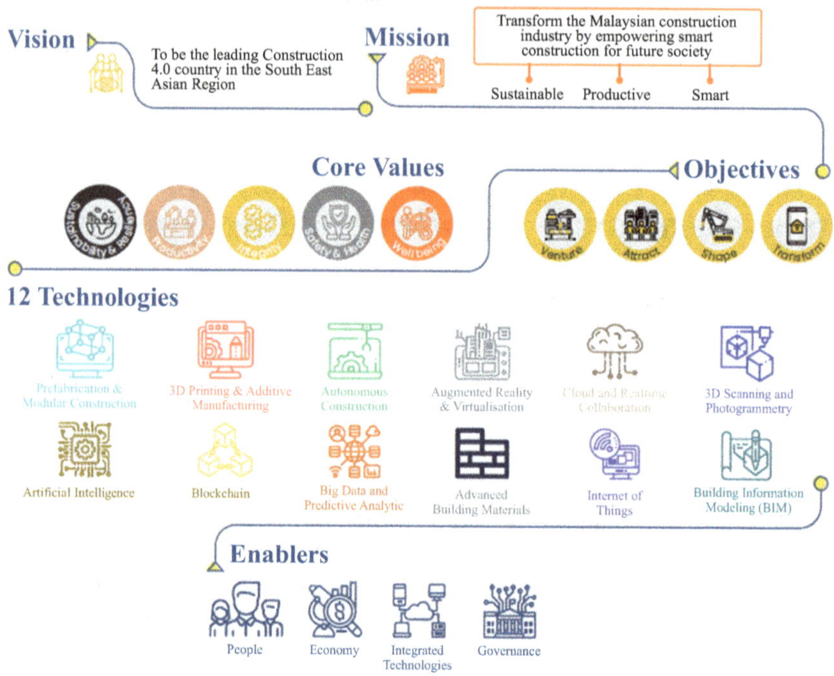

Figure 5.1 *Summary framework of "Construction 4.0 Strategic Plan 2021–2025".* Source*: [1].*

was the digital transformation to enhance new technologies for communication, collaboration among various stakeholders to improve the productivity, safety and sustainability in the whole construction life cycle [1]. Figure 5.1 shows the "Summary Framework of Construction 4.0 Strategic Plan 2021–2025."

"Building Information Modelling (BIM)" is acknowledged as one of the 12 main technologies in Malaysia CIDB "Construction 4.0 Strategic Plan 2021–2025." CIDB has defined the main technologies for Construction 4.0 under "CIDB Construction 4.0 – Strategic Plan" to encompass also "Building Information Modelling (BIM)," "Prefabrication & Modular Construction" and "Advance Building Material."

The future of the construction industry will be highly influenced by the implementation of the emerging technologies and new innovations into the existing processes. The adoption of new emerging technologies such as BIM technologies with new innovative processes will transform the delivery of the medical facilities buildings projects.

5.2 Building information modelling technology

Charles Eastman introduced the concept of BIM in the 1970s and was initially called "Building Description System (BDS)," with the aim to reduce the cost of design by

Table 5.1 Summary of BIM definitions

No.	Building information modelling	References
1	"Building Information Model is the digital representation of physical and functional characteristics of a facility. As such it serves as a shared knowledge resource for information about a facility, forming a reliable basis for decisions during its life cycle from inception onwards"	National BIM Standard – United State [6]
2	"Building Information Modeling (BIM) is the process of generating and managing building data during its design, construction and during the building or assets life cycle"	Hong Kong Construction Industry Council [7]
3	"BIM is a digital representation of physical and functional characteristics of a facility. A building information model is a shared knowledge resource for information about a facility forming a reliable basis for decisions during its life-cycle; defined as existing from earliest conception to demolition"	Building and Construction Authority (BCA), Singapore [8]
4	"Building Information Modelling is a collection of defined model uses, workflows and modelling methods used to achieve specific, repeatable, and reliable information from the model"	NATSPEC BIM Guide, Australia [9]

halves through "drafting and analysis efficiencies" [2]. However, the adoption of BIM only started since mid-2000 [3,4]. The concept of BIM is to virtually construct a virtual model of the building before it physically builds, therefore the problems can be solved and potential impacts can be simulated and analysed.

BIM is the new innovative technologies that can be implemented in the design stage, construction stage, and facility management stage where digital information data representation of the building is created to facilitate the exchange and interoperability of the digital information [5]. Although BIM has been successfully adopted in many countries, there are no specific BIM definition that has been adopted internationally. Every economy has adopted its own definition of BIM based on their own understanding and perceptions. Table 5.1 summaries some of the definitions of BIM.

In Malaysia context, Construction Industry Development Board (CIDB) has defined "Building Information Modelling (BIM), as a modelling technology and associated set of processes to produce, communicate, analyse and use of digital information models throughout construction project life-cycle" [10]

5.3 BIM maturity level

The adoption of BIM varies in the BIM maturity level. Bew [11] studies suggested four different maturity levels in the BIM evolution progress using lenses of data and process sets, where each level required different capabilities of people, process and technologies as shown in Table 5.2 and Figure 5.2.

Table 5.2 BIM maturity level [11]

Level	Description
Level 0	"Use of unmanaged CAD"
Level 1	"Managed CAD in 2D or 3D format where the company engaged industry standard within the process such as BS1192 with commercial data is managed by stand-alone finance and a cost management package"
Level 2	"Managed 3D environment held in separate discipline tools with parametric data and commercial data and managed by Enterprise Resource Planning. During this stage, integration occurs on the basis of proprietary interface or bespoke middleware"
Level 3	"Fully open interoperable process and data integration enabled by IFC. Named as integrated BIM, the data and information are managed by a collaborative model server"

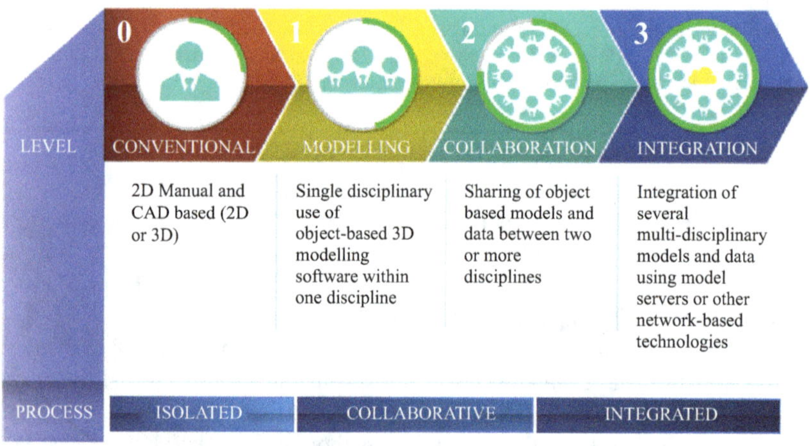

Figure 5.2 BIM maturity level [10]

5.4 BIM level of development (LOD) and level of details (Lod)

LOD defines the extent of the information provided with the geometric details as well as the alphanumeric details and can be associated with a specific design phase [12]. The concept of LOD was first introduced by Vico and Weber in 2005 and subsequently developed in various countries to support BIM development model [13]. The term LOD is distinct and different from the term Lod which emphasises on the geometric appearance and details [12].

The "US-American BIMForum" has defined six standardised LODs (LOD 100, LOD 200, LOD 300, LOD 350, LOD 400, and LOD 500) as published in the LOD Spec 2020 for Building Information Model [14] and summarised in Table 5.3.

Table 5.3 BIM forum definition of LOD [14]

Level of Development	Definition (in BIM Forum – LOD Spec 2020 for Building Information Model)
LOD 100	"The Model Element may be graphically represented in the Model with a symbol or other generic representation, but does not satisfy the requirements for LOD 200. Information related to the Model Element (i.e. cost per square foot, tonnage of HVAC, etc.) can be derived from other Model Elements"
LOD 200	"The Model Element is graphically represented within the Model as a generic system, object, or assembly with approximate quantities, size, shape, location, and orientation. Non-graphic information may also be attached to the Model Element"
LOD 300	"The Model Element is graphically represented within the Model as a specific system, object or assembly in terms of quantity, size, shape, location, and orientation. Non-graphic information may also be attached to the Model Element."
LOD 350	"The Model Element is graphically represented within the Model as a specific system, object, or assembly in terms of quantity, size, shape, location, orientation, and interfaces with other building systems. Non-graphic information may also be attached to the Model Element"
LOD 400	"The Model Element is graphically represented within the Model as a specific system, object or assembly in terms of size, shape, location, quantity, and orientation with detailing, fabrication, assembly, and installation information. Non-graphic information may also be attached to the Model Element"
LOD 500	"The Model Element is a field verified representation in terms of size, shape, location, quantity, and orientation. Non-graphic information may also be attached to the Model Elements"

LOD requirements are usually defined by the clients prior to the project commencement as part of the "Employer's Information Requirements (EIR)" and are usually associated with a specific design phase [12]. The term LOD is different from the term Lod where Ref. [15] defined Lod as "the degree of information details (geometric and non-geometric) throughout the project life cycle." Progress of each Lod carries the details specification as illustrated in the Figure 5.3.

5.5 The adoption of BIM in Malaysia medical facilities building

The idea of the implementation BIM in Malaysia was first introduced by the Director General of Public Work Department (PWD) in 2007 [16,17]. The government has realised the potential of BIM for project efficiency, minimise cost and resolve the design issues during the planning stage particularly for the construction of medical facilities building.

Since 2007, various strategies and initiatives were formulated to execute BIM project in order to enhance government project delivery efficiency and

Family		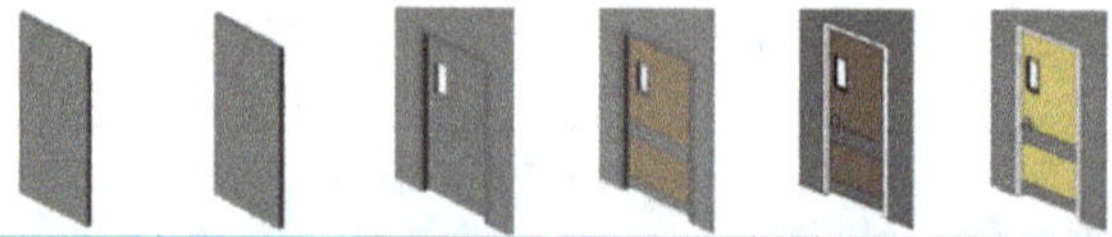					
Stage		Concept	Preliminary	Detailed	Construction	As-Built	Operation
LOD		100	200	300	400	500	600
Dimension	Width	–	900mm	900mm	900mm	900mm	900mm
	Height	–	1800mm	1800mm	1800mm	1800mm	1800mm
	Thickness	–	50mm	50mm	50mm	50mm	50mm
Material		–	–	Wood	Wood	Wood	Wood
Finishing		–	–	Painting	Painting	Painting	Vanish
Identity data	Manufacturer	–	–	–	XY Sdn.Bhd	XY Sdn.Bhd	WZ Sdn.Bhd
	Model	–	–	–	XD 001	XD 001	F 005
	Fire rated	–	–	2 Hours	2 Hours	2 Hours	2 Hours
	Cost	–	–	–	RM200	RM200	RM250
	Installation date	–	–	–	12.08.16	12.08.16	02.03.16

Figure 5.3 Illustration of BIM Lod [15]

productivity. The Malaysian government has realised the importance of BIM technology for the medical facilities building, and the first pilot project that adopted BIM in Malaysia was the medical facilities building known as the National Cancer Institute (NCI) in the 2010 [16]. The successful execution of the pilot project has led to more government public projects that adopt BIM. Between 2007 and 2017, a total of 17 government projects have been implemented using the BIM process [18]. Some of the notable government projects that have implemented BIM technology include the National Cancer Institute (NCI) in Putrajaya, the administration building in Kuala Terengganu City Council, Malaysia Anti-Corruption Commission (MACC) in Shah Alam, and the public health clinic (KK5) in Maran, Pahang [17].

Following the successful BIM technology implementation of the first pilot medical facilities building project "National Cancer Institute (NCI)" that was completed in 31 August 2013, the Malaysian government has realised the benefits of BIM technology for medical facilities building. Subsequently more medical facilities building in Malaysia are constructed using BIM technology by Malaysia Public Work Department (PWD) as shown in Table 5.4.

In 2017, the Malaysian government announced that BIM would be compulsory from 2019 onwards for all public project above RM100 million. This policy was later incorporated as the KPI in the CIDB Construction Industry Transformation Programme [20] where the BIM-related KPI are listed as part of the technology focus areas that include 100% of all government building projects that cost over RM 100 million (for JKR building projects) to adopt BIM Level 2 and 70% of private and public building projects that cost over RM 10 million to implement BIM. In terms of policy, "Malaysia Construction 4.0 Strategic Plan 2021–2025" has specified BIM as one of the 12 main technologies that drive the transformation of Malaysian construction industry [1]

Table 5.4 PWD medical facilities building that adopted BIM technology [19]

Projects	Concept design	Preliminary design	Detailed design	Procurement	Construction	As-build
National Cancer Institute					√	√
Health Clinic Maran Pahang		√	√	√	√	√
Endocrine Complex Putrajaya Hospital			√		√	√
Parit Buntar Hospital			√		√	√
Keamanan Hospital			√		√	√
Pendang Hospital				√		
Pasir Gudang Hospital				√		
Kajang Hospital			√			
Seri Iskandar Hospital			√			

5.6 Benefits of BIM in facilities management

The adoption of BIM technology in the medical facilities building has many benefits particularly on the benefits in terms of facilities management of the medical equipment in the medical facilities building. The study by [21] has indicated various benefits of BIM in terms of facilities management that includes better space management, building life cycle management, building equipment management, fast, effective and efficient facilities management, simpler performance simulation, streamlined maintenance, energy efficiency utilisation, easier and more economical modifications, reduction of waste and enhance project safety.

Other researcher has also concluded the similar benefits of BIM for facilities management as shown in Table 5.5. The studies from various literature have indicated the benefits of BIM technology for facilities management that includes accurate as build and building information, better information for life cycle of asset management, information for scheduled maintenance and operation as well as enhance evaluation of maintenance approach based on cost.

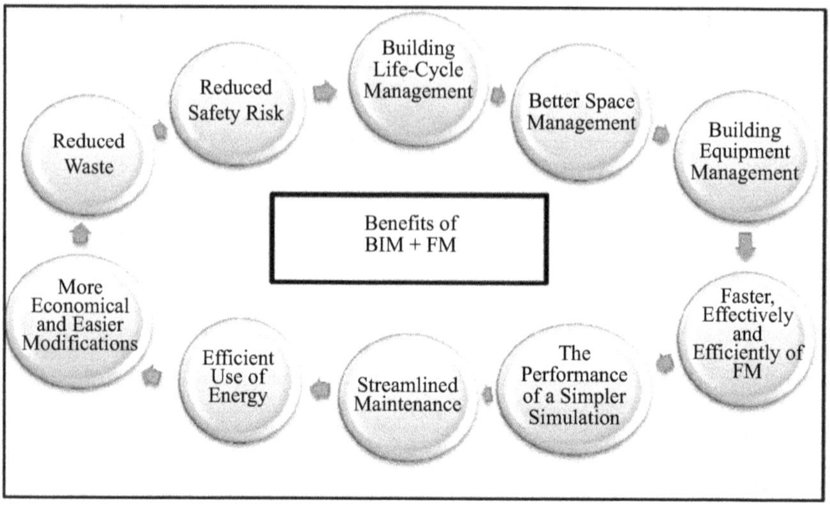

Figure 5.4 Benefits of BIM in facilities management [21]

Table 5.5 Summaries of the benefits of BIM in facilities management

No.	**Benefits of BIM in facilities management**	**Author**					
		[22]	**[21]**	**[23]**	**[24]**	**[10]**	
	Facilities Management and Project Life Cycle						
1	Accurate as built and building information		√		√	√	3
2	Better information for life cycle of asset management	√	√	√	√	√	5
3	Information for scheduled maintenance and operation		√	√	√	√	4
4	Enhance evaluation of maintenance approach based on cost			√	√	√	3

5.7 Case study – National Cancer Institute (NCI) – Malaysia's first medical facilities building adopting BIM technology

BIM is new emerging technology that manages the construction project activities throughout the project life-cycle that includes the project design and planning phase, construction phase as well as facilities management phase [2]. Malaysia's Public Work Department (PWD) has introduced the concept of BIM technology since early 2007 [16,17]. The NCI is the first medical facilities building in Malaysia that adopted the BIM technology by PWD. The NCI project that cost RM 690 million is the brainchild of the late Datin Seri' Endon Mahmood (who died of breast cancer in 2005), the wife of former Prime Minister of Malaysia, Tun Abdullah Ahmad Badawi in 2004. The NCI is Malaysia's first medical facilities

Table 5.6 Summary of NCI medical facilities building project [16]

No.	Description	Details
1	Project owner	Ministry of Health, Malaysia
2	Site procession	1 Sep 2010
3	Completion date	31 Aug 2013
4	Contract duration	36 months
5	Total site areas	10.65 acres (4.31 hectare)
6	Total gross floor area (GFA)	75,555 sq m
7	BIM consultant	Precision Design Solution(M) Sdn. Bhd.
8	BIM tools	Autodesk Revisit (Architectural, Structure, M&E) and Naviswork
9	Project consultant	Perunding Alam Bina Sdn. Bhd.
10	Project contractor	Kiara Teratai Sdn. Bhd.

building that has implemented the "Total Hospital System" (THIS) that includes the element of "Oncology Information System" (OIS) [16].

According to the study by [16], the NCI design concept has utilised the BIM tools of Autodesk Revit (Architecture, Structure, M&E) and Naviswork with the focus to provide state-of-the-art specialised diagnostic and treatment facilities in a cheerful, user friendly and functional ambiance. The details of the NCI medical facilities building are summarised in Table 5.6.

With the implementation of BIM technology in the construction of the NCI medical facilities building, the project was completed 2 weeks ahead of the project schedule on 31 August 2013. The study by [16] through the interview with the stakeholders of the project owner, consultant and contractor for the NCI medical facilities building project has concluded the following benefits of BIM implementation for medical facilities building:

1. BIM minimises the delay in constructions (the project is completed 2 weeks ahead of schedule)
2. BIM avoids construction cost overrun and provides saving to the project cost
3. BIM provides a better project construction quality
4. BIM technology allows crash analysis to be conducted prior to the construction commencement thus resolving the design issues during the planning stage
5. BIM provides a clear 3D visualisation for the design and structure of the medical facilities building thus resolving the fabrication issues at the early stage
6. Minimise the construction waste

5.8 Conclusion

The Malaysian government has realised the importance of BIM technology for the construction of medical facilities building. The facilities management of medical facilities building is paramount important and the BIM technology has demonstrated the benefits that it can be derived from the adoption of BIM for medical facilities building construction. The successful implementation of the first pilot medical facilities building of the NCI using BIM technology has paved the way for the other medical facilities building to adopt and implement BIM technology. The Malaysian government has included the BIM technology as the national policy in "CIDB Construction Industry Transformation Programme" where the BIM is made compulsory for all public projects above RM100 million from 2019 onwards. Subsequently, Malaysian government has also incorporated BIM technology as a new innovation under "Malaysia Construction 4.0 Strategic Plan 2021–2025" to drive the transformation of Malaysian construction industry [1].

References

[1] CIDB, *Construction 4.0 Strategic Plan (2021–2025).* Kuala Lumpur: Construction Industry Development Board (CIDB), 2020.

[2] E. Chuck, T. Paul, S. Rafael, and L. Kathleen, *BIM Handbook: A Guide to Building Information Modelling for Owners, Managers, Designers, Engineers and Contractors*, 2nd ed., New York, NY: John Wiley & Sons, Inc., 2011.

[3] S. Azhar, M. Khalfan, and T. Maqsood, "Building information modeling (BIM): now and beyond," *Austral. J. Constr. Econ. Build.*, vol. 12, no. 4, pp. 15–28, 2012, doi:10.5130/ajceb.v12i4.3032.

[4] S. K. Z. Xiong, *The Actual Implementation Level of BIM and the Strategies to Increase Adoption of BIM,* Iskandar Puteri: Universiti Teknologi Malaysia, 2018.

[5] CREAM, *Issues and Challenges in Implementing BIM for SMEs in the Construction Industry*, Kuala Lumpur: Construction Research Institute of Malaysia (CREAM), 2014.

[6] National BIM Standard – United State, "NBIMS-US-3: 3 – Terms and Definitions," *National BIM Standard – United States – Version 3*, 2015. https://www.nationalbimstandard.org/files/NBIMS-US_V3_3_Terms_and_Definitions.pdf.

[7] HK CIC, "What is BIM?," 2020. https://www.bim.cic.hk/en/bim_in_hk/what_is_bim.

[8] BCA, "BIM Guide for Asset Information Delivery," 2018. https://www1.bca.gov.sg/docs/default-source/docs-corp-buildsg/integrated-digital-delivery-(idd)/bim_guide_for_asset_information_delivery_v1.pdf.

[9] NATSPEC, "National BIM Guide v1.0 Sep 2011.doc," 2016. www.natspec.com.au.

[10] CIDB, *BIM Guide 1: Awareness*. Kuala Lumpur: Construction Industry Development Board (CIDB), 2016.

[11] G. Bew, M. Storer, J. Underwood, and J. Wix, "Going BIM in a commercial world," in *eWork and eBusiness in Architecture, Engineering and Construction*, 2008, London: Routledge, pp. 139–150.

[12] A. Borrmann, M. König, C. Koch, and J. Beetz, "Building information modeling What? Why? How?: Technology foundations and industry practice," *Build. Inf. Model. Technol. Found. Ind. Pract.*, no. February 2019, pp. 1–584, 2018, doi:10.1007/978-3-319-92862-3.

[13] I. Grytting, F. Svalestuen, J. Lohne, H. Sommerseth, S. Augdal, and O. Lædre, "Use of LoD decision plan in BIM-projects," *Procedia Eng.*, vol. 196, no. June, pp. 407–414, 2017, doi:10.1016/j.proeng.2017.07.217.

[14] J. Bedrick, W. Faia, P. E. Ikerd, and J. Reinhardt, *Level of Development (LOD) Specification Part I & Commentary for Building Information Models and Data*, 2020. www.bimforum.org/lod.

[15] CIDB, *BIM Guide 2: Readiness*. Kuala Lumpur: CIDB, 2016.

[16] A. A. Latiffi, S. Mohd, and J. Brahim, "Application of building information modeling (BIM) in the Malaysian construction industry: a story of the first government project," *Appl. Mech. Mater.*, vol. 773–774, no. May 2012, pp. 943–948, 2015, doi:10.4028/www.scientific.net/amm.773-774.943.

[17] CIDB, *Handbook for the Implementation of Building Information Modelling in Construction Industry Transformation Programme 2016–2020*, Kuala Lumpur: CIDB, 2018.

[18] CIDB, *BIM Guide 4: BIM Execution Plan (BEP)*. Kuala Lumpur: Construction Industry Development Board (CIDB), 2017.

[19] I. Othman, Y. Y. Al-ashmori, Y. Rahmawati, Y. H. M. Amran, M. Ali, and M. Al-bared, "The level of building information modelling (BIM) implementation in Malaysia," *Ain Shams Eng. J.*, vol. 12, no. 1, pp. 455–463, 2021, doi:10.1016/j.asej.2020.04.007.

[20] CIDB, *Construction Industry Transformation Programme 2016–2020*. Kuala Lumpur: Construction Industry Development Board (CIDB), 2015.

[21] S. A. Abdullah, N. Sulaiman, A. A. Latiffi, and D. Baldry, "Building Information Modelling (BIM) from the perspective of Facilities Management (FM) in Malaysia," no. April, 2014, doi:10.13140/2.1.4886.0164.

[22] D. W. M. Chan, T. O. Olawumi, and A. M. L. Ho, "Perceived benefits of and barriers to building information modelling (BIM) implementation in construction: the case of Hong Kong," *J. Build. Eng.*, vol. 25, no. August 2018, p. 100764, 2019, doi:10.1016/j.jobe.2019.100764.

[23] K. Ullah, I. Lill, and E. Witt, "An overview of BIM adoption in the construction industry: benefits and barriers," *Emerald Reach Proc. Ser.*, vol. 2, pp. 297–303, 2019, doi:10.1108/S2516-285320190000002052.

[24] M. A. Aziz, *Building Information Modelling (BIM) for Power Plant Projects in Malaysia: The Perspective of Clients and Way Forward*, Selangor: Universiti Putra Malaysia, 2020.

Chapter 6

Medical equipment engineering standards for design and risk management of immersive virtual reality for in-clinic and home used

Lee Poh Foong[1]

Virtual reality (VR) refers to a computer-generated three-dimensional environment that can create a virtual world, tricking the human brain through visual, auditory, and tactile stimuli. It provides users with a sense of mental and physical immersion by responding to their movements and interactions in the real world. In recent years, the use of immersive VR technology in medical rehabilitation has become increasingly prevalent. Consequently, it is crucial to examine the ergonomic design of VR systems tailored for different target populations, whether for in-clinic or home use. Additionally, conducting risk analyses and implementing effective management strategies are vital to ensure the safe and reliable use of VR as a medical device.

6.1 VR devices as medical equipment and its benefit

Virtual reality (VR) is classified into three main categories as shown in Figure 6.1. A non-immersive simulation provides the least immersive implementation that lets for outer alertness of the real world outside the VR. Consumers involve in 3D computer-generated environments through a window by exploiting ordinary great resolution monitors. On the other hand, semi-immersive simulation enables the user to partially immerse in a virtual environment (VE) powered by high-performance graphical computing systems, together with multiple televisions projection structures, purposely to appropriately stimulate the user's images. Finally, a fully immersive simulation brings the most immersive execution simulation. It is able to deliver a widespread view, great resolutions, and improved update rates. Therefore, by sending extraordinary contrast to the consumer's head-mounted display, it delivers supreme realistic consumer experiences.

[1]Mechanical & Material Department, Lee Kong Chien Faculty of Engineering & Science, Universiti Tunku Abdul Rahman, Malaysia

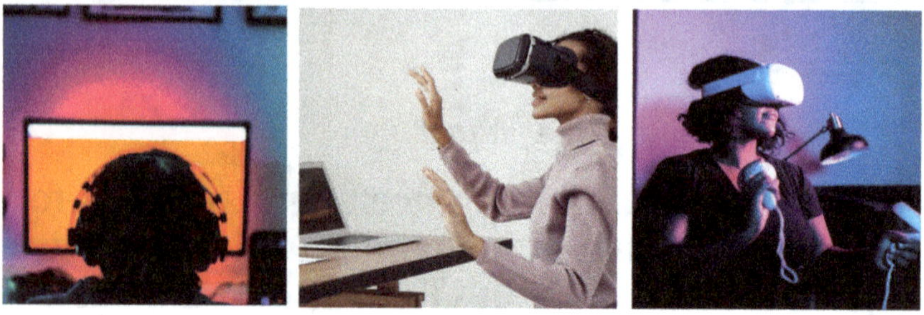

Figure 6.1 Three categories of virtual platform

For performing full-immersive VR simulations, one of the most important components is a personal computer or smartphone. They act as the data center, processing all inputs and giving outputs. Next, a head-mounted display is a device that provides visual content to the users. It normally fully covers the user's view and is accompanied by audio stimulation (*What is Virtual Reality (VR)? Ultimate Guide to Virtual Reality (VR) Technology*, 2019). Input devices such as joysticks, data gloves, tracking balls, motion trackers, and controlled wands are necessary to perform interactions between users and VR. They are also the key component to provide a sense of immersion to the users.

In the era of the fourth industrial revolution, virtual reality (VR) systems have emerged as crucial tools for enhancing human lifestyles. VR finds applications in various fields such as education, scientific visualization, medicine, industrial design, architecture, as well as games and entertainment. Prior to the introduction of VR systems, physical methods were employed for motion and behaviour rehabilitation, necessitating precise setup and arrangement of the treatment environment for patients. While extensive research has been conducted on VR systems specifically designed for motion rehabilitation, there is a significant lack of completed research on behaviour rehabilitation using VR. Traditional rehabilitation methods still exist and are utilized today, but they often require prolonged periods of treatment with no guaranteed improvement. Moreover, the traditional rehabilitation process is time-consuming and costly, involving specialized equipment, controlled environments, and professional therapists. Additionally, traditional rehabilitation may expose patients to unsafe conditions, necessitating the expensive construction of specialized environments to minimize the risk of injuries.

One of the limitations of traditional rehabilitation is the repetitive nature of the environments, leading to patient boredom and apathy. However, with the advent of VR systems, the potential for behaviour rehabilitation opens up new possibilities. While research in this area is scarce, the immersive and interactive nature of VR holds promise for revolutionizing behaviour rehabilitation. Overall, the integration of VR systems into rehabilitation processes has the potential to overcome the limitations of traditional methods, offering more engaging, cost-effective, and personalized treatment options for patients. However, further research and development are needed to explore the full potential of VR for behaviour rehabilitation.

Traditional rehabilitation does exist and is still in use today. However, the rehabilitation processes require years, and no improvement is guaranteed. A long period of rehabilitation with special equipment, environment, and professional rehabilitators will also end up in high-cost consumption. Traditional rehabilitation may also expose patients to unsafe environments where they are required to. Hence, to minimise the risk of injuries, traditional rehabilitation is limited to certain environments and surroundings that require a high cost to build. The environments may be the same for the whole rehabilitation process which will cause patients to feel bored and antipathy.

6.2 Uses of VR in healthcare

The advance technology integrating VR with the current healthcare system has brought in numerous benefits for the physician and patients. For instance, 3D visualization of CT results can be shown to the patients while physician explaining the conditions through using 3D models in VE [1] as shown in Figure 6.2.

On the other hand, employing VR for detecting different mental state condition offers feasible VR treatment. When the VR technology merges with artificial intelligence, accuracy in assessing and reliable treatment plan can be offered to more people, which AI-driven precision medicine tools in mental health care are currently missing [2]. According to research studies, VR can be effectively applied in psychotherapy as a method of treating various phobias and other mental health conditions [3]. VR provides a safe and controllable environment for doctors to situate patients in uncomfortable conditions present individually for each case to train them to overcome their fears and gain confidence [4]. There are abundant of phobias such as fear of open or confined spaces, fear of various living beings, stage fright, fear of heights or water, and spider with VR that potentially be treated in such a way.

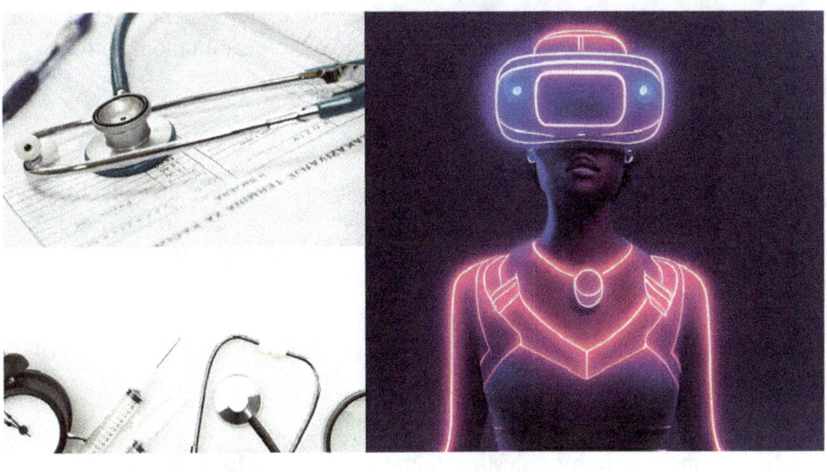

Figure 6.2 Application of VR to medical area

Table 6.1 Interacting modules in rehabilitation platform [7]

Modules	Description
Physical system	Hardware platform (computer, webcam, and controllers such as handgrip)
Tracking system	Receive information from tracking system and controller (location and pressure)
Simulated environment	Present the game and interact with user. To provide feedback and database for adjustment and improvement
Trunk compensation	By stalking user head with elementary head features and several classifiers. To provide alarm or block the game when non-causal association occurred
Adaptation module	Adjust the 3D space where the implementation happens Adjust task difficulties according to partly observable Markov decision

VR-based interventions for stroke rehabilitation are rising over the time although the efficacy of this intervention is under vigorous investigation. However, VR-based intervention is in favour due to its ability to mobilize recovery mechanism. A prior study on evaluating the effect of specific design VR and nonspecific VR for rehabilitation of the post stroke patients indicates that the specific design shows better outcome [5]. Moreover, VR as a medical tool for patients to receive therapy either in clinic and home used is currently serving as enhancement for patients with various conditions ranging from musculoskeletal issues to cognitive deficits [6].

For home use, the VR-based intervention is namely telerehabilitation. VR intervention can enhance patient's motivation, adaptability, and variability based on patient baseline, transparent data storage, online remote data access, economy of scale, and reduced medical costs. However, there remain a few challenges in VR use for rehabilitation such as lack of computer skills on the part of therapists, lack of support infrastructure, expensive equipment (initially), and patient safety concerns [6]. Table 6.1 has displayed the interacting modules in rehabilitation platform.

6.3 Human factors design with VR

VR is a virtual world created by a computer system that makes users feel that they are in an environment, but they are not. They give a false image to the users' brains by cheating them through human senses and interactions. According to another gesture therapy research done previously, the rehabilitation platform comprises five interacting modules [7].

6.4 VR system in rehabilitation

According to the research on gesture therapy, there are four principles to follow to increase the effectiveness of rehabilitation. A prior project reported the effectiveness of VR-based intervention for post-stroke patients for a continuous following up for 4 weeks. The rehabilitation training involves motor and balances rehabilitation. They have developed two applications in this project to serve motor dysfunction and balance impairment. The aim to promote the use of VR headsets enables an individual to expose to a 3D VE. Then, the immersive VR is capable to offer mirror therapy in post-stroke rehabilitation and thus aids in recovery. The system related to the leap motion sensor and Kinect sensor enabled the patient to interact with the virtual world. This project proves that VR can enhance physical rehabilitation training [8]. The pick and placed task in VR is shown in Figure 6.3.

There are potential advantages and disadvantages of involving VR systems in rehabilitation therapies. The counts on advantages are including the VR-designed intervention that can alter the setting according to customer requirements and improvement which account for its dosages, frequencies, difficulties, and mission changeability. Besides, VR-based intervention for rehabilitation involves very little clinical observation that enables home use, is cost-effective, and makes available for telerehabilitation. VR design for medical use can provide the enhancement of ecology validity in VEs which may increase the efficiency of the rehabilitation process [9].

On the other hand, a few challenges or drawbacks have also been reported for the usage of VR in the medical field such as the requirement of specialist expertise in giving training and operation which also indirectly increases the cost. There is cyber-sickness reported after the use of VR, this is a great setback for participants who suffered from motion sickness because of the usage of VR. In addition, some users are unfamiliar with the VR system and do not enjoy the VEs by perception. However, VR systems can provide patients with any environment they need for rehabilitation. The system activates different regions of the brain and boosts the efficiency of rehabilitation [8]. Cybersickness is a common and unpleasant side effect of VR immersion. A study measured physiological changes that were experienced by seated subjects who interacted with a VE first while viewing a display monitor and second while using a head-mounted display (HMD) and was then compared. The outcome of the results showed that half of the subjects exited the VE after 6 min of HMD use and reported feeling some nausea. This research also discovered that changes in stomach activity, blinking, and breathing can

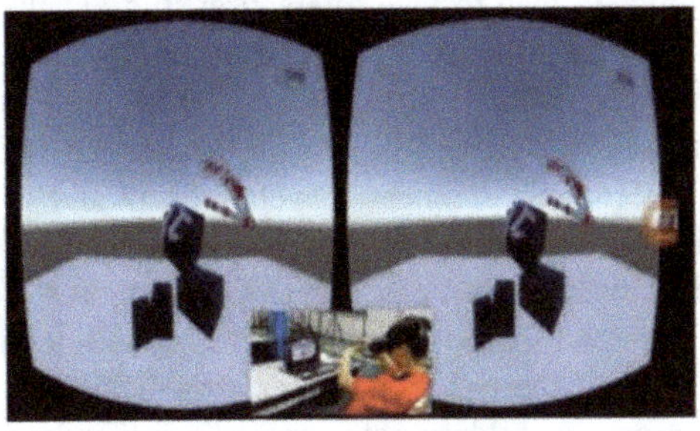

Figure 6.3 Pick and place task in VR [8]

estimate post-immersion symptom scores, with R2 values reaching as high as 0.75. The work concluded that the HMD use by seated subjects is strongly correlated with the development of cyber sickness. Therefore, cyber-sickness is a great challenge for VR systems to widen their usage to a wider population or target participants [10]. A VR headset is a head-mounted device that provides simulated images to the user. They comprise a stereoscopic head-mounted display that provides separate images for each eye, stereo sound and may be a head motion sensor.

In these recent years, the technique has been studied to reduce cybersickness through incorporating spatial blur in VR systems with the technique that makes use of concepts from foveate imaging and depth-of-field. The experimental analysis highlighted the aptness of our foveate depth-of-field effect in reducing cybersickness in VEs obtained a reduction of sickness scores by approximately 66% [11]. There are a few more suggestions from studies to create a more compiling VE for users, for instance, to place the virtual objects at a comfortable viewing range at 0.75–3.5 m, avoid linear oscillations at 0.2 Hz and off vertical axis rotation [11].

6.5 Risk analysis and concerns about VR-based intervention

The usage of VR-based intervention in-clinic and at home used especially for rehabilitation has its risks and concerns. There are a few concerns about the application of VR in the medical field such as the concern about reducing face-to-face communications, education on learning how to use the system, and the user's attitude toward using the system for medical use.

VR system intervention in the clinic may still be able to maintain communication between physicians and patients. However, the home user or out of the care of healthcare organization may affect the efficiency of applying VR as a telerehabilitation tool which the direct supervision from the physician to the patient is missing. Therefore, evaluation should be established for the protocol for ensuring the effectiveness of the VR-based system. Meanwhile, VR-based education or training provided to the caregiver, patients, and physicians are essential. The good news in recent study shows that the design considered the aim to increase the VR system that embodies a high level of social presence with conversation patterns reported to be as similar to face-to-face interaction study [12].

VR-based applications in medical usage especially in the mental health area required a comprehensive manual that specifies the detailed steps of the technology. The identifying individual who is suitable to use VR includes gender, age, personality, history of motion sickness, psychological and a variety of clinical conditions should be assessed. Sensitivity in some patients needs to be considered, including apprehensiveness to using a HMD [13], the real test itself, learning capacity to act in a VE, and the potential side effects and duration. Each variable can contribute to a risk for the usage of VR as a medical tool. A fascinating outcome with VR on distracting children with cancer from pain has been reported to be efficient and the setup of the experiment included VR distraction intervention, non-VR distraction or normal treatment without distraction [14]. Therefore, in obtaining more details on how the VR will work for a specific aim, more data must be collected to optimize its usage.

VR application in mental health has raised more concern as report shows that patient who suffers from severe anxiety, and psychosis may trigger negative effects or else must be used in special care. However, prior research shows that the use of VR demonstrated a promising tool to cope with anxiety-related disorders [15]. Hence, it is depended on the design of the VR-based intervention for the specific targeted group who can help in reducing the risk of triggering the negative side effect from this intervention. Meanwhile, the age of the patients who engage in this intervention for healing may be suitable for a certain age range, for instance, children but may not be reaping similar effects from older populations. A study focused on youth for their presence effects in VR on attention, enjoyment and memory and the outcome showed that there is no evidence that attention is associated with enjoyment or memory [16].

The setup of the VR system comprises high-quality hardware, high-speed computers, efficient graphics cards, accurate tracking systems, high-resolution displays, and highly specialized accessories. Therefore, it is a high cost of design and implementation, which slow down using these tools. However, VR has been established as a simple tool for its application even with mobile App, this gives a bright direction into VR as medical device for in-clinic and home-used tools. Besides, the design content of VR for specific apply fields acquires skills from different professions and hence increases its cost. A study has reported on the evaluation of a low-cost 3D sound simulation in a virtual training environment [17]. Although the initial study of lowering the cost of VR systems in a general way is not specific to medical usage areas, however, it is hopeful that VR installation can be more affordable in different areas. Besides, VR-based interventions or applications with the purpose of medical use must be interesting and attractive to be designed for increasing their efficiency for users. Thus, in the design process, the involvement of the end-users and engaging their views and opinions is a key factor to make it more effective.

The user's attitude towards VR technology plays a crucial role in its successful implementation as a medical intervention. The level of acceptance by users significantly influences their willingness to adopt VR systems as part of their medical care. If users have a negative attitude or perceive the technology as difficult to use, it may lead to system abandonment or refusal to learn how to operate it effectively. While virtual environments (VEs) can elicit similar sensations to real environments, users may not experience the same emotional reactions. This raises concerns about using VR-based interventions for patients who may have unpleasant emotional responses, as they may face obstacles in accepting and engaging with the technology. To address this challenge and promote optimal utilization of VR systems, close and periodic monitoring of users is essential. By closely observing users' experiences and reactions, healthcare providers can identify any barriers or challenges they face in using the technology. This monitoring allows for personalized adjustments and interventions to ensure a positive and comfortable user experience. Furthermore, providing comprehensive education and support to users is crucial. Offering clear instructions, user-friendly interfaces, and ongoing assistance can help alleviate concerns and enhance users' confidence in utilizing VR systems as part of their medical care. In summary, user acceptance and attitude towards VR technology are critical factors in its successful implementation. By closely monitoring users, addressing their concerns, and providing adequate support, healthcare providers can maximize the benefits and effectiveness of VR systems as medical tools.

One significant challenge in utilizing VR for rehabilitation is the requirement for users to adapt and familiarize themselves with manipulating 3D objects in the virtual world before the rehabilitation session can commence. This necessitates the study of cognitive models that consider individual behaviour within the VR simulation. Effective system design should consider cognitive aspects to establish an applicable and efficient manner of interaction. Research indicates that long-term usage of VR may potentially affect cognition, including human experiences, judgment, and memories. Extended exposure to VR could blur the user's perception of the real world and the virtual environment, leading to difficulties in making accurate judgments and maintaining a clear sense of self-identity. Consequently, managing the health and safety implications of VR systems in medical applications requires careful consideration. One approach to addressing this concern is to adopt a proactive approach, continuously conducting empirical studies to gather convincing evidence that can guide the usage of VR.

Home-based VR systems for rehabilitation also come with multiple risks and concerns. These include monitoring the learning curve of patients, providing remote technical support for systems used outside of healthcare centres, addressing logistical challenges, and ensuring a stable internet connection. Designing home-based rehabilitation programs with VR systems should prioritize user-friendliness and ease of installation, ideally offering a plug-and-play experience. These concerns become more critical for participants with physical or mental disabilities and for the elderly. Nevertheless, it's important to note that VR is considered an alternative treatment and should be prescribed by appropriate clinical experts after conducting proper assessments to mitigate potential risks. Overall, while challenges exist in utilizing VR for rehabilitation, addressing cognitive implications and ensuring user-friendly designs for home-based systems can contribute to maximizing the benefits and minimizing the risks associated with VR technology in medical settings.

Risks and concerns of VR-based systems inducing cyber-sickness and perceptuomotor after-effects have been reported as the potential side effects of VR [10]. Long duration of exposure to the VR system can cause headaches and eye-strain [18]. Physical illnesses after using the VR system such as nausea, vomiting, eye fatigue, dizziness, ataxia, and dizziness [19] are also reported. Some cyber-sickness cases persist such as when the real gravity is in contrast with the scene environment. However, not every user will experience motion sickness from the VR system exposure, but this issue has remained a serious threat to the development and wide usage of VR in treatment. Meanwhile, although there is currently no evidence of the additive nature of VR in medical use, it contains a hidden risk if the user is addicted to the VR environment which is like the addition to the games. Therefore, the sign of excessive use of the program has been alerted.

In the future, the VR-based system intervention may need not to acquire from a physician but rather download easily from the Internet or purchase VR-based training, rehabilitation or diagnostic games from mobile applications or websites. The potential risks for patients who download the system from the Internet may have their data hard to be kept as confidential. In short, VR systems in the medical field provide great benefits for improving the rehabilitation system but it is good to remain as an option for patients and physicians who are preferred actual physical training.

References

[1] J. Marescaux, J. M. Clément, V. Tassetti, *et al.*, "Virtual reality applied to hepatic surgery simulation: the next revolution.," *Ann. Surg.*, vol. 228, no. 5, p. 627, 1998, doi:10.1097/00000658-199811000-00001.

[2] N. Koutsouleris, T. U. Hauser, V. Skvortsova, and M. De Choudhury, "From promise to practice: towards the realisation of AI-informed mental health care," *Lancet Digit. Heal.*, vol. 4, no. 11, pp. e829–e840, 2022, doi:10.1016/S2589-7500(22)00153-4.

[3] S. Weech, S. Kenny, and M. Barnett-Cowan, "Presence and cybersickness in virtual reality are negatively related: a review," *Front. Psychol.*, vol. 10, no. FEB, p. 158, 2019, doi:10.3389/FPSYG.2019.00158/BIBTEX.

[4] C. Botella, R. M. Baños, H. Villa, C. Perpiñá, and A. García-Palacios, "Virtual reality in the treatment of claustrophobic fear: a controlled, multiple-baseline design," *Behav. Ther.*, vol. 31, no. 3, pp. 583–595, 2000, doi:10.1016/S0005-7894(00)80032-5.

[5] M. Maier, B. Rubio Ballester, A. Duff, E. Duarte Oller, and P. F. M. J. Verschure, "Effect of specific over nonspecific VR-based rehabilitation on poststroke motor recovery: a systematic meta-analysis," *Neurorehabil. Neural Repair*, vol. 33, no. 2, pp. 112–129, 2019, doi:10.1177/1545968318820169/ASSET/IMAGES/LARGE/10.1177_1545968318820169-FIG2.JPEG.

[6] G. C. Burdea, "Virtual rehabilitation – benefits and challenges," *Methods Inf. Med.*, vol. 42, no. 5, pp. 519–523, 2003, doi:10.1055/S-0038-1634378/ID/BR1634378-14.

[7] J. I. Vasquez-Gomez, L. E. Sucar, R. Murrieta-Cid, and E. Lopez-Damian, "Volumetric next-best-view planning for 3D object reconstruction with positioning error," *Int. J. Adv. Robot. Syst.*, vol. 11, no. 10, p. 159, 2014, doi:10.5772/58759/ASSET/IMAGES/LARGE/10.5772_58759-FIG2.JPEG.

[8] S. K. Swee, L. Z. You, B. W. W. Hang, and D. K. T. Kiang, "Development of rehabilitation system using virtual reality," in: *Proceeding 2017 International Conference on Robotics, Automation and Sciences (ICORAS 2017)*, vol. 2018, pp. 1–6, March 2018, doi:10.1109/ICORAS.2017.8308045.

[9] L. Sucar, R. S. Leder, D. Reinkensmeyer, *et al.*, "Gesture therapy – a low-cost vision-based system for rehabilitation after stroke," in: *Proceedings of HEALTHINF 2008/BIOSTEC*, pp. 107–111, June 2008, doi:10.5220/0001044001070111.

[10] P. Caserman, A. Garcia-Agundez, A. Gámez Zerban, and S. Göbel, "Cybersickness in current-generation virtual reality head-mounted displays: systematic review and outlook," *Virtual Real.*, vol. 25, no. 4, pp. 1153–1170, 2021, doi:10.1007/S10055-021-00513-6/FIGURES/1.

[11] R. Hussain, M. Chessa, and F. Solari, "Mitigating cybersickness in virtual reality systems through foveated depth-of-field blur," *Sensors (Basel).*, vol. 21, no. 12, p. 4006, 2021, doi:10.3390/S21124006.

[12] H. J. Smith and M. Neff, "Communication behavior in embodied virtual reality," in: *Proceedings of the SIGCHI Conference on Human Factors in Computing Systems*, 2018, doi:10.1145/3173574.

[13] T. Baniasadi, S. M. Ayyoubzadeh, and N. Mohammadzadeh, "Challenges and practical considerations in applying virtual reality in medical education and treatment," *Oman Med. J.*, vol. 35, no. 3, p. e125, 2020, doi:10.5001/OMJ.2020.43.

[14] J. Gershon, E. Zimand, M. Pickering, B. O. Rothbaum, and L. Hodges, "A pilot and feasibility study of virtual reality as a distraction for children with cancer," *J. Am. Acad. Child Adolesc. Psychiatry*, vol. 43, no. 10, pp. 1243–1249, 2004, doi:10.1097/01.CHI.0000135621.23145.05.

[15] T. Oing and J. Prescott, "Implementations of virtual reality for anxiety-related disorders: systematic review," *JMIR Serious Games*, vol. 20, no. 11, p. e10965, 2018, doi:10.2196/10965.

[16] S. J. Kim, T. H. Laine, and H. J. Suk, "Presence effects in virtual reality based on user characteristics: attention, enjoyment, and memory," *Electronics,* vol. 10, no. 9, p. 1051, 2021, doi:10.3390/ELECTRONICS10091051.

[17] K. U. Doerr, H. Rademacher, S. Huesgen, and W. Kubbat, "Evaluation of a low-cost 3D sound system for immersive virtual reality training systems," *IEEE Trans. Vis. Comput. Graph.*, vol. 13, no. 2, pp. 204–212, 2007, doi:10.1109/TVCG.2007.37.

[18] J. B. F. van Erp and A. Toet, "Social touch in human–computer interaction," *Front. Digit. Humanit.*, vol. 0, p. 2, 2015, doi:10.3389/FDIGH.2015.00002.

[19] J. P. Stauffert, F. Niebling, and M. E. Latoschik, "Latency and cybersickness: impact, causes, and measures. A review," *Front. Virtual Reality*, vol. 1. Frontiers, p. 31, 2020. doi:10.3389/frvir.2020.582204.

Chapter 7

Medical equipment engineering in industrial revolution

Mohankumar Palaniswamy[1,2]

Technological advancements alter the way humans generate goods. The industrial revolution refers to the transition from primitive to advanced manufacturing technologies. The First Industrial Revolution is regarded as a major breakthrough in human history since it affected nearly every area of everyday living throughout the world. Societies all across the world were barely surviving prior to the First Industrial Revolution. The disease was pervasive, famines were widespread, poverty was ubiquitous, and trade was restricted to adjacent geographic regions. The First Industrial Revolution brought about significant social transformation. One significant development was the transition from handwork done at home in cottage industries to work done in factories.

7.1 Industrial revolutions

The First Industrial Revolution was followed by three additional industrial revolutions till the end of the twentieth century. A name is linked with each one. The first is known as the Mechanical Revolution, the second as the Electrical Revolution, the third as the Automated Revolution, and the fourth as the Digitized Revolution. A storm of technical and scientific discoveries has come in the twenty-first century. Nobody is sure what to name them. The Fourth Industrial Revolution (FIR) has been renamed Industry 4.0 [1].

The utilization of steam power and mechanization of industry kicked off the First Industrial Revolution in the eighteenth century. The First Industrial Revolution was a milestone moment in history, influencing practically every area of everyday life in some manner. Average income and population, in particular, began to demonstrate an exceptional persistent rise. What was previously generated on simple spinning wheels accomplished multiple times the volume at the same time with the automated version. Steam power was already well understood. The utilization of it for industrial purposes

[1]INTI International University, Malaysia
[2]Department of Physiotherapy, School of Allied Health Sciences, Hindustan Institute of Technology and Science, India

was the most significant advance in enhancing human productivity. Steam power and machine tools came to dominate the world, while steamships and railroads transformed how people traveled from point A to point B. And what became the new focal point of communal life? Manufacturing facility – The Factory [2].

The Second Industrial Revolution began in the nineteenth century with the invention of electricity and assembly line manufacturing employing new technology (refer Figure 7.1). The Second Industrial Revolution, often known as the Technological Revolution, occurred between 1870 and 1914 and was characterized by rapid standardization and industrialization. Electric illumination, radio, and telephones revolutionized how people lived and socialized [2].

The Third Industrial Revolution began in the 1950s, just a few years after World War II ended, with partial automation employing memory-programmable controllers and computers. Since the emergence of these technologies, a complete manufacturing process may be automated without the need for human intervention. The automation revolution is another name for the Third Industrial Revolution [2].

The FIR is distinguished by the use of Information and Communication Technology (ICT), primarily to industry, but also to the operations of the rest of society. It builds on the Third Industrial Revolution's advances, particularly the digital revolution. It is also known as the Digitation Revolution. The US Department of Labor reports that between 1960 and 2014, the number of manufacturing workers in America fell by two-thirds, while productivity rose significantly. In addition, new employment was generated in new industries, and the average hourly salary climbed by 85% between 1973 and 2014. The manufacturing sector lost workers to the service sector during the Third Industrial Revolution. Not simply the quantity of tasks but also the type of labor that must be done will probably alter as a result of the FIR [4].

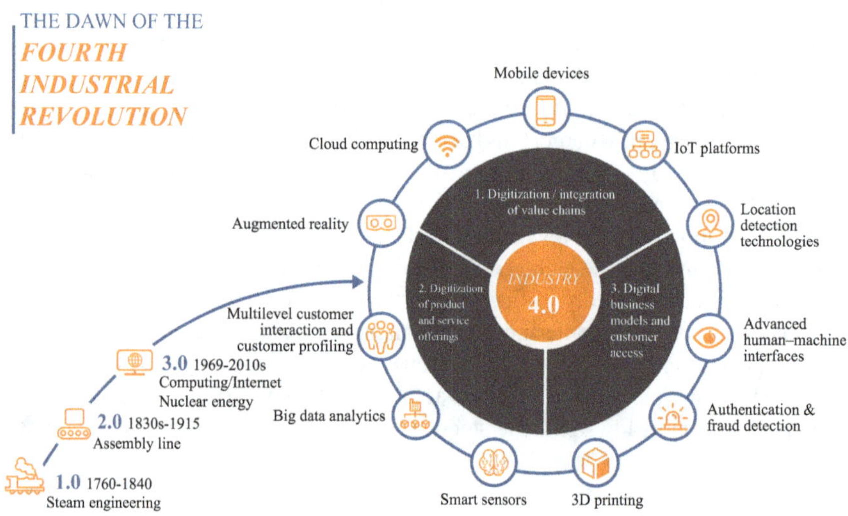

Figure 7.1 Industrial revolutions [3]

7.1.1 IR 4.0 in COVID

As the development of tools expands, healthcare systems undergo dramatic changes and technological standards related to Industrial Revolution 4.0 (IR 4.0). During the onset of COVID-19, the Industrial Revolution 4.0 emerges substantially. Social separation and lockdown in diverse nations have a substantial impact on practically every country's economic and industrial area [5]. As a result, a mandatory integration of IR 4.0 was noticed more frequently during the beginning of COVID-19 years than in prior decades. Nevertheless, technical progress is crucial during this epidemic. Several healthcare professionals are leaning toward new technology, such as smartphone applications and remote monitoring, to enhance the level of patient care they deliver in order to stay up with the needs of their patients. Telemedicine, for example, enables nurses and physicians to contact patients in remote or distant places who may otherwise struggle to receive proper medical treatment, while wearable technology aids in the long-term monitoring of heart diseases and other disorders [6]. These new tools enable more efficient solutions that can give medical treatments to remote communities while reducing the burden on hospitals and emergency departments.

The COVID-19 epidemic has resulted in a significant loss of human life worldwide and has had a significant impact on healthcare systems [7]. IR 4.0 technology has enabled excellent supply chain management in the healthcare area, allowing for the fulfilment of personalized requests. Furthermore, the Internet of Things (IoT), artificial intelligence (AI), big data analytics, and 3D printing have been widely employed to battle the COVID-19 epidemic and provide value-added services in the healthcare industry. The FIR has fundamentally restructured the traditional healthcare field organization. The sophisticated Information and Communications Technologies (ICT) of Industry 4.0 have been extensively utilized to restrict the spread of the COVID-19 pandemic [8]. The notion of Cyber-Physical Systems (CPS) underpins Industry 4.0. It is also referred as Medical Cyber-Physical Systems (MCPS) in the healthcare profession. Through the integration of new technologies, it is possible to regulate and monitor physical processes. MCPS are future systems that give effective functions for dealing with emergency circumstances as well as externally controlling and monitoring medical care.

AI is recognized as a powerful tool in Industry 4.0 and has been extensively used in this pandemic, such as analyzing complicated health data, reducing the impact of the infodemic, assisting in the discovery of best treatment, and assessing the clinical signs of suspects employing medical imaging such as computer tomography scan and X-ray imaging for virus detection [9].

In the FIR, IoT is responsible for automated production. It is one of the new trends arising from the Industry 4.0 revolution. IoT allows diverse medical equipment in the healthcare industry to communicate with one another. It links all gadgets to the Internet and uses sensors to collect patient health data. In the COVID-19 tragedy, IoT is utilized for real-time patient testing and monitoring, tracing infectious patients, and surveillance of crowded locations to guarantee quarantine implementation [10].

Big data analytics is utilized to organize vast amounts of data so that it may be quickly accessible and analyzed for improved decision making. Big data has been heavily employed in the pandemic crisis to gather real information from Internet sources such as social media and anticipate the trajectory of COVID-19 cases. Furthermore, big data is utilized to keep patient information, which aids doctors in determining the best therapy for them [11].

3D printing is a key pillar of the FIR, offering exceptional design and production flexibility [12]. During the COVID-19 period, 3D printing technology was frequently used to treat medical situations. It is used to meet the COVID-19 patients' urgent need for ventilators. It manufactures reusable and recyclable face masks as well as other health devices aimed at preventing the spread of COVID-19.

ICT trends indicate the evolution of new technologies across time. ICT trends depict the most recent technology that writers heavily rely on in their study. The most productive nations and the frequency of ICT terms is seen in Figure 7.2 and Table 7.1. According to the findings of Sandeep Kumar Sood *et al.* [13], the most popular ICT keywords in 2019 are e-learning, data analytics, and privacy, in 2020, it was deep learning, machine learning, and medical imaging, in 2021, it was text mining, fuzzy set, and face recognition. The most productive nations were China, United States, and India. Countries like Germany, Brazil, Czech Republic, and Australia are some notable mentions too. Similarly, researchers have deployed a flood of technologies to address the pandemic's numerous concerns. Deep learning, machine learning, medical imaging, AI, the IoT, and other technologies are among the technologies anticipated for 2020. Likewise, innovations launched in 2021 are depicted as the most recent ICT developments are used to tackle COVID-19. Text mining, fuzzy sets, facial recognition algorithms, 5G mobile network systems, and medical computing are just a few examples.

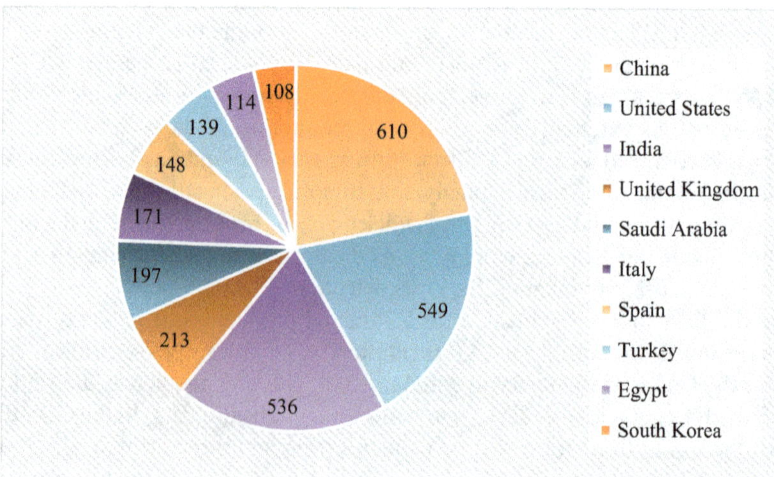

Figure 7.2 Most productive nations in ICT [13]

Table 7.1 Frequency of ICT terms used in the literature [13]

2019	2020	2021
Data Analytics (52)	3D Printing (8)	3D Printer (15)
Data Privacy (28)	AI (336)	5G Technology (28)
e-Learning (121)	Big Data (101)	Bio Sensor (14)
	Blockchain (78)	Bluetooth (14)
	Cloud Computing (51)	Data Science (21)
	Data Mining (71)	Face Recognition (29)
	Deep Learning (777)	Fuzzy Logic (21)
	Feature Extraction (133)	Fuzzy Set (32)
	IoT (165)	Industry 4.0 (23)
	Language Processing (64)	Intelligent System (17)
	Machine Learning (509)	IoT (22)
	Medical Imaging (345)	Language Processing (22)
	mHealth (41)	Medical Computing (24)
	Personnel Protective Equipment (45)	Supervised Learning (22)
	Random Forest (49)	Telehealth (16)
	Social Distance (77)	Text Mining (35)
	Social Media (152)	
	Telemedicine (54)	
	Virtual Reality (45)	

The FIR has evolved as a topic of rising attention in academic and industry disciplines in the healthcare sector. Sandeep Kumar Sood *et al.*'s [13] study is a representation of 4,763 citation data points relying on COVID-19 research published between 2019 and 2021 that was taken from the Scopus database. The analysis results show that deep learning technology has been widely employed for COVID-19 diagnosis. It suggests that researchers, politicians, and academic institutions should continue to expand research collaborations and focus new technologies in the healthcare sector (such as 5G, deep learning, machine learning, 4D printing, and IoT). Under the worldwide profile of technological breakthroughs, Industry 4.0 is an important basis for futuristic healthcare. China and the United States of America made significant early contributions to Industry 4.0-assisted COVID-19 research. However, because each nation has its unique historical growth path and future dynamics, all countries must establish indigenous plans.

7.1.2 IR 4.0 in healthcare

Health technology is described by the World Health Organization as "the use of systematic knowledge and expertise in the form of equipment, medications, vaccines, procedures, and systems devised to address a health issue and enhance the quality of life." In order for a piece of technology to function, at least three elements must be present at once, according to researchers from the science technology society: (i) hardware (tools, machines, devices); (ii) knowledge (knowledge and wisdom embodied in the hardware); and (iii) organization (systematic procedures or flow of work which describes the use of the hardware and facility) [14].

Healthcare has existed since the dawn of humanity, but it has developed tremendously in the previous several decades. Healthcare 1.0 was primarily concerned with providing basic health services such as vital sign monitoring and natural childbirth. Then, with the introduction of modern technology, Healthcare 2.0 expanded its repertory to include mechanical services such as surgery and medical machinery. Healthcare 3.0 focuses on the patient, whereas Healthcare 4.0 addresses cloud computing, fog computing, and IoT. With an increasing population and technology capabilities, it is becoming increasingly important to provide better healthcare services in a more dynamic way. Healthcare 4.0, according to Jayaraman *et al.* [15], is a fairly recent term derived from Industry 4.0. Innovative health, mHealth, eHealth, mobile health, online health, Wi-Fi health, ubiquitous health, telehealth/telemedicine, medical information technology, digital medicine, health informatics, and health information systems are examples of data-driven digital health technologies used in healthcare 4.0 (refer Figure 7.3). The majority of smart healthcare services are hospital-based. Furthermore, patient records are disorganized and program dependent, resulting in attention lags in several circumstances. Bedon *et al.* [17] created a home-based smart health model that takes into account the IoT, the Internet of medical things, and smart medical apps to address such situations. When compared to current healthcare facilities, the suggested health service minimized attention lags.

Business process digitalization and the IoT have already begun to revolutionize the worlds of manufacturing, shipping, and supply chain management. Healthcare, on the other hand, has lagged behind in terms of digitization and innovation [18]. Healthcare technology can now communicate and exchange data

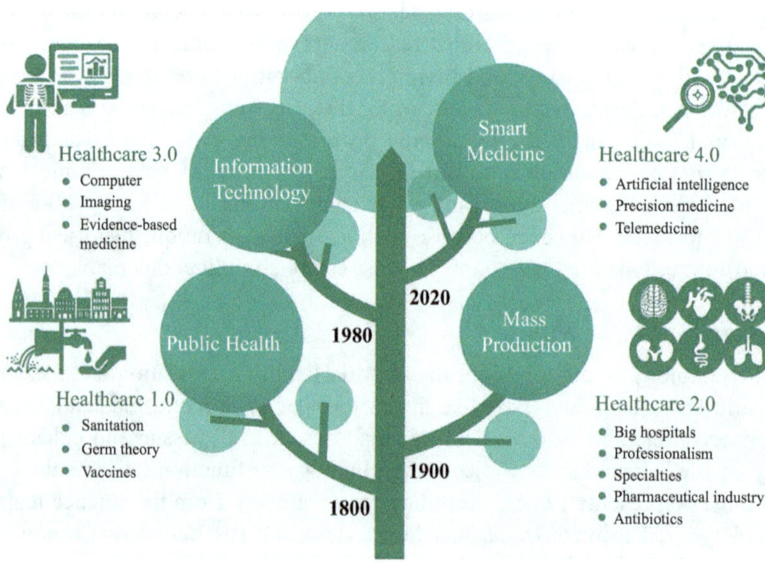

Figure 7.3 Revolutions in healthcare [16]

on an unprecedented scale because to the spread of mobile devices and medical equipment. Over the last several decades, the healthcare sector has seen numerous important upheavals, from the introduction of vaccinations and antibiotics to the development of patient-centered care and, most recently, next-generation genomic medicine. We have witnessed an explosion of innovation at each level of this development, changing how patients and doctors engage with one another.

Advance diagnostic technologies (precise diagnostic scanners), medical equipment, procedures, treatments, new medications, surgical robots, AI developments, and drug delivery systems have significantly enhanced the treatment process. Furthermore, as a result of these improvements, health care is today less expensive, less disruptive, and pleasant than it was previously [19]. Health innovation is critical for increasing health and alleviating poverty. Furthermore, health innovation is critical to human evolution. Health innovation has boosted efficiency and improved health care tremendously.

According to Schwab [20], the FIR will have far-reaching ramifications for life expectancy and health. Significant technological innovation has enhanced the healthcare system's capacity to deal with health concerns and is projected to advance it further. Better data collecting allows the globe to develop worldwide and produce cross-sector ideas. Given the trend of population growth and ageing, the current healthcare system is insufficient to address health-related challenges. As a result, governments throughout the world are formulating ways to strengthen the existing healthcare system to cope with this demographic transition.

Another research [21] looked at the influence of health innovation, health technology, and healthcare spending on the wellness of G7 countries from 1990 to 2017. They investigated the influence of panel data on health, innovation, health technology, and healthcare cost. The research was carried out for G7 nations with varying levels of healthcare spending as a proportion of GDP and life expectancy. They postulated that health outcomes are affected by health innovation, healthcare spending, and medical technology. Furthermore, they investigated if there is a relationship between health innovation and healthcare spending in G7 nations. According to the study's findings, G7 countries should develop initiatives like health innovation to enhance existing medical technologies. Health innovation expands the potential for the recipient of care, the patient, and stakeholders. Furthermore, it is crucial in promoting health and alleviating poverty. As a result, in order to increase social development, G7 countries must prioritize health innovation, which is directly tied to efficiency and health care. Given the trend of population growth and ageing, as well as the need to address health concerns, it is essential to look for effective alternatives to improve the present healthcare system. Furthermore, in order to deal with this demographic shift, the G7 nations need to boost their healthcare spending to at least 20% of GDP, which will have far-reaching repercussions for public health, human development, and economic growth. Spending on healthcare expands options for the recipient of treatment, the patient, and the stakeholder. Continued investment in healthcare and medical innovation is more likely to enhance overall health status on both a micro and macro scale.

7.2 Medical technology

Historically, healthcare providers have depended on technology to help them provide the finest care possible to their patients, but substantial improvements in the last decade have enhanced therapy quality and patient outcomes. Healthcare is always evolving, though one factor remains: the need for a safe healthcare system that is immune of security breaches. Electronic medical records, personal health records/digital health records, clinical data repositories, and health information exchanges all contain patient data nowadays. These repositories contain crucial data that should be safeguarded, although cybercriminals often attack them. Because cybercriminals are increasingly targeting healthcare facilities and healthcare companies are discovering that their Information Technology (IT) resources are no longer secure and sufficient [22]. The FIR represents the next phase of effective and efficient health technology that allow hospitals and other health professionals to monitor infection rates more accurately, safeguard their patients from severe diseases, and get real-time support whenever it is most required.

One of the most pressing challenges in the healthcare industry is the protection of patient data. Based on a 2020 research published in cybercrime magazine, 93% of healthcare businesses in the United States had experienced a significant security breach resulting in data breaches, denial-of-service attacks, malware, or other cyber-intrusions. Without conducting an audit of an individual's electronic health record system, it is hard to establish how frequently their electronic health record system has been hacked [23]. Because the majority of healthcare systems save patient information in the cloud, cloud settings have emerged as one of most appealing locations for cybercriminals. Various research offered numerous protective measures to safeguard cloud-based clinical information in light of the security challenges in healthcare. As a response, the healthcare industry is developing a cloud server that demands a greater level of protection and reliability.

Signcryption, for example, a hybrid of signature and encryption, has shown promising results in cloud-based network access. Unfortunately, the majority of them are particularly appropriate to monotonous rather than diverse environments. Chute *et al.*'s [24] Care 4.0, a comprehensive care paradigm, promises to give patients the most authority over their clinical records. The primary goal of Care 4.0 is to create credible and interconnected networks which are connected to digital care and health services. The projected Care 4.0 networks and technologies may help people to manage and use their resources, both within their primary care circle and across the broader society.

To counteract virus spread, mobile apps, robots, Wi-Fi cameras, scanners, and drones are being used [25]. Industry 4.0 has had an influence on digital technology's substantial role in pandemic containment. At the height of COVID-19, the planet was caught in the hands of an unparalleled healthcare catastrophe. As a result, researchers and practitioners create a diverse set of tools and strategies to modernize systems in order to reduce the transmission of pathogens and expand the range of healthcare facilities.

The medical technology in healthcare constitutes of sectors like telemedicine, sensors, AI, virtual reality, wearable gadgets, intelligent apps, data science, IoT, robotic automation, edge computing, 3D scanning & printing, big data, tissue engineering, 5G, nanomedicine, cyber security, drones, Internet of behaviors, and blockchain [26].

Robotics in medicine and healthcare is a growing industry with significant development potential. They are first categorized as service robots by Japanese regulatory bodies. Healthcare robots can also be categorized as service robots for home usage as an aid or medical robots for use in a hospital setting [27]. However, the divisions are vague because the industry is still in its infancy, and new goods might fall under either group. The firms listed in Table 7.2 employ the latest technology to promote a healthy living [28,29].

Table 7.2 List of companies and their products in healthy living

Brands	Devices
Abbott	Microneedle patch – to measure glucose level from interstitial fluid
Alcon	Contact lens – to measure glucose level
Backbone Labs	Posture correcting harness – to correct the posture
Breathometer	Mint – IoT-enabled breath analyzer to measure oral health & hygiene
Carre Technologies	Hexoskin – IoT-enabled clothing to monitor heart rate, breathing, and sleeping pattern
Cyberdyne	Hybrid assistive limb – wearable healthcare robot for mobility
Dexcom	Microneedle patch – to measure glucose level
GE Healthcare	IoT framework – auto/Smart bed
Integrity Applications	Finger clip – to measure glucose level from blood using ultrasonic, electromagnetic, and thermal waves
Keriton	KeritonKare Nurse app – an IoT-enabled app that helps to reduce the workload of the Neonatal Intensive Care Unit (NICU) nurses
LifeFuels	Smart bottles – to monitor the hydration level of a user and recommend fluid intake
Meru Health	Ascend – a digital software program for people who undergo depression
Naya Health	Breastfeeding pumps – display milk volume in the pump and other data
Nemaura Medical Inc.	Patch – to measure glucose level using reverse iontophoresis
OpenAPS	Glucose monitoring device – inject insulin
Orbita	Voice app – collects data from smart devices and shares with healthcare professional
Propeller Health	Smart inhalers – provide allergen forecast and track record
Roche	Bluetooth-enabled device – to measure blood coagulation
Semeoticons	Wize Mirror – noninvasive device for monitoring human wellbeing
Senseonics	Subcutaneous small stick – to measure glucose level using fluorescence
Sensimed	Contact lens – to measure eye dimensions
Takeda Pharmaceuticals	Cognition kit – to measure cognitive health
TruInject	Human model – to train healthcare workers on how to inject
Verily	Contact lens – to measure glucose levels for peoples with diabetes

7.2.1 IoT in healthcare

When Kevin Ashton sought to use RFID tags to link devices to the Internet in 1999, the IoT was created [30]. The IoT is a collection of network-connected devices that can send information without human involvement. Smartphones, wearables, and other medical gadgets are substituting conventional glucometers, pedometers, calorie counters, and sphygmomanometers. These gadgets will eventually be included in a doctor's handy kit. The interconnected device environment will allow medical practitioners to customize therapies for patients. The IoT ecosystem will empower healthcare practitioners to forecast, protect, and treat diseases or infections, which in turn potentially boost the life expectancy (refer Figure 7.4). IoT is a rapidly expanding subject in the healthcare sector. But the IoT concept has just become more popular in the last 6–10 years. With a maximum of 62 papers in 2014 alone, scholarly output on IoT in healthcare has risen extremely slowly throughout the 15 years from its inception (1999–2014). As a result, IoT studies in the healthcare industry are a relatively new area of study. The number of publications from 2015 to 2020 has progressively grown, reaching a peak in 2020 at 1458 articles [32] (refer Figure 7.5). A significant number of publications suggest that scholarly work is becoming more prolific. This is perhaps also because businesses have just recently become interested in creating fresh and enhanced IoT ideas for the healthcare industry. Between 2015 and 2020, there was a considerable rise in the number of patent applications for IoT advancements in the healthcare industry. About 818 patents were produced during the first period (2015–2017), as opposed to 3,390 during the second period (2018–2020). India, the United States of America, China, and the United Kingdom are the top five nations for IoT-related publications in the healthcare industry. Instead, when it comes to patents, South

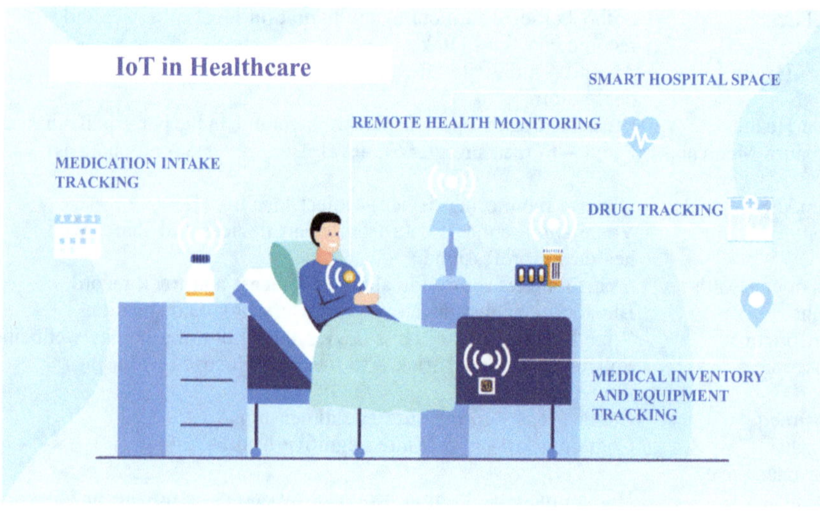

Figure 7.4 IoT in healthcare [31]

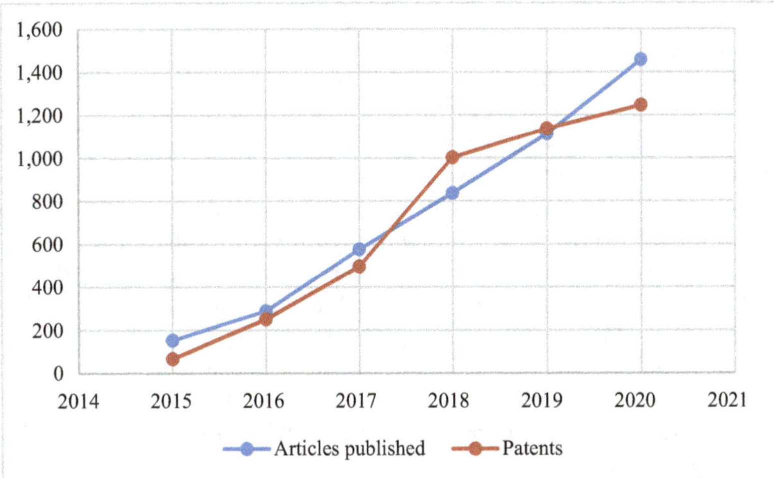

Figure 7.5 IoT-related articles and patents in healthcare [33]

Korea leads the pack and is particularly focused on the IoT, followed by India, China, and the USA [33].

The main organizations that produce publications and patents were examined. Analyses of national scientific productivity were also conducted. Indian universities like Anna University, Vellore Institute of Technology University (VIT), King Saud University, Visvesvaraya Technological University (VTU), and Qatar University are among the most prolific academic institutions. Samsung, a major participant in mobile telecommunications, was identified as one of the companies generating IoT patents in the healthcare industry. The top-ranking South Korean business produced 87.7% of the Health IoT patents. The market for wearable technology and linked products in the healthcare industry is dominated by this business. IBM, a US-based company, is the second patent generator. Watson Health, one of its products, uses IoT and big data analytics to help healthcare practitioners. Other sources of patents include the wireless telecom company Qualcomm, public research institutions like the South Korean Electronics and Telecommunications Research Institute (ETRI) and the Indian Council of Scientific and Industrial Research (CSIR), and private universities like the Indian Lovely Professional University and the South Korean Sungkyunkwan Research and Business University [33].

Patients have been presented to IoT devices in various ways during the last decade or so. Following up on various indicators, such as temperature, fetal, ECG, and blood glucose, is critical for some patients, but it must be handled by healthcare practitioners. The emergence of IoT devices has significantly altered this paradigm by eliminating the requirement for direct interaction with healthcare personnel. IoT has paved the road for medical practitioners to access real-time and more critical data. Some basic IoT applications in healthcare included smart beds that could recognize whether or not a bed was unoccupied or whether a patient was attempting to get up without the need for human assistance. Another example is home medicine dispenser, which could send notifications when medicines were not taken or alarms and send the information to the cloud for suitable action. Remote observation and disease prevention technologies will aid in improved care coordination throughout the whole healthcare system. Intel is teaming with the Michael J. Fox Foundation to enhance remote care facilities for Parkinson's disease [34]. They are developing a platform that will gather information via wearables and notice signs that might otherwise go unreported. IoT can lessen the need to admit elderly individuals to nursing facilities. IoT can offer real-time patient connectivity to healthcare specialists, addressing two of today's most pressing issues in the healthcare system: time and accessibility. Current challenges in the healthcare system are geriatric patients, more number of patients with long lasting illness, failing to follow the medications, shortage of healthcare services, high medical expenditure, and increased waiting period. These are the areas where IoT can be implemented through mobile health or mHealth, IoT-assisted living for geriatric and specially abled people, IoT-assisted medication, IoT-enabled implants, and IoT-installed medical emergency rooms. An IoT ecosystem consists of several components. They are as follows:

Sensor: A sensor is a piece of equipment that detects variations in the environment. A sensor is useless unless it is connected to an electronic system. Once connected, it becomes the critical element. Sensors can measure physical variables, such as heat, cold, pressure, movement, and transform it to a digital signal. Rain sensor, proximity sensor, infrared sensor, touch sensor, heartbeat sensor, temperature sensor are to name a few. Sensors are categorized based on a few parameters. They are range, resolution, sensitivity, electrical, chemical, active/passive, and analog/digital [35]. With respect to the healthcare, there are several wearable biosensors like epidermal-based, tear-based, exercise sweat-based, saliva-based, iontophoresis-based, microfluid-based, and implantable biosensors [36].

Gateway: Gateways serve as a connection between IoT devices, tools, systems, and sensors. Gateways connect IoT systems to the cloud as well. By connecting the field and the cloud, these devices enable local processing and storage. They also provide sensor-based autonomous field equipment control. For a wide range of reasons, it is usually hard for devices to communicate directly with systems. Many sensors and equipment do not support technologies such as Wi-Fi or Bluetooth because they consume additional power. Some gadgets must aggregate data, since it is massive and useful in its raw form. The IoT gateway is responsible for a variety of vital duties such as protocol translation, encryption, processing, data management, data filtration, and so on. It simply lies between devices, sensors, and cloud communication systems. A Gateway device is required in an IoT due to various reasons such as to reduce the gap between operational technology and information technology, to add more security, and to provide a real-time field update.

Communication network: IoT refers to the interconnection of gadgets, in which smart devices interact with one another, share data, and execute activities without the assistance of humans. Connectivity between smart devices is critical in IOT since it allows these devices to acquire and share data that leads to the effectiveness of that IOT product. There are six wireless communication protocols that are commonly used to connect the smart devices. They are Bluetooth, RFID, near-field communication (NFC), radio frequency, Wi-Fi, and satellite.

Bluetooth is a wireless technology used for exchanging data across short distances. Because the frequencies are the same as in Wi-Fi, these two technologies look to be quite similar. There are three different Bluetooth technologies available. They are Bluetooth, BLE, and iBeacon. Bluetooth is an outdated technology. This technology has a greater battery drain and a higher security risk. These are seldom seen anymore. Nokia pioneered BLE (Bluetooth Low Energy), which is now utilized by all major operating systems. This technique is quick and saves electricity. iBeacon is Apple's trademark for a streamlined Bluetooth-based communication technology. It is a Bluetooth 4.0 transmitter that emits an ID called UUID that iPhone can identify. For suppliers, this simplifies implementation. Although technically distinct, this is similar to NFC on an abstract level. In general, Bluetooth is energy efficient and inexpensive. But it fails to support long-distance data transmission. Bluetooth can be found in mobiles, laptops, and other gadgets.

Radio frequency identification (RFID) is a cordless technique that recognizes items by using electromagnetic fields. They work with the help of a tag and a reader. An active reader can read or scan the information (confirmatory message) from a passive tag. This method is called Active Reader Passive Tag (ARPT). In some cases, the tag gets activated by the signal received from the reader to pass information. This method is called Active Reader Active Tag (ARAT). The data transmission of RFID can range from 10 cm to 200 m. RFID requires very minimal power and also it is very insecure. RFID can be found in toll booths and industry warehouses.

The underlying technique in NFC is an electromagnetic induction across two-loop antennas positioned somewhere within each other's near field, resulting in the functional creation of an air-core transformer. It operates on the ISO/IEC 18000-3 air interface at speeds ranging from 106 kbps to 424 kbps inside the globally open and unregulated RF ISM band of 13.56 MHz. NFC is made up of an activator and a receiver. The activator actively generates a radio frequency field capable of powering a passive receiver, such as an unpowered chip. As a result, NFC devices can have very basic form factors. Peer-to-peer connection is feasible when both gadgets are powered. NFC can function under two modes, active and passive communication modes. In active, both the activator and the receiver are connected with their respective radio frequencies and they have their own power supply. Whereas, in passive, the activator generates an electromagnetic field, through which the receiver responds. Here, receiver receives power from the activator. NFC has a very simple setup which even support encryption, but have a very limited range. NFC are available in the latest android mobiles and iPhones.

Radio frequency (RF) are certainly the most user-friendly modes of communication among gadgets. Protocols like ZigBee and Z-Wave use a low RF radio that is installed or connected to equipment and gadgets. Every country has its own RF band. For example, US with 908.42 MHz, New Zealand with 921.42 MHz, Israel with 916 MHz, and India with 865.2 MHz. ZigBee has a range from 10 to 100 m and Z-Wave ranges till 30 m. RF is a simple technology which use less power. An example of RF is the connection between a television and its remote.

Wi-Fi is a wireless local area network (WLAN) that operates at 2.4 GHz UHF and 5 GHz ISM frequencies in accordance with the IEEE 802.11 standard. This enables gadgets within a 70-foot range to connect to the Internet. Wi-Fi has a global compatibility, easily accessible, and has good security features. Most homes, universities, and offices use Wi-Fi to access Internet.

Cell phones can communicate across a distance of 10–15 miles, thanks to the satellite connections. Based on the connection speed, they are named as GSM, GPRS, CDMA, EDGE, 2G/GSM, 3G, 4G/LTE, and others. This sort of communication is known as "M2M" (machine to machine) in the field of IoT because it allows devices, such as phones, to transmit and receive data over the mobile network. Satellite connects are very stable but the power and maintenance are high. Communication through cell phone is the classic example of satellite communication.

Data analytics: IoT and data analytics are totally opposite concepts. As data grows rapidly over time, the value of big data analysis grows correspondingly. According to research, there were 31 billion IoT-connected devices in 2020. Data analytics will be critical in comprehending the data collected by all of these devices. Data analytics represents the only way to extract meaning from the data supplied by IoT devices [37]. It is the transformation of data sets into clear ideas and practical findings. These assessments take the shape of indicators and forecasts, which assist big businesses in acting strategically. The sustainability and progress of IoT projects are strongly based on data analytics. Technologies with analytical skills are influencing how firms make choices. The many ways in which these analysis techniques help businesses make better decisions are outlined below (refer Figure 7.6).

- Prescriptive analysis – descriptive + predictive
- Spatial analysis – geographic patterns
- Streaming analysis – real time
- Time series analysis – time based

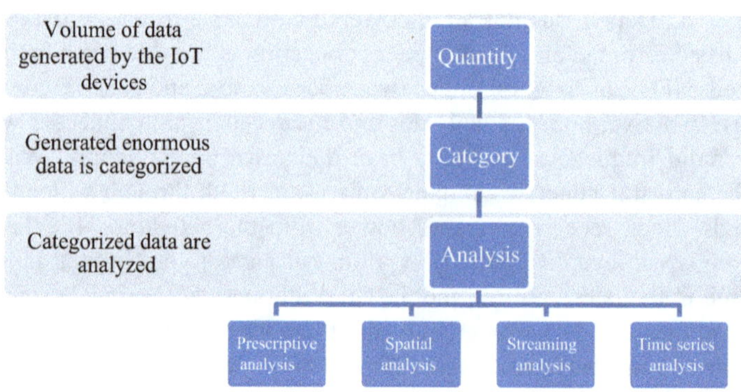

Figure 7.6 Data analytics in IoT

According to predictions, IoT can help cut down on yearly healthcare expenditures. Savings of $300 billion may be possible. Here are some examples of the places where employing technology may cut costs. In a typical system, keeping track of hospital employees, patients, and equipment comes at a significant financial expense. Here, sophisticated tracking devices can be used. This will enhance workflow generally, which enhances the hospital environment. Reducing trips to the doctor's office is made possible by real-time patient monitoring technologies [38]. This also guarantees treatment compliance, which lowers the likelihood of having to redo the entire course of therapy, including all prescriptions, transportation, and waiting periods. This thus results in lower costs and financial savings.

7.2.2 Challenges in implementing IoT

There are several examples where businesses using smart technology failed to comprehend the complexity of the total process. A couple of the causes of these failures include incorrect application deployment, and a lack of knowledge and training. Understanding and expertise in embedded systems, App development, analytics, Big Data, cloud, sensors, and many other topics are necessary for the progression of the IoT. The following are a handful of difficulties that must be addressed for an IoT-based healthcare strategy to succeed.

- Vast amount of information
- Obstacles in regulations and standards
- Privacy and safety
- Inadequate skill set
- Outdated infrastructure and equipment

In order to adapt and implement e-health systems in the future, the following categories are vital [39].

Human capital: It comprises the information, skills, as well as the stakeholders in medical health system that are aware of and competent in using Health 4.0 technologies. As said before, human capital includes personal safety and education.

The phrase also encompasses end users' access to IT pros and their level of digital literacy. It also covers other forms of literacy, such as numeracy and health literacy, which, along with digital literacy, significantly limit older individuals' ability to utilize ICT [40].

ICT: It consists of the equipment required to share e-health data. "Phone lines, fiber trunks, submarine cables, T1, T3, and OC-xx, ISDN, DSL, and other high-speed services are all parts of the ICT infrastructure, along with satellites, earth stations, teleports, telecommunications, electricity, computer access, a number of Internet hosts, a number of Internet service providers, and available bandwidth and broadband access." Such a framework is referred to as the national health information infrastructure for the entire nation. The privacy and security of electronic health records should be also supported by ICT [41].

Social capital: It includes property rights, ethical conduct, cooperative tendencies, openness to employ cutting-edge solutions, and patient attitudes and perceptions. The motivation to share health information is influenced by social capital. The technology acceptance model, theory of planned behavior, and unified theory of acceptance and use of technology are just a few of the ideas that have been established to describe how patients behave when it comes to embracing technology. This topic covers the societal factors that affect how people use technology [42].

Financial resources: Money and wealth are mentioned. Considering the high cost of e-health solutions, this concept is self-explanatory. The development of a regulatory framework, the next factor, and the scaling up of e-health in low- and middle-income nations are both hampered by a lack of financial resources. E-health solution providers have observed that their desire to invest more is constrained by financial concerns [43].

Governance: Institutional relationships, sovereignty, decision-making procedures, executive authority, institutions, rules, and form of government are all included. Representation, involvement, adaptability, networks, experience, dedication, use of data and understanding, equality of decision-making and knowledge accessibility, education, and income are some of the ways they are demonstrated. Coordination, however, necessitates a more centralized strategy, i.e., leadership [44].

Legal regulations: Local, regional, and national laws make up regulations. Patients' worries about personal information and privacy in cloud-based health informatics have an impact on their decision to use e-health solutions as well as their confidence and perception of the privacy risk. After the General Data Protection Regulation (GDPR) was implemented in 2016, the problem of data protection became more significant in the European Union [45]. The government, employers, and employees all have Occupational Health Safety (OHS) responsibilities under the Korean Occupational Safety and Health Act [46]. The establishment and enforcement of OHS regulations, the advancement of technology for safety and health, and the setup and maintenance of facilities are all responsibilities of the government when it comes to disaster prevention in the workplace. The Industrial Safety and Health Act, the guidelines for preventing industrial accidents, and the provision of a pleasant working environment are all requirements that the employer must follow. Workers must take the steps needed to prevent workplace accidents and adhere to measures taken to prevent workplace accidents.

IoT in healthcare is fairly new, with most of the scientific and patent creation occurring just in the recent past. While it is restricted to patents, health IoT is presently a global research concern. Private sector businesses own the majority of health IoT patents, yet public research institutions appear to be crucial to the advancement of IoT research. Partnerships between business and academia should consequently be encouraged from a policy perspective. The healthcare industry has evolved and is continually evolving as a result of IoT. Despite all of the difficulties, IoT is rapidly expanding in the healthcare industry. Patients are starting to accept the use of IoMT devices for maintaining their health. A growing number of businesses are entering the IoT-based healthcare services market. To provide patients with a good healthcare service, professionals have begun to employ linked devices to enhance clinical outcomes. Researchers, healthcare practitioners, technological experts, and device designers are collaborating to increase the quality and quantity of living beings.

7.2.3 AI in healthcare

AI, or artificial intelligence, has been received positively in the medical and healthcare sectors. AI is rapidly expanding in the field of medicine and is now regarded to be one of its most important applications [47,48]. With many healthcare organizations now implementing such technology, it is clear how crucial it will be in industrial 4.0 and healthcare. Many virtual reality-based tools are already being used to assist professionals in illness detection, whereas other equipment employs complex algorithms that operate with datasets collected from medical files while maintaining them protected at all times [49,50]. Hospitals have also made widespread use of handwriting recognition machines, which are used to prescribe medication to patients after examining their medical data. An AI system could also be employed with neuroimaging studies of individuals with Alzheimer's disease, dementia, or stroke victims whom might no longer recall their identities or how they appear. Professionals are rapidly incorporating AI systems to undertake surgical procedures such as tumor removal, and knee replacement surgeries, while physicians commonly employ virtual reality technology for physical training. Young doctors can also adopt similar technology to gain a deeper knowledge about how the human body functions during a treatment. Ambulances now have access to accurate information about the swiftest routes to crisis situations via using intellectual software solution in conjunction with GPS trackers installed on vehicles, and also some healthcare facilities even engage robotic systems that function 24/7 by loading patient records into their framework whilst also monitoring their therapeutic demands [51].

7.2.4 Personalized healthcare

7.2.4.1 Ambient assisted living (AAL)

The term AAL refers to ICT solutions that are integrated into the living space to continuously observe the surroundings and actions of its residents.

AAL systems can extend beyond monitoring; they can transform into engaging by prompting the user, calling for help from emergency agencies, and giving relatives and caregivers the most recent information. The three primary goals of AAL are:

- Observing human action and behavior patterns, from basic movement tracking and human activity identification up to long-term psychosocial assessment.
- Tracking human biological signs like physical, clinical, vital, and emotional parameters (refer Table 7.3).
- Overseeing environmental conditions (such as lights, temperature, doors, and gas detection) for the users' security and comfort.

The main goal of AAL solutions is to improve the environment through the use of a distributed sensor network. The sensors include wearable or body sensors that

Table 7.3 Parameters measured in AAL systems

Vital signs	Posture & movement	Anthropometrics
Heart rate	Gait analysis	Height
Heart rate variability	Fall detection	Weight
Respiratory rate	Rehabilitation	Skin-fold thickness
		Triceps skin-fold
		Neck circumference
		Waist circumference
		Hip circumference
		BMI

are attached to the wearer's body or clothes, as well as ambient sensors. Often, a vast network of sensors is required to collect sufficient data to carry out the challenging tasks necessary for AAL applications.

7.2.4.2 Wize Mirror

The SEMEOTICONS project, funded by the European Community's Seventh Framework Programme, created a unique AAL solution that significantly integrates computer vision techniques into a noninvasive gadget for health monitoring. The Wize Mirror, a multimodal device that resembles a regular mirror, was designed as an efficient technology-assisted intervention to avoid cardiometabolic disorders [52]. The Wize Mirror seamlessly combines a contactless sensor framework with several cameras and a data processing platform that can examine the subject ahead of it and analyze physiological risk indicators for cardiometabolic disease. The Wize Mirror examines the visual and emotional characteristics of the facial and the pattern of the inhalation and exhalation to find both overt and covert correlations. The Wize Mirror framework consists of depth-based 3D scanner, multispectral imaging (MSI) system with five monochrome cameras, computer-controlled LED strips, high-resolution RGB cameras, and a portable gas sensor device.

- 3D scanner: Used for face detection, recognition, track head pose, facial movements, 3D reconstruction, detect signs and symptoms related to obesity.
- MSI: Analysis of skin composition, detect signs and symptoms related to glucose dysmetabolism, endothelial dysfunction, and dyslipidemia.
- RGB cameras: The mirror calculates vital indicators and emotional signals associated with negative psychological states by analyzing 2D videos.
- Gas sensor: Examines the breath's chemical makeup and provides information on how bad behaviors are having an impact. The Wize Sniffer is a device that can identify compounds including carbon dioxide, ethanol, hydrogen, oxygen, and carbon monoxide.

While users are either standing or sitting in front of it as part of their everyday routine, the mirror scans their faces in just a few seconds without needing too much effort. Overall, data collecting for face morphometry, skin composition, vital signs, and emotional assessments takes 1 min (refer Figure 7.7). Deep breathing is

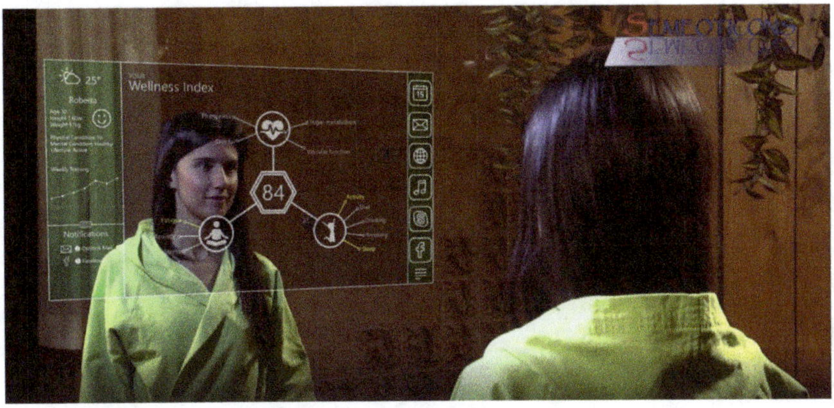

Figure 7.7 Wize Mirror [52]

required for breath analysis, which just requires the straightforward action of inhaling into a mouthpiece. Results are delivered in real time, in only a few seconds, thanks to a parallel implementation on a multiprocessor board. Only endothelial function and heart rate variability need acquisition times of 5 and 6 min, respectively. The Wize Mirror conducted a validation study to confirm the precision, consistency, efficacy, and repeatability of its measures and to assess user acceptance. Three prototypes were used in three clinical settings in France and Italy. Seventy-two people participated in a human research and received mirror scans every 15 days for 3 months. Baseline data were gathered contextually using diagnostic tools for body composition, metabolism, homeostasis, and vital indicators in clinical practice. Comparisons between mirror readings and conventional clinical readings revealed a statistically substantial association.

7.2.4.3 Computer-aided facility management (CAFM) in healthcare

Modern hospitals must manage a large quantity of data, which is directly tied to how they are organized. In order to perform their clinical and medical obligations, hospitals must adhere to a wide number of standards. In order to meet minimum sanitary, quality, and organizational standards, structures must adhere to these requirements, which are imposed by national and international agencies. Over the years, several technical instruments have been created to oversee the hospital by taking measurements of quantitative, architectural, technological, and personnel-related data. Integrated Healthcare Facility Management Models (IHFMM), which give indices on those activities that might impact the performance of the healthcare structure, are the foundation for CAFM systems, which can be thought of as decision-support tools. For the top management's performance, risk evaluations, company management, and development, these tools can be quite helpful. There are several CAFM systems developed earlier. Whereas, most recent systems were based on the "everything inside DWG" approach [53].

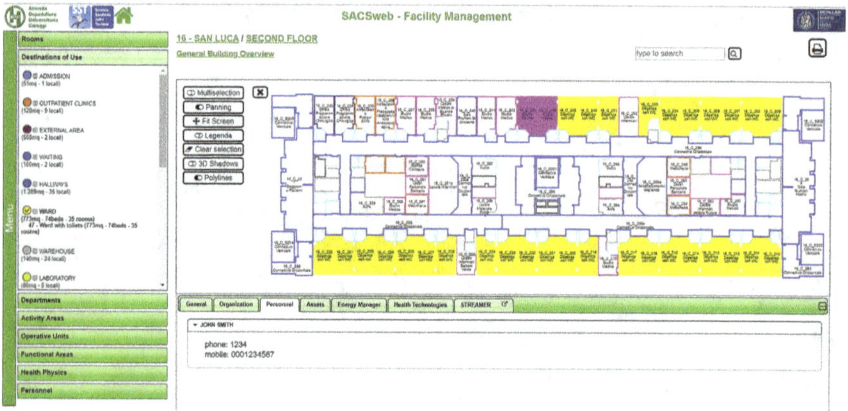

Figure 7.8 Everything inside DWG – multi-section view [53]

Hospital buildings' electronic floor plans are managed and analyzed by the systems, which record the data on a central MS SQL Server database connected to the Hospital Information System. The primary core program features built-in CAD drivers that enable direct use of CAD applications like Autodesk AutoCAD and enables automation directly on DWG files, preserving the data inside the map itself by utilizing the XData extension for every CAD item (refer Figure 7.8). With this method, users may edit DWG files straight from the main program and, in addition, recreate data about a hospital's internal structure, usage locations, and ambient comforts using nothing but DWG maps. This everything inside DWG approach in healthcare consists of a web viewer, search engine, sanitation management, fire evacuation, energy management, and bed management.

7.2.4.4 Parametric optimization and control

Massive volumes of biomedical data, or "big data," are produced when electronic health records are widely used. Precision medicine has a lot of potential now that researchers can access a vast quantity of information on a patient's medical history, genetic profile, etc., thanks to big data. How to make use of the data abundance and extract information for individualized treatment is thus an urgent and important subject. Big data analytics and statistical techniques can be quite useful, given the growth in modern computer power. Using high-fidelity, dynamic mathematical models as the foundation, complex optimization and control studies may be executed and designed using the parametric optimization and control (PAROC) program [54]. PAROC consists of four steps.

1. High-fidelity modeling and analysis – A thorough, dynamic model built on fundamental principles is developed and validated in the framework's initial stage.
2. Model approximation – Large sets of partial and/or regular differential and algebraic equations with highly nonlinear components are included in the models created in the preceding stage, necessitating computationally costly

simulations. Because of this, it is sometimes required to replace the model formulation with a linear system representation in order to properly conduct control experiments.

3. Model-based system validation – The control issue is formulated utilizing receding horizon rules and the state-space model created in the previous stage.
4. Moving horizon estimation techniques – When the processes are noisy or there is little feedback information available, the framework also permits the application of moving horizon estimate approaches. When it occurs, the Kalman filter is frequently used.

The framework was used to evaluate the suggested in silico tools against patient case studies in three different biological systems. The creation of a unique chemotherapy treatment plan for leukemia patients was the first example. After leukemia, the framework was used to create sophisticated control mechanisms for situations involving intravenous and volatile anesthesia. Advanced blood glucose controllers for people with diabetes were being developed. The case studies discussed above showed the potential of computational tools in biological systems and their capacity to deal with various difficulties. It is obvious that integrated strategies need to be used, incorporating both robust in silico platforms and experimental and/or clinical data.

7.2.4.5 Graphene-based wearable e-textiles

E-textiles are lightweight, pleasant, and long-lasting while yet maintaining the required electrical qualities, in contrast to the current bulky and stiff wearable gadgets. In order to create the next generation of multifunctional wearable clothing, a study was done employing highly conductive, flexible, and machine-washable graphene-based e-textiles [55]. High-conductivity and machine-washable e-textiles are made possible by easy and scalable screen printing of graphene-based ink on textiles, followed by fine encapsulation of conductive track. These wearable e-textiles exhibit remarkable flexibility when bent and squeezed in forward and reverse directions. Thanks to a reproducible response in the electrical resistance change. Furthermore, they were able to record the motions of several body parts, including the joint in the knee, the elbow, and the index finger, to show their potential as activity sensors. The fabrics' capacity to create a more comfortable biosensor than the present rigid clinical electrodes was demonstrated by their application to record EEG bio-signals with performance equivalent to regular commercial Ag/AgCl electrodes (refer Figure 7.9).

High conductive e-textiles: The idea of completely printed, multipurpose wearing e-textiles that can store energy in the form of flexible textile supercapacitors while also monitoring human activity and other vital indications like heart rate, temperature, and oxygen saturation level. The printing of highly conductive graphene-based inks utilizing a popular, scalable, high-speed screen-printing technology can be employed to develop such e-textiles.

Machine washable and flexible e-textiles: One of the main obstacles to the widespread commercial adoption of e-textile goods is thought to be their low

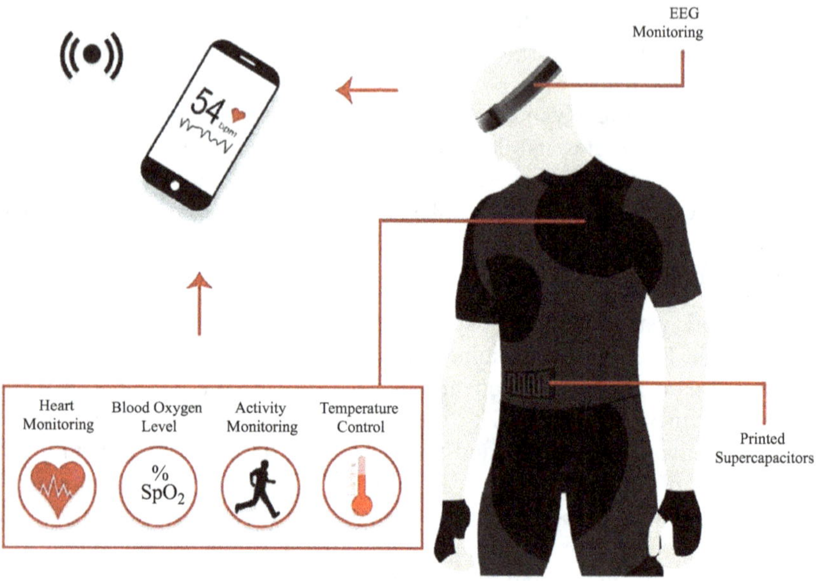

Figure 7.9 Graphene-based e-textiles [55]

stability after repeated washings in the washing machine. To withstand severe mechanical deformations and water intrusion during washing cycles employed throughout their life cycles, e-textiles must have strong washability. The performance of graphene-printed e-textiles was evaluated during 10 simulated home laundry washing cycles using the British Standard (BS EN ISO 105C06 A1S) (ISO, 2010).

Activity monitoring e-textiles: Due to its ongoing and non-invasive nature, wearable sensors for physiological and movement data collection may be used to monitor both an individual's and a patient's health problems. The piezoresistivity mechanism is used by strain-type sensors, which are made of conductive networks of active materials and behave as resistors when a voltage is applied. The tunneling effect, disconnection mechanism, inherent resistive response of active materials, length and/or cross-sectional area variations, and mechanical strain imparted during stretch or compression all affect the electrical resistance of the conductive track.

Energy storage e-textiles: Using the same screen-printing method, a printed solid-state symmetrical supercapacitor device on the fabric was prepared. On both the cathode and anode sides of the printed device, there are five branches, each measuring 33 mm in length and 2 mm in width. Each branch on the cathode is 2 mm apart from its neighboring branch on the anode. Cyclic voltammetry and galvanostatic charge-discharge were used to evaluate the in-plane supercapacitor's electrochemical performance. Based on long-term charge-discharge curves, the supercapacitor's electrochemical stability was examined. After 10,000 cycles, the devices still retained 5% of their initial capacitance, showing outstanding stability.

The graphene-based textiles can also be used to record EEG. These research discoveries could result in a genuinely versatile wearable garment for applications in customized healthcare.

7.2.4.6 The CARE algorithm

Many illness prediction algorithms have been created in recent years to perform a variety of jobs. While some algorithms concentrate on predicting a person's likelihood of having a particular diagnosis, such as heart disorders, others can be used in a more-broad way to pinpoint people's high-risk future diseases. The creation of systems to simulate jobs like the course of degenerative illnesses as well as extensions into the genomic area, identifying target regions exploited in biomarker and drug discovery, have seen further development of these prediction tasks over the last few years. The Collaborative Assessment and Recommendation Engine (CARE) Algorithm is one of the early generic illness prediction algorithms for customized healthcare that takes advantage of patient similarities [56]. In order to predict future diagnoses with a high chance for a patient, CARE collaboratively filters the patient's medical history. Historically, a method called collaborative filtering has been used to find people who have similar tastes or characteristics. The goal of collaborative filtering is to find new preferences for a person based on non-shared preferences found amongst people who are similar to that person. These methods have been used for a long time in online applications like book, movie, and product suggestions, but more recently they have also shown potential in the healthcare industry.

There are three main stages in CARE. The method starts with a preliminary filtering of all patients in the database for patient p, excluding only those who share at least one ailment with p. This is done because comparing patients with complete differences would just increase the calculation time and provide no prospective information about similarity. The collaborative filtering process is then completed using this selection of patients. The collaborative filtering process used by CARE uses binary diagnosis codes, with 1 denoting an actual diagnosis and 0 denoting an absence or unidentified condition. In order to give less prevalent diagnoses more weight, the inverse frequency of each diagnostic is also considered. A chronological component of CARE also shows when a patient's condition first manifested itself in their medical history. Then, for each comparable group of patients discovered for each illness of p, an array of these collaborative filtering models is produced. After that, the findings are combined to provide an ordered list of high likelihood illnesses for p.

7.2.5 Mobile health

Digital health solutions have the potential to improve personalized healthcare delivery and boost the ability to diagnose and treat disease efficiently. Furthermore, new ways for patients to keep track of their health and access information are made possible by technology like cell phones, social networks, and Internet apps. With the use of mobile technology, doctors, and experts will be able to converse remotely and keep in touch wherever they are. In order to improve patient satisfaction and speed up interaction involving hospitals and patients, several healthcare software applications are being developed [57].

The use of mobile devices in medical and public health is known as "mobile health." The use of mobile phones, tablet computers, personal digital assistants, and wearables for health services, information, and data collecting is included in this subcategory of electronic health. Robert Istepanian defined "developing mobile communications and network technologies for healthcare systems" as the phrase "mobile health." "Medical and public health practice assisted by mobile technology, such as mobile phones, patient monitoring devices, PDAs, and other wireless devices," is how the World Health Organization defines mobile health. A mobile device aids a patient or user in finding different mobile health systems that may be utilized for self-managing health and illness conditions through interaction or knowledge searching. i.e., a patient can make direct contact with a doctor or healthcare provider to make an appointment or in the event of an emergency [58]. This solution assists healthcare providers in providing patient-centered treatment and ongoing healthcare monitoring. It has been discovered that individuals in certain locations utilize simple mobile phone apps, such as calling and texting to convey health information, despite the fact that this has a substantial influence on raising the quality of the healthcare system and governance.

Telehealth, telemedicine, telecare, virtual health, digital health, and other technologies are also used to assist the practice of healthcare [59]. Telehealth is the utilization of medical data that may be transmitted from one location to another through electronic communication to improve patients' health status. A wide range of other technology and services are also included in order to provide patient care and improve the whole healthcare delivery system. The definition of telemedicine is the delivery of distant healthcare services to patients without a face-to-face encounter using electronic communication tools (computers, video, phone calls, texting, and both auditory and virtual forms of voice). Telecare is the term used to describe the delivery of healthcare remotely using technology to assist vulnerable individuals. Telecare establishes a continuous contact between people in their houses and qualified Carelink call-handlers at a round-the-clock monitoring facility [60]. The use of wearable technology, mobile health, health information technology, telehealth, and telemedicine to boost the patient quality of care while lowering costs and inefficiencies is known as digital health. Virtual health means linking doctors, patients, care teams, and other healthcare professionals via telehealth, telemedicine, and remote collaboration in order to provide clinical services, support patient self-management, and coordinate treatment.

According to a Canadian study [61], mHealth apps have been used for COVID-19 case detection, identification, and tracking. Applications for mobile health are being deployed in several high-income countries to track down contacts of COVID-19 cases as part of the worldwide effort to stop this epidemic. mHealth has been recognized as a strategy for COVID-19 patient detection and therapy in previous studies conducted in China [62], helping to lower the risk of spreading to other patients and healthcare workers. When compared to the conventional methods of illness diagnosis and treatment, studies have shown that mHealth apps have the potential to improve the early identification of the highly contagious COVID-19 disease.

7.2.5.1 Alzheed

Alzheed, a mobile application, is suggested for monitoring Alzheimer's disease patients at day centers in order to make ongoing patient monitoring easier [63]. A "mobile health" tracking system of this kind is called Alzheed. Alzheed relies on mobile devices for caregivers at day centers to monitor patients with Alzheimer's disease. The type of data gathered and the method used to collect it give Alzheed's tracking program its distinctive characteristics. The types of information gathered by Alzheed include: (i) behavioral information, such as roaming, hostility, and extreme tiredness; (ii) clinical and health information; (iii) activities performed; (iv) performance in intellectual and physical therapies; (v) attitudes and crises, such as frustration, imaginings, changes in mood, and nervousness; (vi) sanitary practices; (vii) eating patterns; and (viii) administrative information, such as arrival time to the day center (refer Figure 7.10). Manual data registration, consistent tracking, noninvasive patient monitoring, and contextual data input are characteristics of Alzheed's data-gathering technique. It is crucial to note that Alzheed might be used to track and collect information on people who have conditions including Lewy Body dementia, Parkinson's disease, and vascular dementia, which are all associated with Alzheimer's disease. Memory loss, confusion, language impairment, personality changes, and sadness are common symptoms and behaviors among patients with these disorders. In order to avoid misconceptions made by healthcare experts and day center employees, it can be acknowledged that Alzheed should carefully perform observation activities there.

7.2.5.2 Brain4U

A frequent chronic neurologic condition affecting children is epilepsy. Controlling seizures while avoiding negative side effects from anti-seizure medication is the

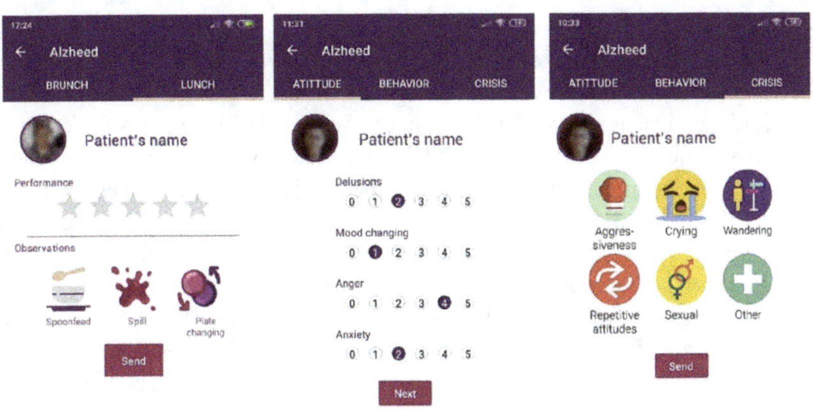

Figure 7.10 Screenshots from Alzheed's app [63]

main goal of epilepsy treatment. As a result, it is critical to document seizures, assess drug compliance, and monitor side effects when receiving therapy for seizures. In addition to recording seizures, determining the unique seizure triggers for each patient can aid in controlling seizures. The hospital electronic health record has been connected with a mobile epilepsy management software named "Brain4U" [64]. A seizure journal, prescription reminder that may track patient adherence, comorbidity self-screening tools, a customizable dashboard for each patient, and instructional content are just a few of the features of this app. Users can enter date and time, seizure types, numbers of each kind, durations, and timings, as well as provide short seizure descriptions. Users can create reminders for when they intend to take medications, based on the medication data provided by the practitioner. Brain4U gives users a reminder when they activate the medication reminder, such as "[7:30 am] Take your medications and record your dosage." In order to preserve these occurrences as an adherence rate, users can respond to reminders by checking the box that reads, "Yes, I have taken medicine." Reminders that go unanswered by the users are regarded as having had low compliance. An alarm is present to notify people of impending doctor visits. Additionally, there are educational resources that address more than 80 queries about epilepsy in general, identification, and management, problems with daily living brought on by epilepsy, as well as video examples of each kind of seizure. Along with a QOL survey, it also includes comorbidities self-screening tools for depression, anxiety, and attention deficit hyperactivity disorder (ADHD). The Korean short version of the Children's Depression Inventory is used to measure depression. For kids under the age of 13, the State-Trait Anxiety Inventory is used to measure anxiety. For caregivers and patients, the Conners Rating Scale and ADHD Rating Scale-IV is used to assess ADHD. The Quality of Life in Childhood Epilepsy Questionnaire is used to evaluate QOL. Brain4U's mobile application was able to collect specific seizure records, seizure-triggering variables, and side effects of anti-seizure medication in comparison to data obtained by merely questioning patients or caregivers at the clinic [65].

7.2.5.3 CalcVAN

Due to multi-drug resistance strains, *Staphylococcus aureus* is a significant pathogen that can cause severe infections in inpatients, such as osteomyelitis, endocarditis, and bacteremia. Vancomycin continues to be the medication of choice for so many infections among the available choices. Vancomycin does, however, have a limited therapeutic index, which is the minimal difference between beneficial and hazardous dosages. Therefore, it is necessary to customize medication dose regimens depending on the clinical details of each patient, such as bodyweight and anticipated creatinine clearance. For Android-powered smartphones, the CalcVAN [66] app was created. Vancomycin dose calculators for adult and pediatric patients, working team details, and literature references are all included on the mobile app's six Portuguese-language panels. For the vancomycin dosing schedule to be shown automatically, the healthcare practitioner must provide numbers for the patient's actual weight and predicted creatinine clearance. The smartphone app was created to compute dose schedules for patients with severe illnesses, which is vital to keep in mind.

An individual's health is directly impacted by their use of mobile health applications and services. A customized, comprehensive system has to be developed in collaboration with healthcare experts by technology entrepreneurs and software engineers, who then execute it through the proper channels by enlisting doctors or specialists. In order to guarantee the integrity and security of data at every step of health management, these apps and systems should be monitored and controlled by standard organizations.

References

[1] M. Bonner, "What is Industry 4.0 and What Does it Mean for My Manufacturing?" 2 March 2017. https://blog.viscosity.com/blog/what-is-industry-4.0-and-what-does-it-mean-for-my-manufacturing. [Accessed 12 September 2022].

[2] P. P. Groumpos, "A critical historical and scientific overview of all industrial revolutions," *IFAC-PapersOnLine*, vol. 54, no. 13, pp. 464–471, 2021.

[3] G. Moore, "3 ways to be a good leader in the Fourth Industrial Revolution," World Economic Forum, 3 January 2019. https://www.weforum.org/agenda/2019/01/the-fourth-industrial-revolution-needs-new-forms-of-leadership/. [Accessed 9 September 2022].

[4] S. H. Ahn and M. H. Lee, "The impact of the fourth industrial revolution on jobs," in *Proceedings of the Korean Management Association*, 2016.

[5] H. F. Anjum, Z. A. Rasid, H. Khalid, *et al.*, "Mapping research trends of blockchain technology in healthcare," *IEEE Access*, vol. 8, pp. 174244–174254, 2020.

[6] M. M. Ahsan, P. M. Mahmud, P. K. Saha, K. D. Gupta and Z. Siddique, "Effect of data scaling methods on machine learning algorithms and model performance," *Technologies*, vol. 9, no. 3, p. 52, 2021.

[7] G. Aceto, V. Persico, and A. Pescape, "Industry 4.0 and health: Internet of Things, big data, and cloud computing for healthcare 4.0," *Journal of Industrial Information Integration*, vol. 18, p. 100129, 2020.

[8] S. K. Sood and K. S. Rawat, "A fog assisted intelligent framework based on cyber physical system for safe evacuation in panic situations," *Computer Communications*, vol. 178, pp. 297–306, 2021.

[9] R. Sandhu, S. K. Sood, and G. Kaur, "An intelligent system for predicting and preventing MERS-CoV infection outbreak," *The Journal of Supercomputing*, vol. 72, pp. 3033–3056, 2016.

[10] M. Bhatia and S. K. Sood, "Exploring temporal analytics in fog-cloud architecture for smart office healthcare," *Mobile Networks and Applications*, vol. 24, no. 4, pp. 1392–1410, 2019.

[11] H. Kaur, S. U. Ahsaan, B. Alankar, and V. Chang, "A proposed sentiment analysis deep learning algorithm for analyzing COVID-19 tweets," *Information Systems Frontiers*, vol. 23, no. 6, pp. 1417–1429, 2021.

[12] M. Palaniswamy, “3D processing for human-machine interaction and additive manufacturing,” in W. Y. Leong (ed.), *Human Machine Collaboration and Interaction for Smart Manufacturing: Automation, Robotics, Sensing, Artificial Intelligence, 5G, IoTs and Blockchain*, UK: IET Digital Library, 2022, pp. 193–222.

[13] S. K. Sood, K. S. Rawat, and D. Kumar, “A visual review of artificial intelligence and Industry 4.0 in healthcare,” *Computers and Electrical Engineering*, vol. 101, p. 107948, 2022.

[14] D. Baines, L. S. Norgaard, Z. U.-D. Babar, and C. Rossing, “The Fourth Industrial Revolution: will it change pharmacy practice?” *Research in Social and Administrative Pharmacy*, vol. 16, no. 9, pp. 1279–1281, 2020.

[15] P. P. Jayaraman, A. R. M. Forkan, A. Morshed, P. D. Haghighi, and Y.-B. Kang, “Healthcare 4.0: a review of frontiers in digital health,” in: *Wiley Interdisciplinary Reviews: Data Mining and Knowledge Discovery*, 2020.

[16] C. Chen, E.-W. Loh, K. N. Kuo, and K.-W. Tam, “The times they are a-Changin’ – Healthcare 4.0 is coming!” *Journal of Medical Systems*, vol. 44, no. 40, 2020.

[17] J. Bedon-Molina, M. J. Lopez, and I. S. Derpich, “A home-based smart health model,” *Advances in Mechanical Engineering*, vol. 12, no. 6, 2020.

[18] D. Golinelli, E. Boetto, G. Carullo, A. G. Nuzzolese, M. P. Landini, and M. P. Fantini, “Adoption of digital technologies in health care during the COVID-19 pandemic: systematic review of early scientific literature,” *Journal of Medical Internet Research*, vol. 22, no. 11, p. e22280, 2020.

[19] L. Kimble and R. M. Massoud, “What do we mean by innovation in healthcare?” *European Medical Journal Innovations*, vol. 1, no. 1, pp. 89–91, 2017.

[20] K. Schwab, “The fourth industrial revolution,” World Economic Forum, 2017. https://www.weforum.org/about/the-fourth-industrial-revolution-by-klaus-schwab. [Accessed 12 September 2022].

[21] X. Xiong, “Bring technology home and stay healthy: the role of fourth industrial revolution and technology in improving the efficacy of health care spending,” *Technological Forecasting and Social Change*, vol. 165, p. 120556, 2021.

[22] M. M. Ahsan and Z. Siddique, “Industry 4.0 in healthcare: a systematic review,” *International Journal of Information Management Data Insights*, vol. 2, no. 1, p. 100079, 2022.

[23] S. Calif, “Healthcare industry to spend $125 billion on cybersecurity From 2020 to 2025,” *Cybercrime Magazine*, 8 September 2020. https://cybersecurityventures.com/healthcare-industry-to-spend-125-billion-on-cybersecurity-from-2020-to-2025/. [Accessed 14 September 2022].

[24] C. Chute and T. French, “Introducing Care 4.0: an integrated care paradigm built on industry 4.0 capabilities,” *International Journal of Environmental Research and Public Health*, vol. 16, p. 2247, 2019.

[25] G. Narayanamurthy and G. Tortorella, “Impact of COVID-19 outbreak on employee performance – moderating role of industry 4.0 base technologies,” *International Journal of Production Economics*, vol. 234, p. 108075, 2021.

[26] A. Haleem, M. Javaid, R. P. Singh and R. Suman, "Medical 4.0 technologies for healthcare: features, capabilities, and applications," *Internet of Things and Cyber-Physical Systems*, vol. 2, pp. 12–30, 2022.

[27] M. Lizuka and Y. Ikeda, "Regulation and innovation under the 4th industrial revolution: the case of a healthcare robot, HAL by Cyberdyne," *Technovation*, vol. 108, p. 102335, 2021.

[28] T. Dutta, S. Pramanik, and P. Kumar, *"IoT for healthcare industries: a tale of revolution," in Healthcare Paradigms in the Internet of Things Ecosystem*, London: Academic Press, 2021, pp. 21–45.

[29] A. Awad, S. J. Trenfield, T. D. Pollard, *et al.*, "Connected healthcare: improving patient care using digital health technologies," *Advanced Drug Delivery Reviews*, vol. 178, p. 113958, 2021.

[30] S. Li, L. D. Xu, and S. Zhao, "The Internet of Things: a survey," *Information Systems Frontiers*, vol. 17, pp. 243–259, 2015.

[31] A. Macsin, "Why IoT in healthcare becomes a priority," IoT Central, 24 March 2021. https://www.iotcentral.io/blog/why-iot-in-healthcare-becomes-a-priority. [Accessed 14 August 2022].

[32] A. Ustundag and E. Cevikcan, *Industry 4.0: Managing The Digital Transformation*, New York, NY: Springer, 2017.

[33] A. Belfiore, C. Cuccurullo, and M. Aria, "IoT in healthcare: a scientometric analysis," *Technological Forecasting and Social Change*, vol. 184, p. 122001, 2022.

[34] H. Dubey, J. C. Goldberg, M. Abtahi, L. A. Mahler, and K. Mankodiya, "Echowear: smartwatch technology for voice and speech treatments of patients with Parkinson's disease," in *Wireless Health*, Bethesda, MD: National Institute of Health, 2016.

[35] H. Kalantarian, B. Motamed, N. Alshurafa, and M. Sarrafzadeh, "A wearable sensor system for medication adherence prediction," *Artificial Intelligence in Medicine*, vol. 69, pp. 43–52, 2016.

[36] D. Verma, K. R. Singh, A. K. Yadav, *et al.*, "Internet of things (IoT) in nano-integrated wearable biosensor devices for healthcare applications," *Biosensors and Bioelectronics: X*, vol. 11, p. 100153, 2022.

[37] I. A. T. Hashem, I. Yaqoob, N. B. Anuar, S. Mokhtar, A. Gani, and S. U. Khan, "The rise of "big data" on cloud computing: review and open research issues," *Information Systems*, vol. 47, pp. 98–115, 2015.

[38] N. Suryadevara, S. D. T. Kelly and S. Mukhopadhyay, "Ambient assisted living environment towards Internet of Things using multifarious sensors integrated with XBee platform," in *Internet of Things*, New York, NY: Springer, 2014, pp. 217–231.

[39] M. Cwiklicki, J. Klich, and J. Chen, "The adaptiveness of the healthcare system to the fourth industrial revolution: a preliminary analysis," *Futures*, vol. 122, p. 102602, 2020.

[40] R. W. Berkowsky and S. J. Czaja, "Challenges associated with online health information seeking among older adults," in *Aging, Technology and Health*, London: Academic Press, 2018, pp. 31–48.

[41] P. Bossuyt, L. Pouillon, G. Bonnaud, S. Danese, and L. Peyrin-Biroulet, "E-health in inflammatory bowel diseases: more challenges than opportunities?" *Digestive and Liver Disease*, vol. 49, no. 12, pp. 1320–1326, 2017.

[42] N. Hossain, F. Yokota, N. Sultana, and A. Ahmed, "Factors influencing rural end-users' acceptance of e-health in developing countries: a study on portable health clinic in Bangladesh," *Telemedicine and e-Health*, vol. 25, no. 3, pp. 221–229, 2019.

[43] C. Cavicchi and E. Vagnoni, "Does intellectual capital promote the shift of healthcare organizations towards sustainable development? Evidence from Italy," *Journal of Cleaner Production*, vol. 153, pp. 275–286, 2017.

[44] L. Ricciardi, F. Mostashari, J. Murphy, J. G. Daniel, and E. P. Siminerio, "A national action plan to support consumer engagement via e-health," *Health Affairs*, vol. 32, no. 2, pp. 376–384, 2013.

[45] Z. Xu, "An empirical study of patients' privacy concerns for health informatics as a service," *Technological Forecasting and Social Change*, vol. 143, pp. 297–306, 2019.

[46] J. Min, Y. Kim, S. Lee, T.-W. Jang, I. Kim, and J. Song, "The fourth industrial revolution and its impact on occupational health and safety, worker's compensation and labor conditions," *Safety and Health at Work*, vol. 10, no. 4, pp. 400–408, 2019.

[47] M. Abdel-Basset, V. Chang, and N. A. Nabeeh, "An intelligent framework using disruptive technologies for COVID-19 analysis," *Technological Forecasting and Social Change*, vol. 163, p. 120431, 2021.

[48] S. Paul, M. Riffat, A. Yasir, *et al.*, "Industry 4.0 applications for medical/healthcare services," *Journal of Sensor and Actuator Networks*, vol. 10, no. 3, p. 43, 2021.

[49] N. Khan and M. I. Qureshi, "Systematic literature review on online medical services in Malaysia," *International Journal of Online and Biomedical Engineering*, vol. 16, no. 6, pp. 107–118, 2020.

[50] N. Sadman, S. Tasneem, A. Haque, M. M. Islam, M. M. Ahsan and K. D. Gupta, "Can NLP techniques be utilized as a reliable tool for medical science? Building a NLP Framework to Classify Medical Reports," in *IEEE 11th Annual Information Technology, Electronics and Mobile Communication Conference*, Vancouver, 2020.

[51] N. Dutte, S. Zaware, M. Shrotri, and N. Konnuri, "Ambulance tracking and patient health monitoring using GPS and GSM with health monitoring system," *International Research Journal of Engineering and Technology*, vol. 8, no. 6, pp. 574–577, 2021.

[52] S. Colantonio, G. Coppini, D. Giorgi, M.-A. Morales, and M. A. Pascali, "Computer vision for ambient assisted living: monitoring systems for personalized healthcare and wellness that are robust in the real world and accepted by users, carers, and society," in *Computer Vision for Assistive Healthcare*, London: Academic Press, 2018, pp. 147–182.

[53] E. Iadanza and A. Luschi, "Computer-aided facilities management in health," in *Clinical Engineering Handbook*, London: Academic Press, 2020, pp. 42–51.

[54] M. M. Papathanasiou, M. Onel, I. Nascu, and E. N. Pistikopoulos, "Computational tools in the assistance of personalized healthcare," in *Computer Aided Chemical Engineering*, New York, NY: Elsevier, 2018, pp. 139–206.

[55] M. R. Islam, S. Afroj, C. Beach, *et al.*, "Fully printed and multifunctional graphene-based wearable e-textiles for personalized healthcare applications," *iScience*, vol. 25, no. 3, p. 103945, 2022.

[56] K. Feldman, D. Davis, and N. V. Chawla, "Scaling and contextualizing personalized healthcare: a case study of disease prediction algorithm integration," *Journal of Biomedical Informatics*, vol. 57, pp. 377–385, 2015.

[57] A. Haleem and M. Javaid, "Medical 4.0 and its role in healthcare during COVID-19 pandemic: a review," *Journal of Industrial Integration and Management*, vol. 5, no. 4, pp. 531–545, 2020.

[58] R. R. Pai and S. Alathur, "Bibliometric analysis and methodological review of mobile health services and applications in India," *International Journal of Medical Informatics*, vol. 145, p. 104330, 2021.

[59] E. Osei and T. P. Mashamba Thompson, "Mobile health applications for disease screening and treatment support in low-and middle-income countries: a narrative review," *Heliyon*, vol. 7, no. 3, p. e06639, 2021.

[60] P. Webster, "Virtual health care in the era of COVID-19," *The Lancet*, vol. 395, no. 10231, pp. 1180–1181, 2020.

[61] M. F. Alwashmi, "The Use of Digital Health in the Detection and Management of COVID-19," *International Journal of Environmental Research and Public Health*, vol. 17, no. 8, p. 2906, 2020.

[62] W. Cheng and C. Hao, "Case-initiated COVID-19 contact tracing using anonymous notifications," *JMIR mHealth and uHealth*, vol. 8, no. 6, p. e20369, 2020.

[63] A. Chavez, G. Borrego, O. G. Garcia, and L. F. Rodriguez, "Design and evaluation of a mobile application for monitoring patients with Alzheimer's disease: a day center case study," *International Journal of Medical Informatics*, vol. 131, p. 103972, 2019.

[64] S. Yoo, K. Lim, H. Baek, *et al.*, "Developing a mobile epilepsy management application integrated with an electronic health record for effective seizure management," *International Journal of Medical Informatics*, vol. 134, p. 104051, 2020.

[65] S. A. Choi, K. Lim, H. Baek, *et al.*, "Impact of mobile health application on data collection and self-management of epilepsy," *Epilepsy & Behaviour*, vol. 119, p. 107982, 2021.

[66] T. d. M. Lima, M. P. d. Silva, L. D. S. Luz, *et al.*, "Development of a mobile application for vancomycin dosing calculation: a useful tool for the rational use of antimicrobials," *Exploratory Research in Clinical and Social Pharmacy*, vol. 5, p. 100115, 2022.

Chapter 8

Medical equipment engineering in industrial revolution

Nantha Genasan[1] *and Wai Yie Leong*[1]

Human beings have seen three industrial revolutions and currently living in a rapid changing world that is undergoing fourth industrial revolution. Started in 1760, the first industrial revolution begun with the invention of steam engine where the society's lifestyle changed from agriculture (farming based) to the manufacturing process. People's lives were based on the feudal system in which landholders provide land to tenants in exchange for their loyalty and service. The revolution period was from 1760 to 1900 and the transition period was from 1860 to 1900. Coal was used mainly as energy resource during this time period as the main transport means was train. Textile as well steel industries started to bloom during this era of the first industrial revolution.

The second industrial revolution period begun in the early of 1900 and went on till 1960 where the transition period was from 1940 to 1960 with the internal combustion engine which was the major achievement of mankind during this era. Mass production occurred during this era of rapid industrialization by using oil and electricity. Cars begun to appear on roads with Benz and BMW pioneering the automation world. This was followed by third industrial revolution from 1960 till the end of millennium 2000. Natural gas and nuclear energy paved the way during the transition period of 1980–2000.

The invention of computers and robots automated the production in companies across the world as more cars and planes started to appear in human lives. Since the beginning of the twenty-first century, a new revolution started to appear as can be seen in Figure 8.1 whereby new technologies such as computer-aided design, 3D printing, genetic engineering, tissue regeneration, Internet of things (IoT) started to appear and are being used. Table 8.1 shows the main characteristics of industrial revolution.

This fourth industrial revolution is expanding based on the strong base of the third industrial revolution's digital revolution which begun in the middle of the last century. The fusion of multiple technologies is going to shape this fourth industrial revolution. Lots of similarities are present between four industrial revolutions and

[1]Perdana University Graduate School of Medicine (PuGSOM), Malaysia

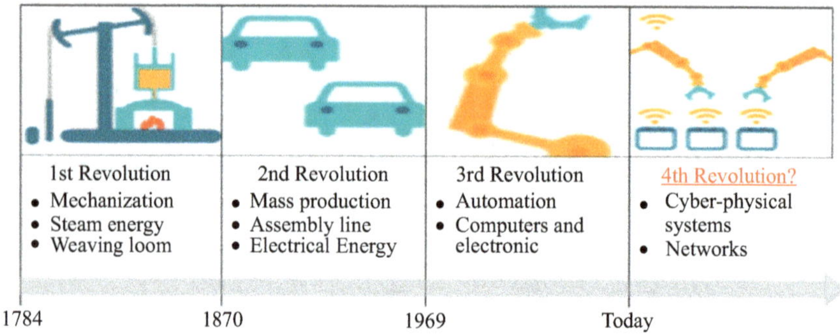

Figure 8.1 Industrial revolutions [1]

Table 8.1 Main characteristics of industrial revolutions [2]

Period	**Transition period**	**Energy resource**	**Main achievement**	**Main developed industries**	**Transport means**
I: 1760–1900	1860–1900	Coal	Steam engine	Textile, steel	Train
II: 1900–1960	1940–1960	Oil electricity	Internal combustion engine	Metallurgy, auto, machine building	Train, car
III: 1960–2000	1980–2000	Nuclear energy Natural gas	Computers, robots	Auto, chemistry	Car, plane
IV: 2000–	2000–2010	Green energies	Internet, 3D printer, genetic engineering	High tech industries	Electric car, ultra-fast train

the five ages of civilization where productivity multiplied 50 times from one age to another and many jobs were replaced by information as well industrial age jobs [2]. Production which used to be done by manual workers was replaced by knowledge workers which become company's investment. No one has the power or capabilities to control or disrupt the changes as well challenges that come with the fourth industrial revolution as we are born to live through it or be left out. Integration of multiple fields with the assistance of IoT will see more active role for artificial intelligence which will enhance our lifestyle. This fourth industrial revolution basically meant to connect every human through lots of system and machines by optimized methods and products. The following nine main pillars of industry 4.0 as can be seen in Figure 8.2 are the one going to change this world for the next few decades. These nine pillars are the one going to change the medical field and future

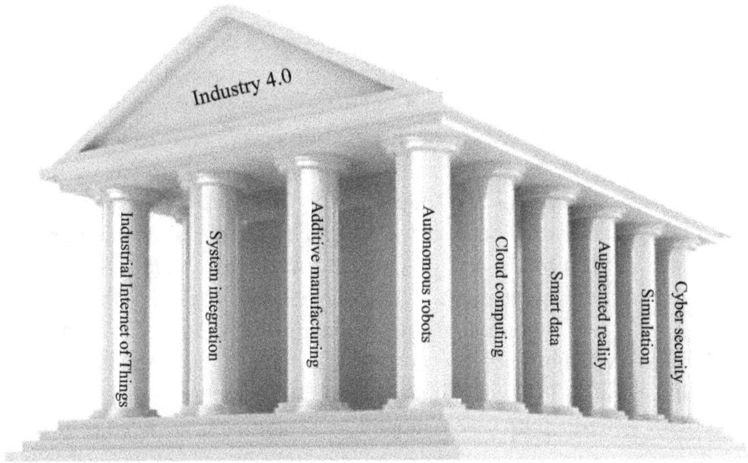

Figure 8.2 Nine pillars of industrial revolution 4.0 [1]

of healthcare whereby the advantages of this revolution depend on the increase agility and productivity.

8.1 Artificial intelligence

Medical technologies based on artificial intelligence are being utilized extensively in healthcare services across the world. The algorithms enable society to get a better healthcare service where early diagnosis of diseases is possible which gives room for optimized treatment options. Less invasive methods are available for patient's treatment and this prevents, induces unwanted medical complications, and also reduces the duration of hospitalization. Complex problems with huge data with many hospital applications can be death with this computer science. According to [3], prediction, prevention, personalizations and participatory are the four models of medicine enabled by artificial intelligence in this industrial revolution 4.0. Utilization of smartphones to fill and distribute patient's electronic health record and using biosensors to monitor patient's vital functions are examples where the 4Ps are involved. Current practices and applications of artificial intelligence in medical field can be classified into the branches of the clinical practice. In cardiology, artificial intelligence is being used to detect atrial fibrillation in patient with cardiac risk. Kardia which is a mobile application created by Alice Cor was given FDA approval in 2014 to allow smartphone-based electrocardiogram (ECG) monitoring and identify atrial fibrillation [3]. Apple Watch 4 also was given green light by Food and Drug Administration (FDA) for the same medical aspect where the data can be shared with patient's consultant through their smartphone.

Apart from this, a company named Medtronic created a system called Guardian and was approved by Food and Drug Administration (FDA) for their functions in endocrinology field to monitor glucose levels in human body. This system continuously monitors glucose levels in diabetic patient and provides information regarding real-time interstitial glucose readings together with the rate of change of it. The investment in artificial intelligence related to endocrinology field was boosted in 2018 when Medtronic joins in hand with IBM developed artificial intelligence called Watson for a new system called Sugar. IQ to assist diabetic patients hypoglycemic episodes. Apart from this, gastroenterologists used artificial intelligence-based deep learning (DL) models such as convolutional neural networks (CNN) to process images from endoscopy and ultrasound as well to detect abnormal structures such as colonic polyps. These artificial neural networks (ANN) play an important role in detecting and diagnosing gastrointestinal diseases such as inflammatory bowel disease, gastritis, metastasis of rectal, and esophageal cancer [3]. In 2018, Food and Drug Association (FDA) approved a wearable device called Embrace developed by Empatica to be used in neurological field for epileptic patient. The pressure of electrodermal captors in this wearable device helps to detect seizures caused by epilepsy and inform the family members as well physician about the patient's localization with the assistance of the mobile application. Some limitations are also present with these artificial intelligence applications in medical field such as unreliable design and lack of expertise to utilize the technologies, algorithm evaluation and adaptation but eventually with progress of industrial revolution 4.0 every problems will be solved with human talents and skills. Not to forget that medical device is a multi-billion dollar market in this era and every countries are investing in it. The need to educate people of medical fraternity is important as innovation and research of artificial intelligence will enhance the quality healthcare services.

8.2 IoT

Apart from artificial intelligence in medicine, IoT which is also knows as Internet of Everything (IoE) and big data analytics has shown promising outcomes with their applications in healthcare services. Uniquely identifiable things such as sensors, computing devices, algorithms, and physical objects are connected together by means of information communication technology (ICT) under IoT [4]. This leads to autonomous data processing as data is connected and transferred without the needs of human intervention. IoT acts as a big element in this industrial revolution 4.0 where it recognizes and trace as well authenticate objects and people, especially in medical devices and patient data for further analysis at which big data analytics get through. Hospital architecture system for IoT consists of three basic elements knows as pacemaker, broker and subscriber as seen in Figure 8.3. Patient's vital information are individually or simultaneously recorded with the assistance of network of connected sensors/medical devices. Heart rate of the patient with blood pressure, ECG, electroencephalogram (EEG) and much more are part of this information. The broker which has the responsibility to process and store the acquired data in the cloud receives this information through a network.

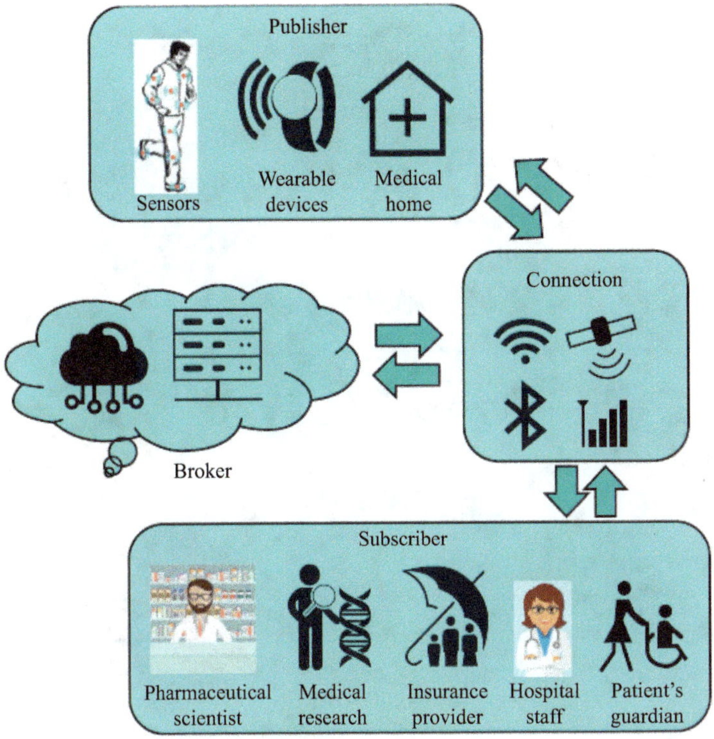

Figure 8.3 Architecture of HIoT framework [5]

Lastly, the patient's information can be accessed, monitored, and visualized through a smartphone, computer, tablet by the subscriber [5]. Real-time analysis that was not done years back is possible in this industrial revolution 4.0 due to the advent of IoT and this helps the medical fraternity to provide better healthcare services at a minimal cost.

Geriatric patient's management utilizes new technology under the branch of artificial intelligence which is known as ambient-assisted living (AAL). Elderly people can live independently at home where this AAL monitor their movement in real-time frame and helps them to receive immediate human service-like assistance in case of medical emergency. Researchers are actively working on the three domains of AAL such as the elderly's activity recognition, their living environment and condition recognition as well their vital monitoring. In another study, patient's fall detection and hear rate control are being monitored with the help of a new sensors in mobile gateway-based HIoT system named "AMBRO." Abnormal heart rate beyond 60–100 beats per minute can be detected by patient they themselves and also the family members whom in turn can reach paramedic immediately. Figure 8.4 shows other HIoT-based noninvasive services and Figure 8.5 shows the applications of HIoT, respectively, in which wearable devices with built-in sensors

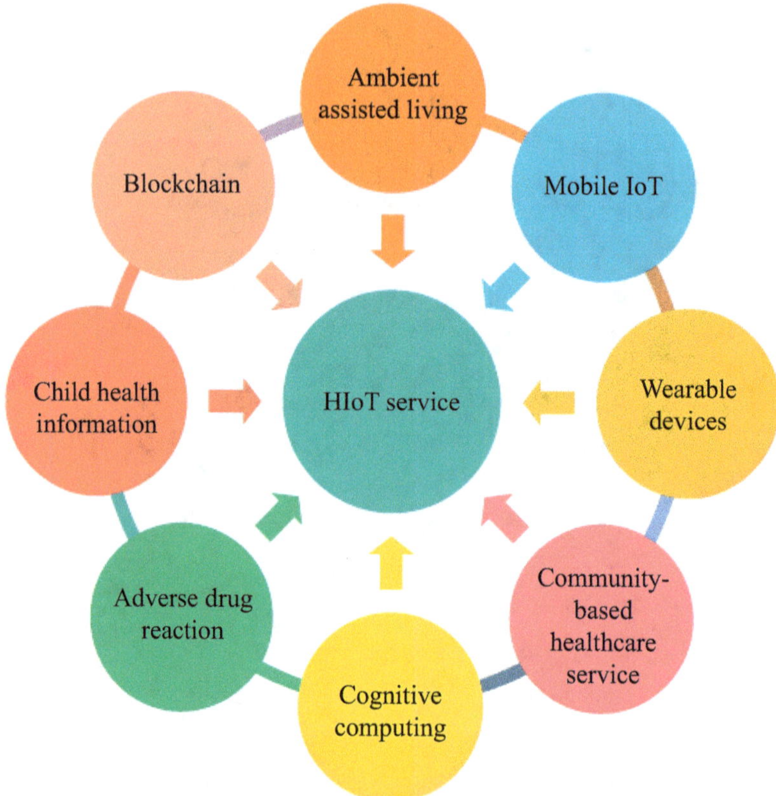

Figure 8.4 HIoT services [5]

connect with the living conditions of the patient and patient's health information are automatically uploaded into cloud networks which are being managed by patient's healthcare services providers. Bio signals from EEG and EMG emitted from these biosensors and analyzed thoroughly with the input from sensors as speech, gesture, and body movement to decide the pathological conditions of a patient. These wearable devices and sensors are getting more cheaper and user friendly due to the rapid development in the IoT technology (Figure 8.6). A system was proposed for IoT-based ECG monitoring system which operates at minimal power of 5.2 mW. The system utilizes a biopotential microchip to acquire ECG data when there's an abnormality in heart beating and the data is transferred to end-users through mobile app which can visualized along [5].

Other than this, a glove was designed by Alarcon Parades to use for real-time blood glucose level with the assistance of Raspberry Pi Camera and a visible laser beam which helps to take diabetic condition pictures from the fingertip. Additionally, double moving average infrared LED and near-infrared photodiode have also been researched for glucose level monitoring. Another study was done by using Arduione

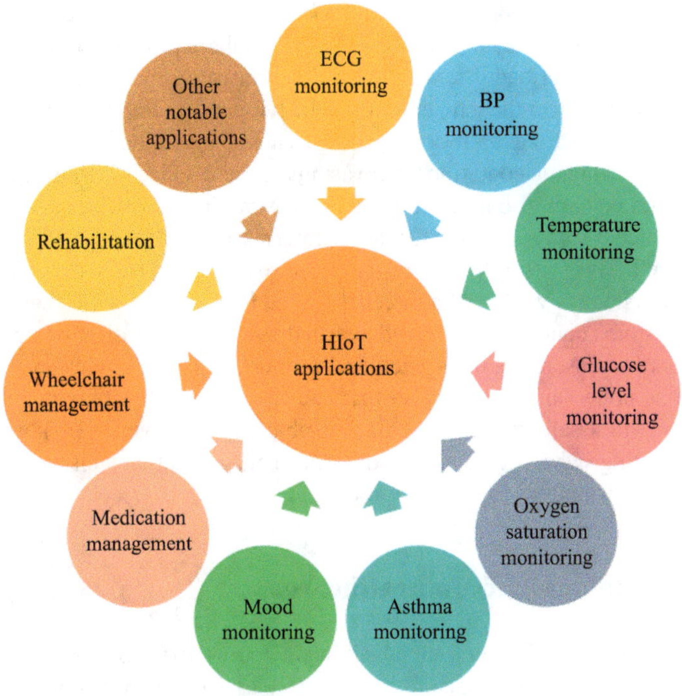

Figure 8.5 Category of HIoT applications [5]

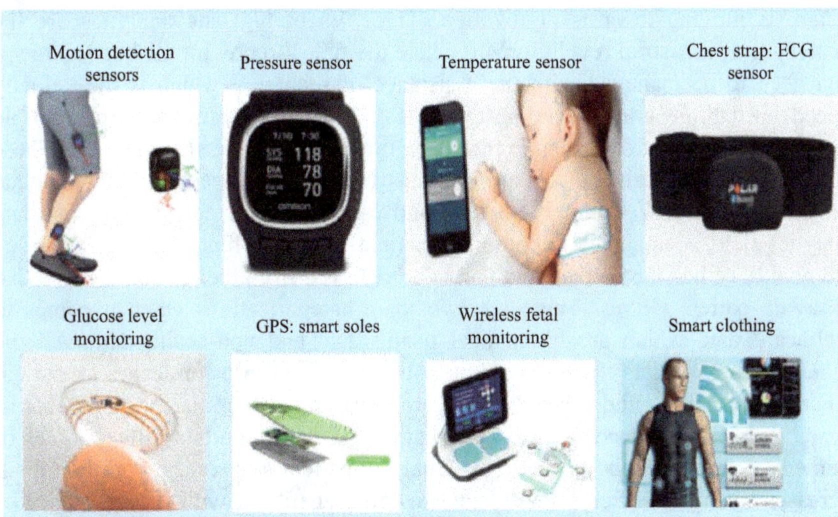

Figure 8.6 Types of wearable sensors [5]

and Raspberry Pi to develop IoT-based temperature monitoring system whereby the tympanic membrane in human ear became the crucial area for temperature detection [5]. The idea was described in a way where 3D-printed wearable device needs to be worn on the ear to detect the temperature on the tympanic membrane with the help of infrared sensor. Swelling of the air passage causes breathing pathway shrinkage which leads to asthmatic condition where asthma patient's faces difficulties to breath, wheezing, and coughing. Inhaler and nebulizer were the only lifesaving options for them but a recent study using LM35 temperature sensors can assist to reduce their burden as well. This sensor detects the temperature of inhaled and exhaled air and act as an alarm system as well once a threshold value is reached. Patients can be valued about their asthma condition and thus they can the necessary medication immediately [5]. Further, the sensors are being modified further to analyze environmental conditions such as pollen and humidity so that can reach the asthmatic patient to move from the side to a safer place [5]. Other notable applications of HIoT are such as mood monitoring, wheelchair, and medication management as well oxygen saturation monitoring (Figure 8.5).

8.3 Big data analytics in healthcare

Set aside artificial intelligence and healthcare IoT (HIoT), big data analytics is going to be a key changer in healthcare industry as previously majority of data in medical networks were stored in hand copy records or single source data storage. The integration of artificial intelligence and IoT in healthcare industry with wearable devices and sensors as well smart medical devices, the data management system is moving towards digitization. Three Vs of big data analytics are the challenges of industrial revolution 4.0 where the first V represent the big volume of data need to be managed with the assistance of second V which is the velocity (speed) of data generation lending to the last "V" namely variety where multiple versions and types of data need to managed, processed, analyzed, and stored. These varieties of data can be structured, unstructured, and semi-structured data. Recently, another 2V's namely veracity and value are being added to the big data analytics field. Veracity is important in-patient care as it represents the accuracy and quality of healthcare data and the value received from the data analytics assist in saving patient's lives. There are two main categorizations when it comes to healthcare data which are biomedical health data and non-health data. All the Omics group of data (genomics, microbiomics, and proteomics) and patient generated data falls under health data category. This electronic medical records, wearable devices, physician entry, and patient's health reports are the sources of biomedical data which are used to analyze patient's disease condition as it increases treatment efficiencies. Physicians are benefitting with the assistance of administrative data such as clinical data, insurance claims, pharmaceuticals, patient's behavior, and life style because this helps them to get a better understanding about patient's health background hence providing better healthcare services [6].

Today's healthcare data analytics are represented by 2Ds namely descriptive and diagnostic and 2Ps which are predictive and prescriptive. When a patient with heart failure is admitted to the hospital possible occurrences related to patient's current condition need to be studied by using descriptive analysis. Factors related to those occurrences are diagnosed followed by predictive analysis of heart failure conditions. Machine learning and advance statistics are used for predictive analysis purposes and, at the end, treatment options are given to the patient by using prescriptive analysis. Additionally, cluster analysis, data mining, graph analytics, machine learning, natural language processing (NLP), neural networks, and spatial analysis are part of big data analytical techniques in this industrial revolution 4.0. In south-east Asia (SEA) region, Singapore has become a key leader to implement big data analytics in healthcare services (Figure 8.7). For a chronic disease such as diabetes, Singapore healthcare providers are using big data analytics in approaching and managing diabetic patients. Diabetes is a disease which is expensive in terms of medication expenses and it has been forecasted that by 2050 about US$1.9 billion need to be spent for diabetic management as it is a major public health issue. Diabetic patient's medical expenses cost two times higher than the prevention measures [6]. The Singaporean government introduced a new task force to manage the disease by early detection of the disease for risky people or the undiagnosed ones and as well control the advancement of the disease.

A diabetic population equation as follows was created as part of the initiative to manage diabetic [6].

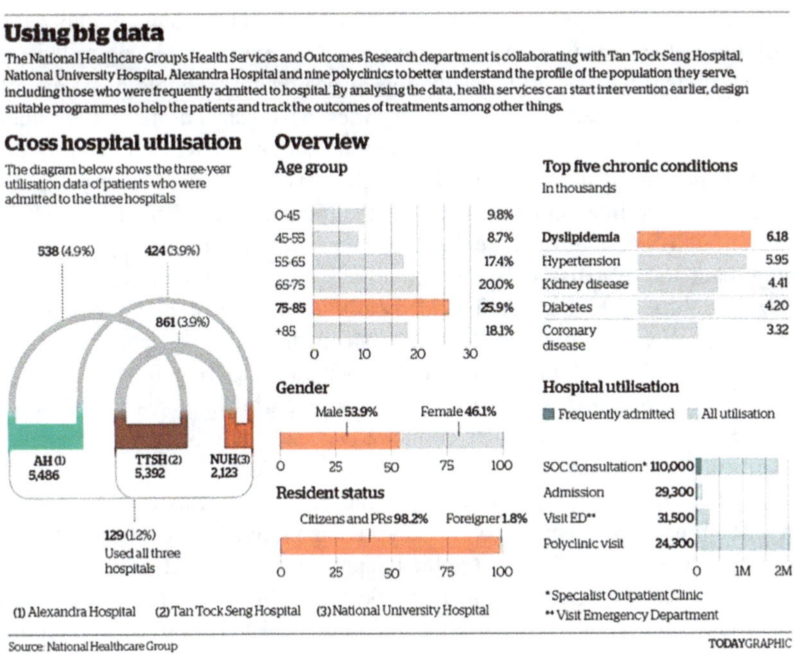

Figure 8.7 Singapore's big data utilization (National Healthcare Group)

Diabetic Population (D) = Early Stage (ES) + Late Stage (LS) + Complex Stage (CS)

Based on this equation, diabetic patients are categorized into different stages of disease and they received different types of healthcare support respectively. Data analytics production was done for each segment of diabetic stage and different strategies for each type of patients are being developed. As prevention is better than cure the main aim of this initiative is on the Early Stage (ES) population as to prevent disease progression to a further harmful stage. Digital intervention can be deployed to reduce disease progression to the late or complex stage. Artificial intelligence-based real-time glucose monitoring wearable devices jumps into this region where patient's daily life can be monitored and assessed. This allows medical staff to intense into patient's wellness data and adjust the treatment accordingly. In 2011, Singapore government created National Electronic Health Record (NEHR) system which tracks all patient's health records from various healthcare service providers. This initiative gives the government to economically monitor the budget/allocation for healthcare sectors and create a healthy wellbeing population of all age [6].

8.4 Wireless network of 5G to 6G

Healthcare services across the world currently rely heavily on fourth-generation (4G) network system to enable smart healthcare applications but in this rapid moving industrial revolution, this limited bandwidth cannot support the requirement of the applications in future. Even though 5G networks are being rolled-out, it is still insufficient to satisfy the evaluation of healthcare technologies. Generally, 5G services are divided into three categories as enhanced mobile broadband (eMBB), Ultrareliable Low Latency Communications (URLLC), and Massive Machine Type Communications (mMTC). 5G services in medical field provide high speed, reliable Internet connectivity to the Internet of Medical Things (ICMT) devices through Massive Machine Type Communications (mMTC) [7]. Enhanced mobile broadband (eMBB) assists in patient's diagnosis and treatment by a better visualization through higher quality video calling for telemedicine and augmented reality (AR) as well virtual reality (VR). Meanwhile, ultra-reliable low latency communications (URLLC) assist drones and autonomous vehicles for emergency medical surveillance and scenarios for example during any diseases outbreak. Figure 8.8 shows the step-by-step comparative analysis of fifth- and upcoming sixth-generation networks from its core plan to user plan.

Nowadays, 6G networks and their applications in healthcare services are being given attention to as many services and technologies are being proposed to improvise the medical field. Holographic telepresence, tactile Internet, autonomous and tele-operated vehicles, aerial networks, and Internet of bio-nano things (IoBNT) are some of the proposed technologies in developing a better communication infrastructure. Futuristic smart healthcare system will have a reliable system with ultra-massive connectivity, connection continuity, network scalability,

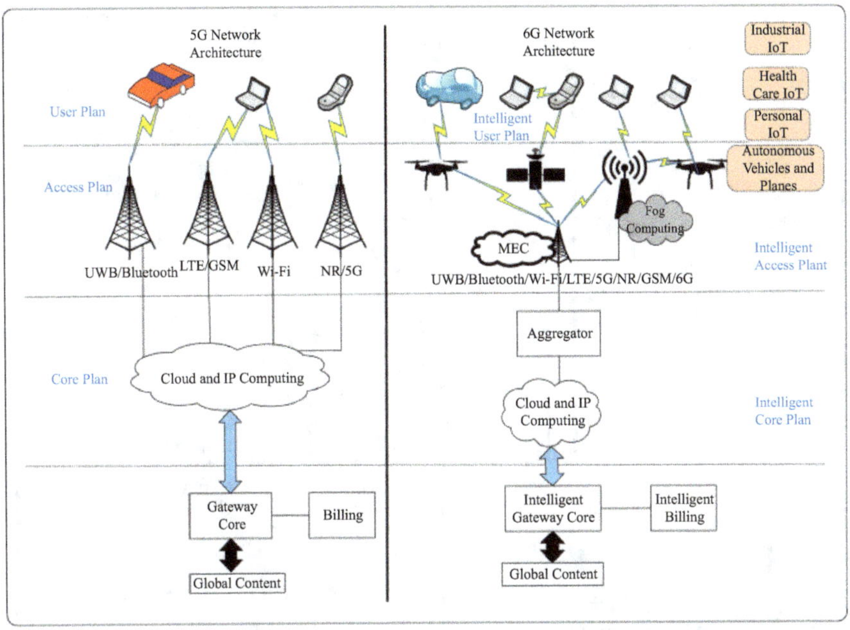

Figure 8.8 Comparative analysis of 5G and 6G network [8]

and secured communication link with physical layer security for e-health applications (Figure 8.9). Artificial intelligence and machine learning are going to be the driver and feature of 6G network systems and their applications.

Sixth-generation (6G) network applications in healthcare services can be categorized into three areas, hospital, remote healthcare, and disaster response unit. Smooth operations of hospitals require constant and effective communication between hospital administrators and their staff consisting of doctors, medical assistants, nurses, and patients at the service receiving end point. In recent years, new methods patient's record followed by introduction of artificial intelligence based services for a better decision in disease diagnosis as well prognosis. High precision in surgeries is being achieved by using robots such as Da Vinci's surgical system [9]. There are situations where hospitals are packed with patients and got out of control due to a limited number of medical staff as well equipment to assist them. During pandemic, these situations get much more serious as infectious diseases can be transferred among medical personnel themselves creating a bigger outbreak circle. Thus, by deploying Internet of medical things (IoMT) and automated robots in hospital environment will help to reduce physical interactions between patients and clinicians. Patients can be monitored with the assistance of IoMT wearable devices and sensors and data can be transmitted to the clinicians over the Internet thus reducing interactions. Furthermore, can help to deliver medical supplies, medical checkups, disinfecting, and sanitizing patients' area.

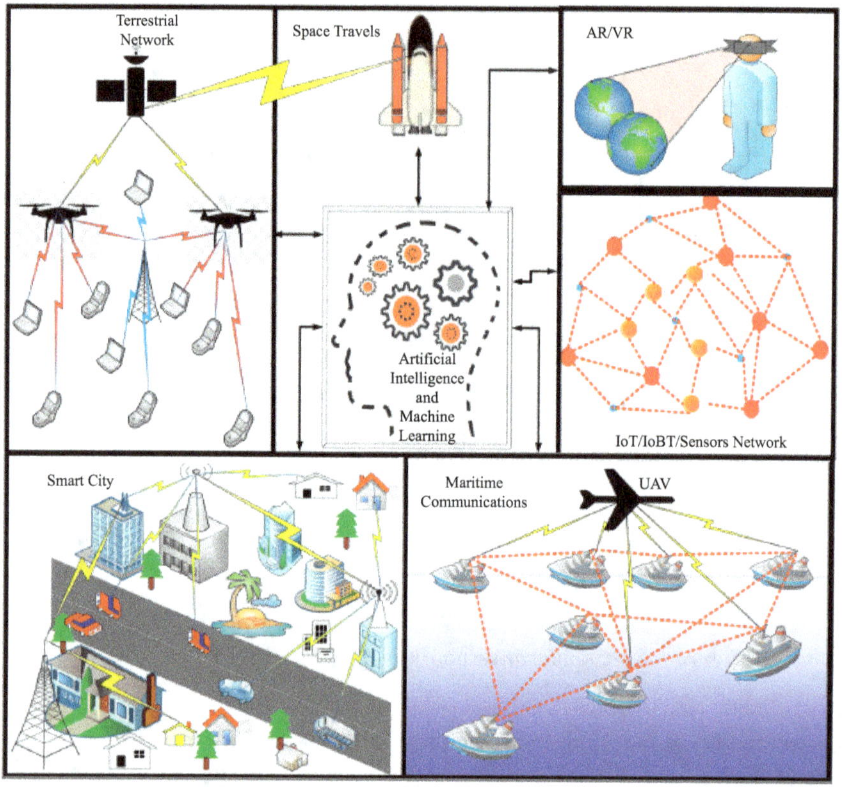

Figure 8.9 Next-generation communication system involving space–air–ground–sea with their applications [8]

These technological advancements are going to be used in massive scale in coming future and thus rely on a secure, reliable, and high data rate communication link. Wi-Fi networks usage is restricted as medical equipment are prone to electromagnetic interference (EMI) and complex architecture of hospital buildings restricts penetration of high-frequency signals causing network covering issues. Implementation of 6G which is an extremely reliable and low-latency communication with advance physical security features will facilitate the communication requirements in terms of capacity and connectivity. Patient's privacy and critical clinical information can be protected from security bridge of hackers and unauthorized personnel's access. Figure 8.10 shows the evolution of security and privacy issues in wireless systems.

Providing a quality health service for people living in interior with limited travel options is a key challenging factor globally for medical fraternity. Tele medicine has been somehow helping the doctors to check on their patients by means of teleconferencing for evaluation and treatment purposes without physical interaction. Rapid development of hologram technology will soon replace the

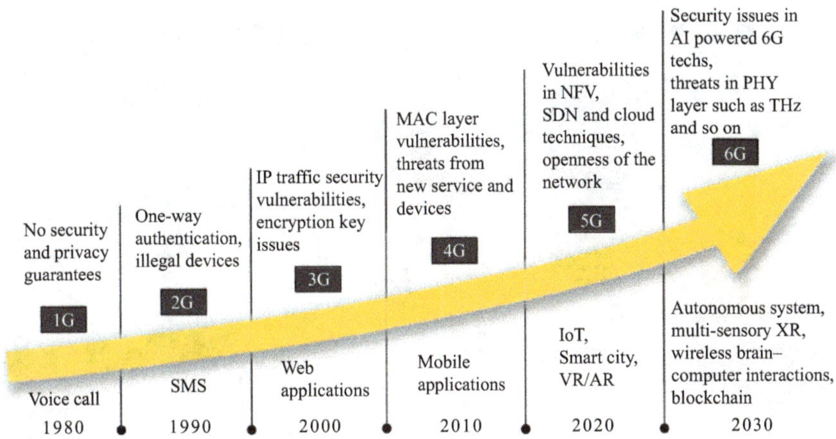

Figure 8.10 Security and privacy issues in wireless systems [9]

current method of high-quality video teleconferencing with holographic representation. Plus, to this, wireless body area network (WBAN) which is based on IoMT wearable device technology is being deployed extensively. This remote health care services depends mainly on extensive, reliable, massive communication infrastructure. With the implementation of 6G network in coming months or years this will ensure further development on these IoMT-based devices, biosensors with ultra-low power communication, and secured network in remote healthcare free from jamming and spoofing. Figure 8.11 shows the future applicability of 6G network system-based technologies in healthcare system where (a) represents wireless sensing in field hospital, (b) represents THz for COVID-19 screening (e.g., of pandemic outbreak), (c) visible light communication (VLC) for localization and capacity enhancement, and (d) smart vest for WBAN security.

When it comes to a medical emergency, disaster response unit acts a frontline mechanism in providing healthcare services to the public through field hospitals, disaster management centers, and emergency mobile services (EMS). Critical services will be provided by EMS outside the hospital arena with prehospital healthcare by ground or air ambulance as per security of the emergency. Sophisticated medical equipment is being installed in smart ambulances nowadays to provide speeder diagnosis and treatment by paramedics where they can consult medical staff through high quality video calling. The disaster response unit also needs to communicate with other departments such as fire brigade, police department, insurance companies, and thus need to have a stronger communication cellular network that is needed. Where there is a field hospital during a pandemic situation, quarantined patients need proper case by which robots and drone technologies are leading the way. These technologies help to deliver the food and medical kits, taking test samples, sanitizing patient areas and so on. High data rate transmission is required in smart ambulances to transfer information collected from medical imaging. Large spectrum bandwidth of 6G network will play a role to change these

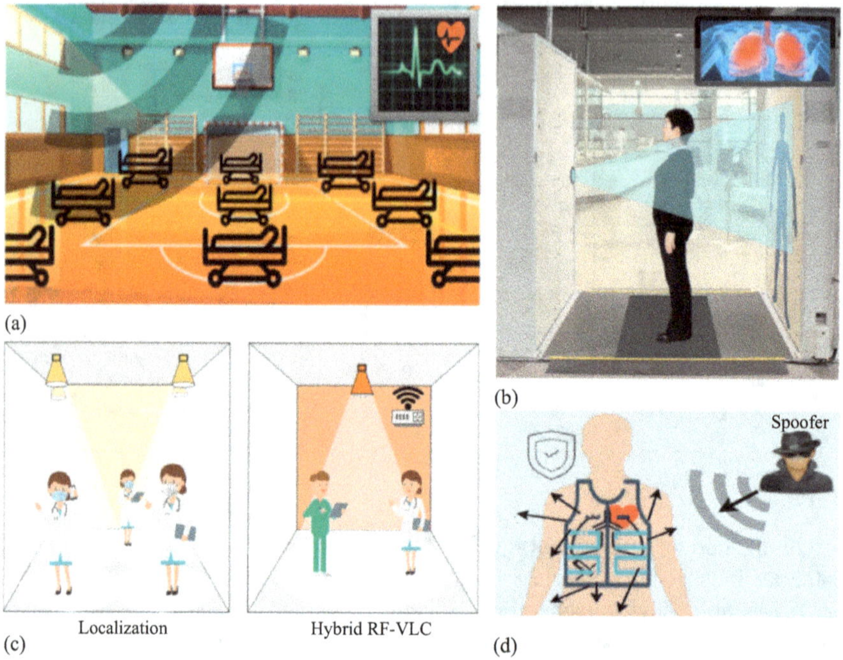

Figure 8.11 Applications of 6G technologies in health care system [7]

challenges present in providing a holistic medical care. High-quality coverage and connectivity with low latency as well high reliability is vital for remote health and disaster response services. The development of medical equipment together with cellular network improvisation needs a precise integration of both into healthcare system for a real-time implementation.

8.5 VR and AR

VR and AR are part of simulated reality technologies that are advancing and being used in fields like military, education, and sports. Originally developed in 1965, VR depends on the creation of an immersive environment. Investments by Japanese giant Sony and California based Google into this VR technology brought new developments such as fish-eye lenses which enhances and creates wider field of view for a more immersive environment [10]. AR technology whereas consists of hologram like entities superimposed on real-world background in comparison with VR. Recent advancement in AR technology's see-through head-mounted displays where the users perceive a 3D object by passing light from micro-projectors onto a wave guide which is then projected back to the wearer's eye. Currently, these AR and VR technologies play an important role in medical field comprising medical education as well medical imaging in radiology training.

Human anatomy which is complex can be conceptualized in the field of radiology with the help of AR for training purposes. Digital Imaging and Communications in Medicine (DICOM) images are connected to 3D object files to train radiology residents. Figure 8.12 shows the examples of a patient's inner ear image through DICOM where the patient went for stapes surgery. Self-directed learning in an immersive environment can be done with VR technology where nine GoPro cameras mounted on a stand can record a contrast agent reaction scenario (Figures 8.13 and 8.14). The recorded module could be played back at a user's own pace with the assistance of immersive headsets since the module mimics events surrounding a contrast material reaction.

Apart from this, low-cost device such as MERGE Cube which is widely available in market can be used to allow anatomic holograms to be affixed with

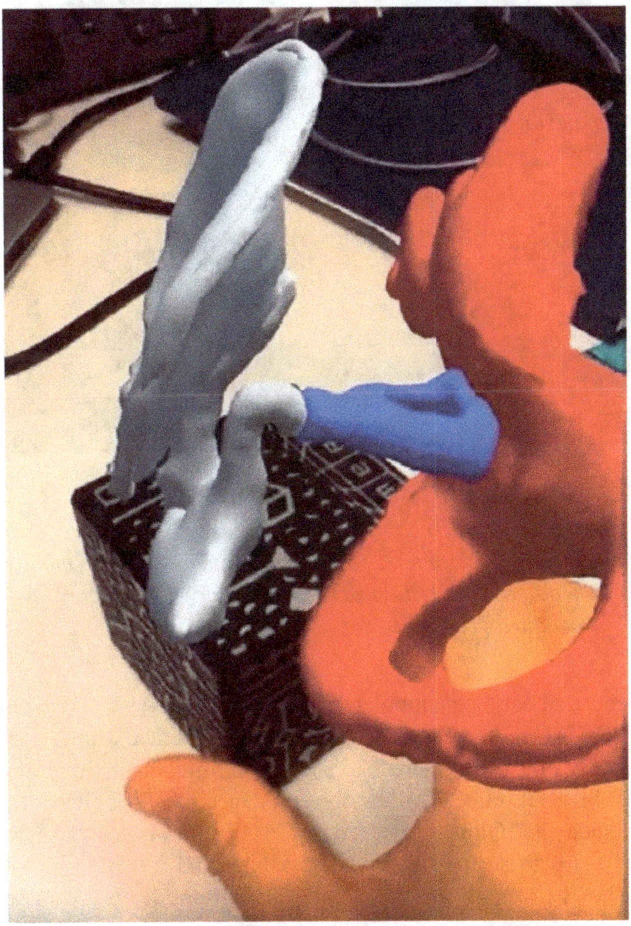

Figure 8.12 DICOM image of the inner ear of a patient who underwent stapes surgery [10]

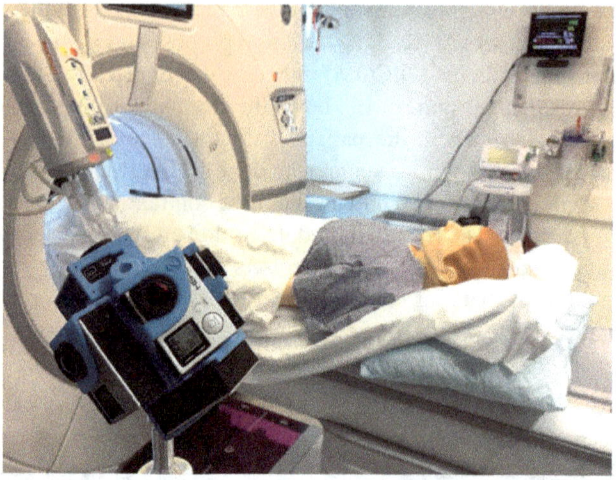

Figure 8.13 *Nine camera apparatus and mannequin used for recording a contrast material reaction simulation module [10]*

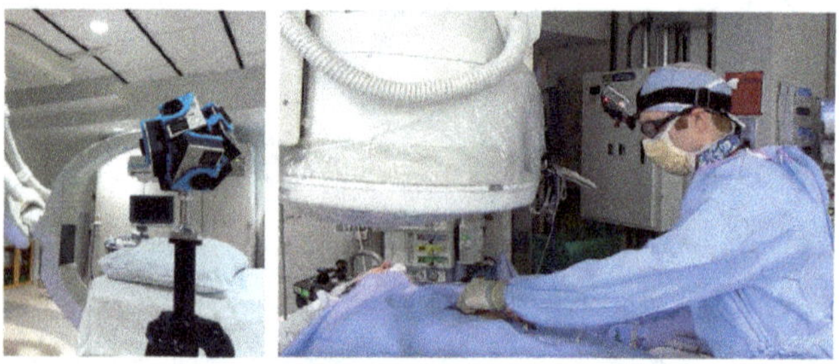

(a) (b)

Figure 8.14 *(a) Seven GoPro cameras on a stand are used to record 360-degree video for VR content. (b) GoPro cameras can be mounted by using a head strap to obtain 3D stereoscopic video recordings of a procedure [10].*

physical objects that can be manipulated. Figure 8.15 shows how the commercially available MERGE Cube can be used to physically interact with AR medical content. The image (b and c) of Figure 8.15 shows the frontal and oblique view of skull with labels in MERGE cube. Further, the assistance of 3D application software in smartphone such as Qlone invented by California-based Eye Cue Vision Technologies helps to scan images in 3D fashion and integrate in AR scenarios. Figure 8.16 shows the application of Qlone, a smartphone app scanner being used to scan an interventional radiology (IR) biopsy gun. As presented in the image A of Figure 8.16, the screenshot shows ease of 3D scanning of IR biopsy gun. A smartphone camera with Qlone software app was pointed 360° around the IR

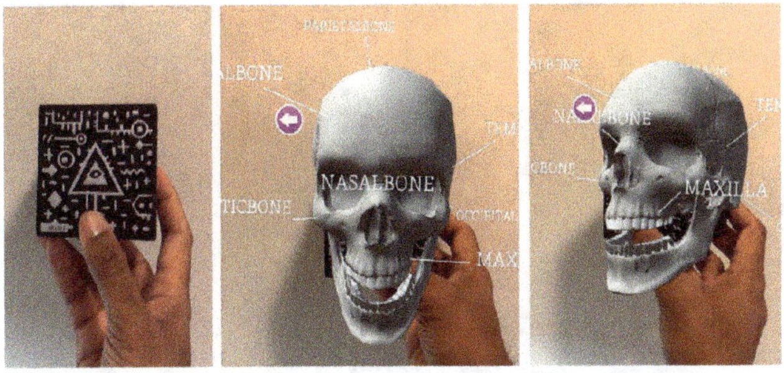

(a) (b) (c)

Figure 8.15 Photographs showing how the MERGE Cube (a) can be used to physically interact with augmented reality medical content. (b, c) Skull with labels overlaid on MERGE Cube that can be rotated from (b) frontal to (c) right oblique view. [10]

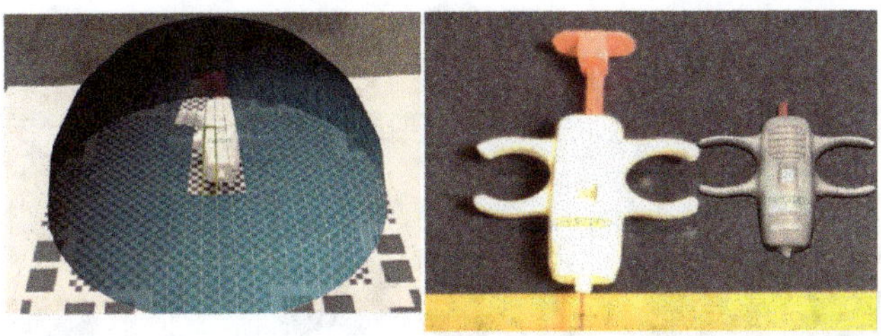

(a) (b)

Figure 8.16 Smartphone screenshot of 3D scanning of IR biopsy gun (a). Real biopsy gun left and virtual augmented reality scanned version of the same biopsy gun right (b) [10].

biopsy gun lying on a paper grid. The differences between the real and 3D scanned version of the IR biopsy gun can be seen in image B of Figure 8.16.

In addition to this, Figure 8.17 shows how medical student's smartphones can be attached with stereoscopic viewers (c) to be used for virtual interventional radiology suite. By scanning into QR code response (a and d), students can access the VR content (b and c). High cost of adoption and implementation use of AR & VR technologies are a matter of concern for many medical schools. Increase in reliability of registration of images with AR and VR will create a pathway for earlier integration for procedural simulation training purposes in anatomy and pathology.

8.6 3D imaging and 3D printing

Besides, 3D imaging technology-based hologram are being used effectively in medical field, medical diagnostics, surgical planning and also to obtain more information about external and internal tissues as well human organs. High-resolution

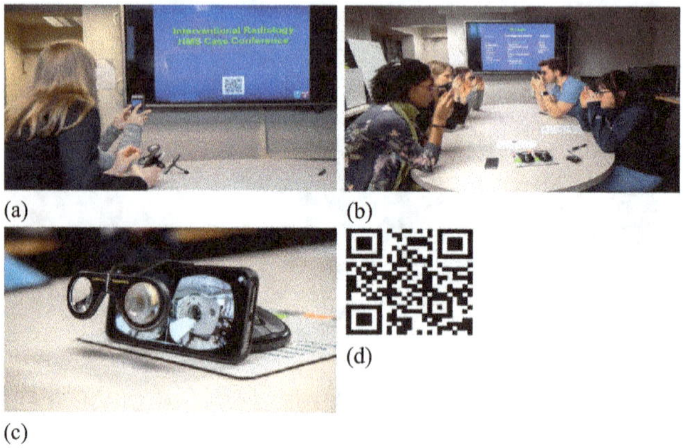

Figure 8.17 Medical students scanning a Quick Response (QR) code to access VR content [10]

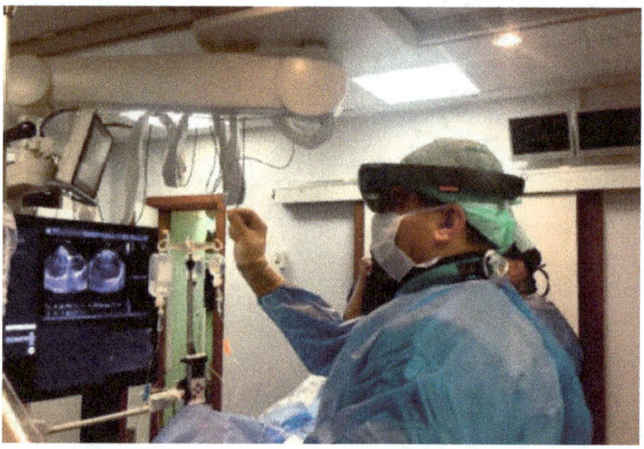

Figure 8.18 Case study – ASD, University Medical College, Krakow, Poland [11]

images can be recorded from various angles such as cavities and deformities in internal organs and holography is a suitable technology for fitting of implants procedure. Complications in imaging can be sorted out as physical testing procedure can be eliminated. Colorful holography gives proper studying of images of vascular, clinic trials, and musculoskeletal systems. The usage of HoloLens goggles technology in real time in operation theatre was done by doctors from Poland for the treatment of atrial speed defect (ASD) (Figures 8.18 and 8.19).

For medical education, this is a best tool for teaching and learning for medical students as detailed, precise information can be seen realistically in real visual field. In future, it is possible for us to have "Holodoctors" for remote healthcare as doctors can visualize the holographic images and provide treatment [12]. In

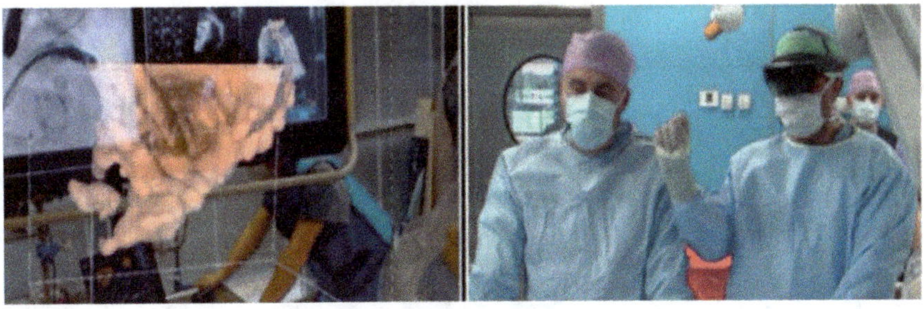

Figure 8.19 Case study – left atrial appendage hologram HoloLens assistance [11]

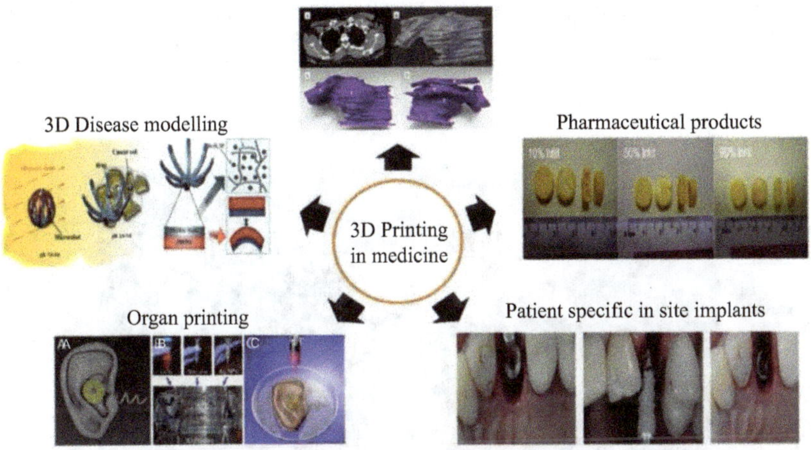

Figure 8.20 Applications of 3D printer in healthcare field [13]

addition to this innovation, 3D printing technology which was used many in aviation as well defense sectors is being used now in surgical field, pharmaceutical industry, biomedical, and veterinary medicine (Figure 8.20). Organ printing, customized implants, and prostheses printing tissue engineering are where the applications of 3D printing being forced mainly for future developments. 3D data designed with CAD programs are used to manufacture the 3D object with a printer where it can be an additive manufacturing (AM) or layered manufacturing. The physical state of main materials such as solid, liquid, or powder is important when we are classifying the 3D printing methods as the technology can be applied to metal, ceramic, composite, and polymer materials. Titanium, stainless steel, aluminum, and magnesium are most commonly used metal materials. The advantages as well disadvantages of these 3D printing methods are shown in Table 8.2. In surgical field, doctors use this 3D printing technology both during and before surgery to get a better visualization of the patient's anatomical structure. The 3D surgical template gives a precisional guidance for surgical procedure to be carried out, to estimate appropriate angles of blade's incision as well to assess blood flow circulation.

Table 8.2 Materials used in 3D printing methods, advantages and disadvantages [13]

Methods	Materials	Advantages	Disadvantages
Fused deposition modeling	ABS, PLA, Wax Blend, Nylon	High speed, high quality, used for a wide range of material	Porous structure for the binder, weak mechanical properties, often required support
Stereolithography	Resin (Acrylate or Epoxy based with proprietary photo initiator)	Large parts can be built easily, high accuracy and surface finish	Expensive, not well-defined mechanical properties due to the usage of photopolymers
Selective laser sintering	Metallic powder, polyamide, PVC	High-resolution, high strength	Only metals can be printed, post-processing required due to its grainy roughness
3D inkjet printing	Photo-resin or hydrogel	Very good accuracy, very high surface finishes	Fragile parts, poor mechanical properties

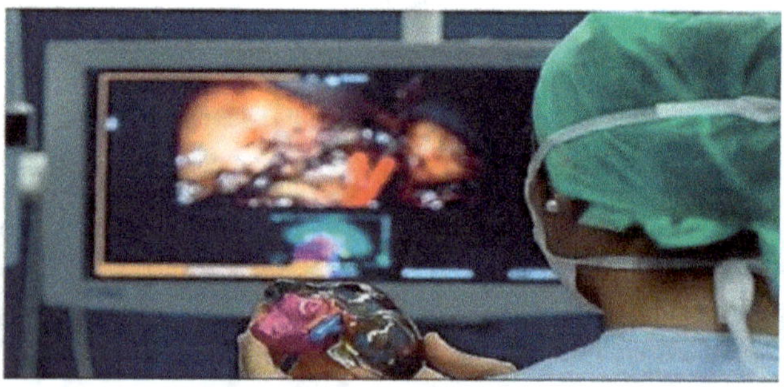

Figure 8.21 Use of 3D printing technology in surgical imaging [13]

Medical students and surgical assistants are being trained with 3D surgical modeling for example in orthopedic surgery to study the structure, direction, and size of the bones. Successful implementation of this technology helps to improvise the accuracy of surgical results, decrease surgical errors, and hence provide a better patient's care. At preoperative planning stage, the 3D anatomical structure of the patient can be viewed, studied so that surgical intervention can be simulated, and surgical instruments can be tested as well with 3D model's assistance (Figure 8.21). Furthermore, nowadays disease modeling such as for kidney diseases is being done with 3D printing technology. High accuracy in kidney modeling assists in planning and simulating complex surgery compared with traditional imaging methods such as tomography. Traditional imaging methods are limited on just flat screen whereas 3D modeling provides a better representation of the anatomy because unexpected findings can be detected. These application areas are expected to increase in near future as shown in Figure 8.22.

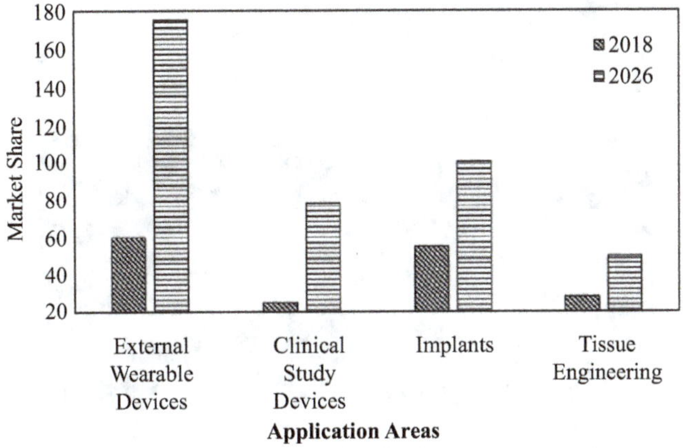

Figure 8.22 Forecast of the increase in the use of 3D printer technology in biomedical applications [13]

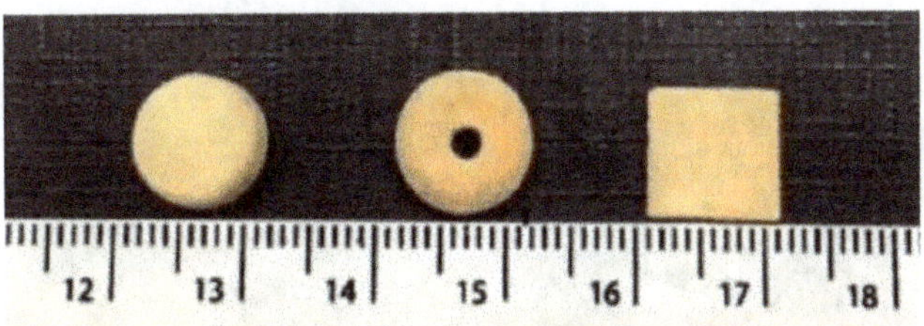

Figure 8.23 Drugs with different geometrics such as cylinder, torus, film, and size produced by 3D printer [13]

Hearing aids are also being printed with 3D printers in a much more shorter time than normal production time at a lower cost. Pharmaceutical production adapted this 3D printing technology in drug designing as per desired dimensions and geometrics (Figure 8.23). This new invention provides a solution for a long studying problem in conventional pharmaceutical manufacturing to develop drugs with complex formulations in terms of cost and time. Besides this, patient-specific implants are being manufactured as well using 3D printers for knee joints, bone, implants, and dental implants (Figure 8.24). Traditional measurement methods are eliminated and this has become convenience for healthcare personnel as well as for patient because of the accuracy, biocompatibility, and shorten waiting time. Once a printed mold can be reversed again for more implant printing and these implants tend to have high fatigue strength and high corrosion resistance. It is also possible to adjust skin tone of the person who is going to use prostheses such as for ear, nose, teeth, bone, hand, and foot according to the person's skin pigmentation. 3D printing prostheses for animals are getting popularity as every year hundreds of animals are disabled through accidents. A damaged bone, tissue, or muscle can be printed and implanted like the original one (Figure 8.25). Replacement of injured or

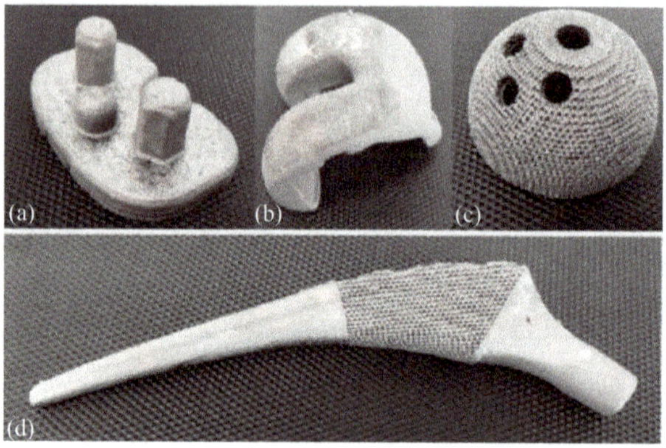

Figure 8.24 *Hip and knee implants manufactured by 3D printer technology; (a) tibial component, (b) femoral component, (c) acetabular cup, and (d) hip stem [13]*

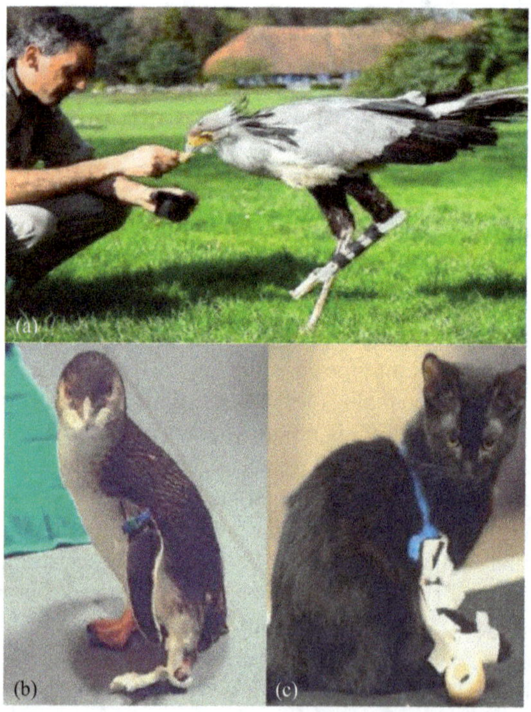

Figure 8.25 *3D printed prostheses for animals: (a) leg prosthesis for Secretary Bird, (b) a prosthesis for a penguin whose foot has been amputated, and (c) prosthesis produced for a kitten who is missing one of the congenital front leg bones [13]*

diseased tissues are being carried out by bioprinting functional tissue structures by means of precise positioning of biological materials and living cells layer by layer.

Changes and developments are happening every day in the current world as per the need and demand of the age of the fourth industrial revolution as well as per the technologies being used to meet our daily life requirements. These developments in medical field are of great benefits for human beings in order to have a better medical care to improve our quality way of living. These miracle technologies are expected to bring revolutionary developments when it becomes widespread. Thus, the future of healthcare relies on mankind's efforts and initiative to work hand-in-hand, to learn, and teach each other with these technologies. If they do not embrace these emerging technologies, they will be left out in coming years. The future might look scary at the moment but mankind cannot evade and escape from any technological revolutions happening in this world. Past revolutions indeed looked scarier for earlier generations but yet they embraced it, they fought together and their hard work as well persistence brought the current generation this mighty development and modernization. As per the saying, "one has to be a master of his/her own home," the sooner the adaptation and realization occurs accordingly to the changes happening around with an open mind, the better will be the quality of human life. Planting a seed today will bring flower one day and a juicy fruit on another day in future.

References

[1] E. Asadollahi-Yazdi, P. Couzon, N. Q. Nguyen, Y. Ouazene, and F. Yalaoui, "Industry 4.0: revolution or evolution?" *American Journal of Operations Research*, vol. 10, no. 06, pp. 241–268, 2020.

[2] M. Xu, J. M. David, and S. H. Kim, "The Fourth Industrial Revolution: opportunities and challenges," *International Journal of Financial Research*, vol. 9, no. 2, p. 90, 2018.

[3] G. Briganti and O. Le Moine, "Artificial intelligence in medicine: today and tomorrow," *Frontiers in Medicine*, vol. 7, p.27, 2020.

[4] J. Y. Khan and M. R. Yuce, *Internet of Things (IOT): Systems and Applications.* Singapore: Jenny Standford Publishing, 2019.

[5] B. Pradhan, S. Bhattacharyya, and K. Pal, "IOT-based applications in healthcare devices," *Journal of Healthcare Engineering*, vol. 2021, pp. 1–18, 2021.

[6] J. Chanchaichujit, A. Tan, F. Meng, and S. Eaimkhong, "Internet of things (IOT) and big data analytics in healthcare," in *Healthcare 4.0*, pp. 17–36, Singapore: Palgrave Pivot, 2019.

[7] M. B. Janjua, A. E. Duranay, and H. Arslan, "Role of wireless communication in healthcare system to cater disaster situations under 6G vision," *Frontiers in Communications and Networks*, vol. 1, Article ID 9195965, 2020.

[8] M. W. Akhtar, S. A. Hassan, R. Ghaffar, H. Jung, S. Garg, and M. S. Hossain, "The shift to 6G communications: vision and requirements,"

Human-Centric Computing and Information Sciences, vol. 10, no. 1, Article number: 53, 2020.
[9] M. Wang, T. Zhu, T. Zhang, J. Zhang, S. Yu, and W. Zhou, "Security and privacy in 6G networks: new areas and new challenges," *Digital Communications and Networks*, vol. 6, no. 3, pp. 281–291, 2020.
[10] R. N. Uppot, B. Laguna, C. J. McCarthy, G. De Novi, A. Phelps, E. Siegel, and J. Courtier, "Implementing virtual and augmented reality tools for Radiology Education and training, communication, and clinical care," *Radiology*, vol. 291, no. 3, pp. 570–580, 2019.
[11] K. Proniewska, D. Dołęga-Dołęgowski, A. Pręgowska, P. Walecki, and D. Dudek, "8 holography as a progressive revolution in medicine," *Simulations in Medicine*, pp. 103–116, 2020.
[12] M. Javaid, A. Haleem, and I. H. Khan, "Holography applications toward medical field: an overview," *Indian Journal of Radiology and Imaging*, vol. 30, no. 3, p. 354, 2020.
[13] Y. Bozkurt and E. Karayel, "3D printing technology; methods, biomedical applications, future opportunities and Trends," *Journal of Materials Research and Technology*, vol. 14, pp. 1430–1450, 2021.

Chapter 9

Ethics, guidelines, and policy for technology in healthcare

Norana Rahman[1], Thirumoorthy Thamotharampillai[2] and Vaikunthan Rajaratnam[3]

This chapter will explore the current body of evidence on the challenges and concerns that various technology has created in healthcare. It will describe the ethical challenges stakeholders face with the commonly embraced technology in healthcare delivery, education, and research. It will examine how the various actors assess and understand the impact of technology on the delivery of care and their outcomes while ensuring the protection of the patients and the community. It will explore how the stakeholders balance technology's universal benefits and risks in healthcare outcomes, value creation, and access. It will describe how frameworks have been developed to guide the ethical and moral use of technology in healthcare and on strategies for regulators to implement. This will ensure the just and ethical use and incorporation of technology in healthcare in advanced and less advanced communities.

9.1 Introduction

Technology has impacted healthcare in many ways. It has helped diagnose and treat diseases, improve patients' quality of life, and reduce healthcare costs. The escalation in its use in healthcare has significantly contributed to the development of our society. However, it has also created some ethical issues that must be addressed.

The first computerized tomography (CT) scan was performed in 1972, and since then, CT scans have become a standard diagnostic tool for many medical conditions. In addition to CT scans, other technologies, such as ultrasound scans, magnetic resonance imaging (MRI), and positron emission tomography (PET), have also become common tools for diagnosis. In addition to these basic

[1]Research Management Centre (RMC), Perdana University, Malaysia
[2]Department of Academic Development, Duke NUS Medical School, Singapore
[3]Senior Consultant Hand Surgeon, KTPH, Singapore

technologies, the current trend of using big data, artificial intelligence, and machine learning (ML) has now impacted healthcare in every aspect of its delivery, collection of data, diagnosis, treatment, and prediction of disease and outcomes. With these advances in medicine, technology implementation in healthcare and biomedical ethics are two of the most challenging topics in the healthcare and technology industry today [1].

Technology's rapid development and use in healthcare are not new, but it has accelerated exponentially. For example, should we allow people with terminal illnesses to use artificial intelligence and deep ML via affective robots as a form of palliative care? These challenges are real and immediate and require a multi-disciplinary approach engaging technology developers, healthcare professionals, bioethicists, and the population, to understand and attempt to resolve them. If left unaddressed, they would significantly impact the safety and security of healthcare and the population at large [2]. As digital technology in healthcare has evolved beyond supporting the treatment of illnesses and injuries into genomics, diagnostics, surveillance and big data and artificial intelligence, key ethical issues have shifted to matters of integrity and equity for individuals, communities and system levels [3].

Despite the various attempts to look at the ethics of technology, there has been a scarcity of research that discussed the impact of these technologies on the health of individuals and their communities. Instead, studies are preoccupied with the intent of using technology in healthcare but avoid studying its impact. This generates more difficult ethical considerations, such as potentially unintended effects, researchers' approaches to ethical issues, and expectations of abiding by regulations and standards. There is a need for a broader approach to ethical issues related to health technology, which should continue from training new researchers to designing and funding new research studies and presenting and publishing new research [4].

It does not do justice to purely look at the ethics of the functions of technology to study its impact on the individuals, community, and healthcare systems and its interactions with the rest of the systems in a community. Hence, going beyond the design ethics and technology studies to the bioethics of digital health. There is a need for a sociotechnical system for digital health technologies that are adopted in healthcare ecosystems. There needs to be a broader perspective with a comprehensive ethical analysis of digital health technologies to study their impact on the people, communities, and the systems by which healthcare is delivered, including all its interactions with other systems. This emphasis on social justice is paramount in the sociotechnical ethical framework for healthcare technology adoption [5].

9.2 Impact of technology on healthcare

The patient journey within healthcare shows the various opportunities (and risks) for technology to impact the whole healthcare process and activities. Figure 9.1

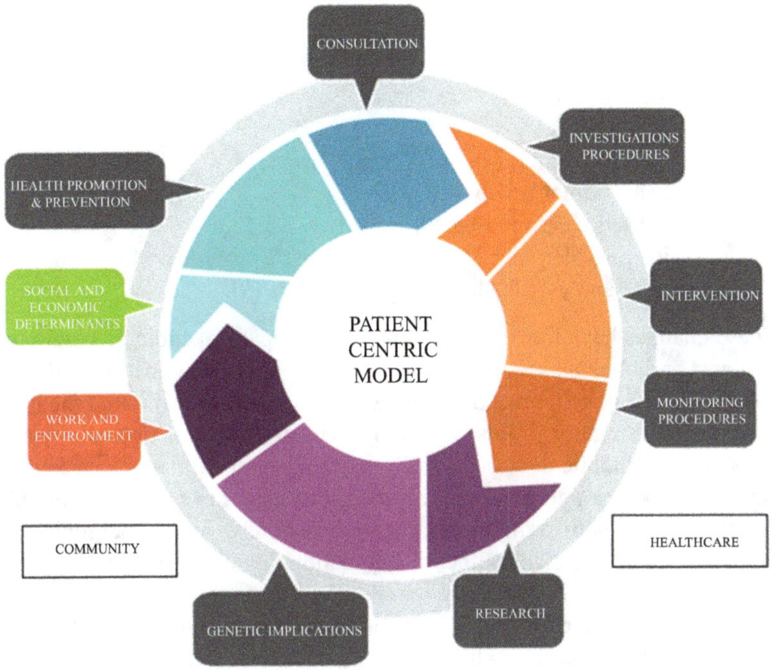

Figure 9.1 The patient journey in modern healthcare. Reproduced, with permission from [7].

shows the patient journey in modern healthcare. It is obvious that there are various environments through which the journey takes the patient, the points of contact with the machine, and the people involved in the care. These are the areas that technology can effectively impact healthcare: from the emergency rooms to the operating rooms and intensive care units, technology enables improving workflow, teamwork, and family engagement. Failure of these technology systems can disrupt human interactions and impede direct patient care. The design of these environments must consider technology integration [6].

Healthcare systems generate large volumes and complex data rapidly, an example of big data. They come from multiple sources like electronic health records, laboratories, government sources, insurers, and medical examinations. They are stored on computer systems and, with sophisticated software, can identify patterns, trends, and associations to guide decision-making, disease surveillance, and planning. The use of the discipline of data science will enable the process of Artificial intelligence (AI) and ML to add value to the healthcare systems. Big data and AI have been extensively used in healthcare in various areas of diagnosis, monitoring, and managing treatment and research [8].

One of the main adoptions of technology in healthcare is focused on its delivery. The ways in which technology will enhance the delivery of healthcare have been described through the adoption of the following information platforms:

1. data collection technology,
2. market intermediaries,
3. services for remote and on-demand healthcare,
4. augmented and virtual reality provider,
5. blockchain-based electronic health record,
6. cloud service provider, and
7. intelligent data analysis for healthcare providers [9].

These changes have transformed how the principal stakeholders communicate with patients and other stakeholders. The advances in communication and wireless technology and the penetrations of broadband globally have facilitated the growing use of remote consultations. This access to broadband wireless technology and the advances in smart mobile devices has allowed the delivery and transmission of data independent of device and platform. Furthermore, they have made it possible for patients to access health professional services remotely, both synchronously and asynchronously, facilitating healthcare interactions and transactions. Apart from wireless connectivity, biometric and secure cloud technologies are paramount for the safe, secure, and credible implementation of these strategies [10]. They are known as virtual healthcare, which includes processes related to telemedicine, mobile apps, and AI-supported patient education systems. They enable remote access and delivery of healthcare and can use the following to enhance healthcare systems:

- general health and fitness-based applications,
- information on medicine-based applications, and
- applications for managing the healthcare process [11].

The introduction of wearable monitoring devices provides another opportunity for connectivity between patients, families, and healthcare providers. All these, while enabling and facilitating the healthcare interactions and processes, introduce and expose areas of concern with the rapid flow of large volumes of data and the potential for breach and manipulation [12].

Some of the challenges that need to be addressed are the following: data interoperability, standardization, privacy, ameliorating systemic biases in algorithms, reimbursement of AI-assisted services, quality improvement, and integration of AI tools into provider workflows [13]. Apart from the biases in AI models, protecting patient privacy is crucial for technology and systems to gain the trust of clinicians and the public. In addition, the ethical integrity and public role of the health professions rely on maintaining broad public trust. The ethics of its use and the operationalization of its use in the community has been raised. As a result, a governance model has been proposed to address these issues [14].

These challenges raise one of the most important ethical issues: data protection. The use of cloud technology in healthcare has made it easier for companies to collect and store information about the users of this data, both directly and indirectly. This knowledge can be used for alternative purposes or transacted without the data generator's knowledge or consent. Hence, this is considered a violation of privacy and can lead to identity theft and compromise, discrimination, and financial impact. The frequency of healthcare data breaches, the extent of records disclosure, and the financial losses resulting from breached records are increasing rapidly. Thus, healthcare data, especially the large volume of patients' demographics and the various transactions, is considered very valuable. This has therefore become a major lure for health record embezzlement and theft [15].

Some AI models used in areas outside of healthcare have shown bias, such as overestimating the risk of repeat criminal offences among members of certain racial groups. Extrapolating these models to healthcare, biased algorithms can also underestimate or overestimate risks in specific patient populations. Despite the complexity of bias and individuals' preferences, developers need to develop AI systems that can help balance human biases and thus lead to fairer outcomes. Therefore, reducing AI biases is necessary to promote better and more equitable health outcomes [14].

9.3 The bioethics framework and healthcare professionals

The principal goal of healthcare is the relief of symptoms of pain and suffering caused by ailments. It includes the process of care and cure of those with sickness. As part of the process, healthcare professionals endeavour to improve the functional status of these individuals. They try to maintain the compromised status of those who cannot be cured as part of their palliative care. Furthermore, beyond the curative function of healthcare is the importance of counselling, care, and support of patients. This extends to the integration of social services to provide the necessary support [16].

Death and dying is also a fundamental process of healthcare. It is crucial that the healthcare process incorporates transparent, realistic, and sensitive end-of-life conversations so that the autonomy and dignity of individuals are preserved in the dying process while ensuring their quality of life as they approach the finality of death [17]. Beyond the curative aspects of medicine, modern healthcare requires consideration of the prevention of disease, the promotion of health, and predictions and mitigation of potential suffering.

This led to the evolution of innovative Predictive, Preventive and Personalised Medicine (PPPM). They are driving efforts in healthcare to curb the prevalence of both communicable and non-communicable diseases such as diabetes, cardiovascular diseases, chronic respiratory diseases, cancer, and dental pathologies. The value-driven healthcare systems and processes and the emerging role of PPPM have been acknowledged as priorities by all stakeholders in healthcare. With this comes greater responsibilities in the hands of the patients, empowerment, and health education. It also requires a multidisciplinary approach and the adoption of innovative technology to develop and deliver healthcare [18].

The secondary important and legitimate goals of medicine that support the primary objectives include medical research, medical education, clinical governance, and professional governance. These are complex issues facing modern healthcare systems with the interactions of diverse stakeholders with their often competing agenda. In developing and adopting new and improving current technology in healthcare, all stakeholders must serve the primary and secondary goals of medicine. In developing technology for healthcare, all stakeholders and technology developers must be cognizant of the undesirable and inappropriate use of medical knowledge and skills as in commercial exploitation of the sick and vulnerable, police or prisoner interrogation, torture, assistance and participation in capital punishment and experimentation or research without consent. They would be considered as serious infractions of the beneficent goals of medicine [19].

In executing their responsibilities, healthcare professionals constantly evaluate the decisions and actions under the professional and ethical framework governing healthcare. Utmost in their consideration is the primacy of the patient's welfare and the avoidance of conflict of interest. This principle is based on dedicating all thoughts and actions in medicine to serving the patient's medical interest. Commercialization, market forces, political and societal pressures, and organizational administrative exigencies must not compromise this principle. Physicians involved in the commercialization of healthcare technology get into financial conflicts of interest regarding data exploitation in ways that violate privacy, support marketing interests, create vulnerabilities, increase surveillance, and compromise both informed consent and patient–clinician relationship. The provision of commercially profitable and medically unnecessary products and services not only exposes one's patients to avoidable harm and expenses but also diminishes the resources available to others. Healthcare professionals have a positive obligation to recognize and disclose to all stakeholders, including the public, and appropriately manage conflicts of interest that arise in their professional duties and activities [20].

At all times, healthcare professionals have a commitment to scientific methods and knowledge. Much of the practice of clinical medicine is based on the integrity and appropriate use of scientific knowledge and technology. Introducing new technology needs to pass not only the test of medical beneficence but also sound and evidenced-based science. Healthcare professionals are obligated to uphold scientific standards, promote research of high scientific value, create new knowledge, and ensure its appropriate use. The professionals and all stakeholders in healthcare are responsible for the integrity of this knowledge, which is based on sound scientific evidence, especially in locations with little broadband and few available devices, poor health services, illiterate populations, or other obstacles to remote or in-person healthcare [3].

The requirements of an elevated level of professional standards in healthcare are the result of the trust bestowed upon them and their influence in the lives of those they care for and their communities. To ensure standardized guidelines and clarity for all stakeholders, the professional organizations and regulators of healthcare professions have provided guidelines and codes of conduct for their practice [1].

These arise from the fact that illness, injury, and interventions impact an individual in more ways than just the physical. The introduction of the biopsychosocial model of medicine by George Engel in 1977 critiqued the preoccupation of medicine with the biological and physical impact of illness and the failure to understand the psychosocial variables and factors that impacted the susceptibility, severity, and course of illness in an individual [21]. It has been further shown that it is not only the psychological and social impact of illness on individuals and their community but also the economics (Figure 9.2) [22] and political [23].

Bioethics is the foundation of civil society and ensures that ethical, social, and legal issues are addressed in the relationship among individuals, their communities, and the environment. It ensures that the good and the right are incorporated into the interactions between individuals and the environment. It has three areas, as shown in Figure 9.3 [24].

Therefore, it shows the importance of a framework to understand and address the impact of technology on individuals in healthcare and the need for comprehensiveness to cover all the areas impacted. We would suggest that the bioethics framework include the social, economic, political, technological, and environmental domains.

The traditional pillars of bioethics (Figure 9.4) are based on the four areas of

- Beneficence
- Nonmaleficence

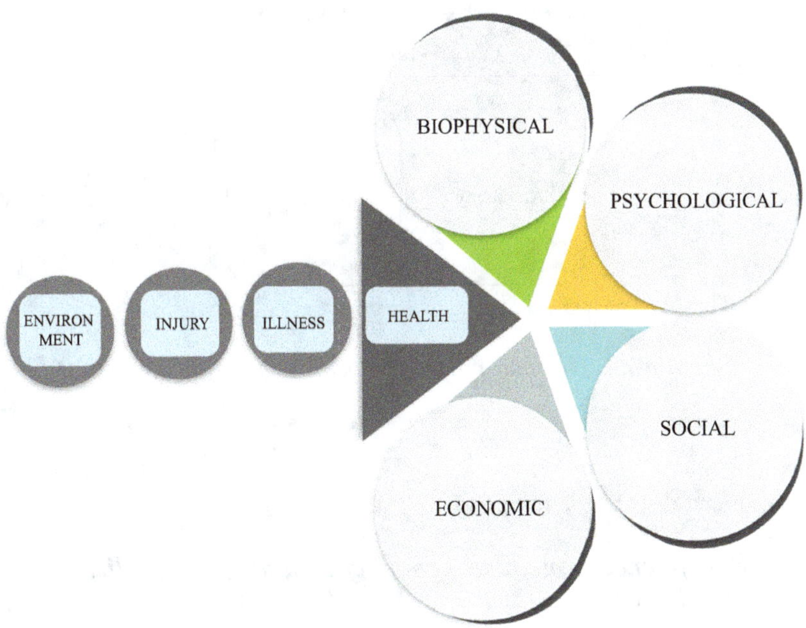

Figure 9.2 Biopsychosocial and economic impact of illness. Adapted from [22].

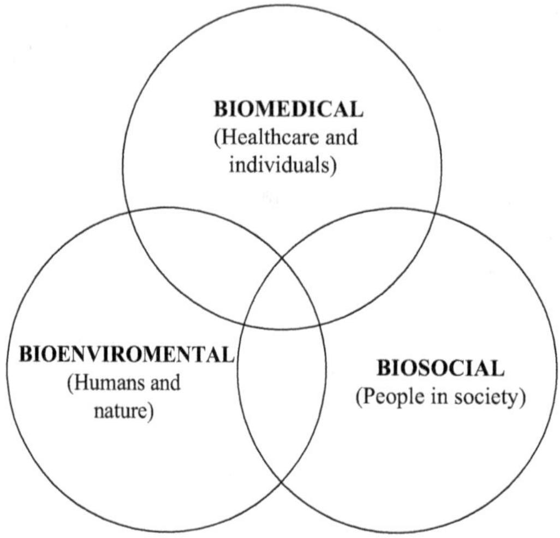

Figure 9.3 The various domains of bioethics in society. Adapted from [24].

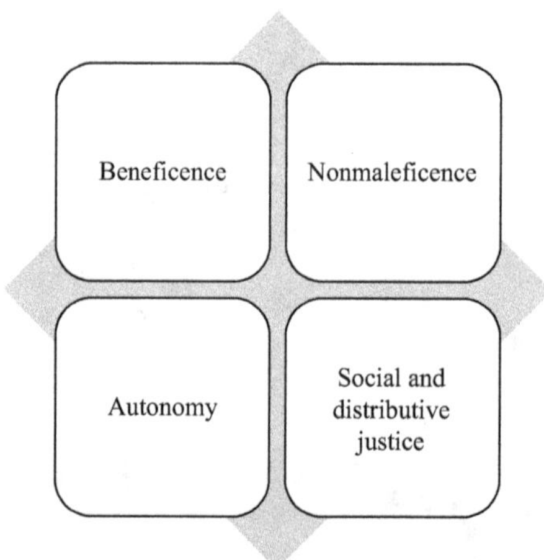

Figure 9.4 The four pillars of bioethics in healthcare [5]

- Autonomy
- Social and distributive justice [5]

9.3.1 Beneficence – medical beneficence and good quality healthcare

The community entrusts healthcare professionals to use various modalities and interventions to help individuals overcome illness and disease and relieve their pain and suffering. Such influence of the health professional on the lives of individuals is founded on the principle that they would always do good. The numerous technological advances and interventions available bring about the opportunity to improve the lives of individuals with professional and ethical practises of the healthcare profession. It is imperative that as they perform their duties of caring, they must always adhere to the call to avoid harm. They must ensure that whatever interventions they apply, they would consider the benefits to the individual and promote the welfare of those they care for in the community. Health professionals must also ensure that they practise a high level of altruism and morality in their practice. The language used in this area of beneficence is to ensure that there is a proactive effort by the professionals to do good and not just merely to avoid harm. So, in summary, the adoption of healthcare technology must include the following:

(a) For technology in healthcare to be ethical, it must contribute to good quality healthcare.
(b) Superior quality healthcare is achieved by a commitment to continuous learning and improvement in areas of patient safety, the effectiveness of care, patient-centred care, timeliness of care, efficiency of care, and equitable nature of care.
(c) Technology in healthcare must bring medical beneficence to the patient's needs to align with the goals of good quality healthcare (medicine). Before a new technology is introduced into the clinical care realm, it must be supported by good evidence to verify that it results in beneficial, effective, and safe outcomes.
(d) In developing and promoting technology in healthcare, healthcare professionals have a duty to work collaboratively with other professionals and related disciplines to reduce medical error, increase patient safety, minimize the overuse of healthcare resources, and optimize the outcomes of care [4].

9.3.2 Nonmaleficence

On the flip side, nonmaleficence is the duty of the physician to avoid any form of harm to those whom they treat and to the community. In terms of harm, this goes beyond the effect of ensuring the avoidance of unnecessary pain and suffering but includes discrimination, offence, and deprivation of opportunity and care. There must be careful consideration by healthcare professionals to ensure that they have carefully weighed the benefits and risks of any intervention so as not to harm the individuals, not only physically but also mentally, socially, and economic aspects.

To adhere to the principle of veracity and fidelity, the following process has to be considered:

(a) Healthcare professionals must ensure that patients are completely and honestly informed (of sufficient, clear and contextualized information) before the patient has consented to treatment and after treatment has occurred.
(b) In the complexity of healthcare delivery, professionals acknowledge that in healthcare, medical errors that injure patients do sometimes occur. Whenever

patients are injured as a consequence of medical care, patients should be promptly informed because failure to do so seriously compromises patient and societal trust. This act is the principle of Duty of Candour as mandated by the General Medical Council of the UK. "Every health and care professional must be open and honest with patients and people in their care when something that goes wrong with their treatment or care, causes, or has the potential to cause, harm or distress."

(c) Reporting and analysing medical mistakes provide the basis for appropriate prevention, appropriate compensation to injured parties, and remediation where needed.

(d) With the widespread use of technology in healthcare and when errors or injuries occur due to technology, hard or software, timely investigations and truthful information sharing are essential in minimizing the ethical and legal fallout [25].

9.3.3 Autonomy

In today's practice, it is expected that all healthcare professionals adhere to the principle that every individual has the right to make decisions about their own body, health, and lifestyle. This respect for the individual's decision-making based on sound judgement is fundamental to the modern-day practice of medicine. This was well captioned by Justice Cardoza in 1914, when he said, "Every human being of adult years and sound mind has a right to determine what shall be done with his own body, and a surgeon who performs an operation without his patient's consent commits an assault for which he is liable in damages." This is true except in cases of emergency where the patient is unconscious, and it is necessary to operate before consent can be obtained. (Cardozo B. Basic right to consent to medical care – Schlendorff vs the Society of the New York Hospital, 211 NY 125 105 NE 92 1914 LEXUS 1028, [1914]). This autonomy needs to be balanced with the circumstances and contacts, as in the case of someone who has no mental capacity to make that decision, or in the event of harm to others, from the actions of an individual.

These aspects of ethics based on autonomy can be challenging in certain societies with a paternalistic approach towards healthcare. This can be quite dynamic in nature, dependent on the community and context, that is grounded on various cultural, religious, and racial norms. Fundamental to this autonomy is the requirement by the healthcare professionals to fully disclose all necessary information so the individual and the family members can make a sound and informed decision based on the available evidence at that time. This is the basis of informed consent with full disclosure of the facts pertaining to an individual, which is required in modern-day practice to ensure that the patient has all the information necessary to make an informed decision as to the treatment or intervention they agreed to. There has been some resistance to this in situations where they are unacceptable in the cultural context. It requires a much more inclusive approach towards informed consent and autonomy [26].

With this comes the confidentiality of personal information, and it becomes more challenging with the introduction of electronic medical records in the movement of data rapidly among multiple users. The maintenance of such confidentiality needs to be incorporated into the structures and systems of electronic medical records and the various technological communication platforms used in healthcare today. However, there have been records of situations where exceptions to patient confidentiality can be challenged based on the overall importance and safety of the community [27].

Thus, the principle of respect for patient autonomy and informed consent requires the following guiding principles:

(e) Patients' decisions about their health and medical care must be respected and upheld as long as those decisions are in keeping with ethical practice and do not lead to demands for inappropriate care.
(f) When patients need treatment, the physician has the duty to obtain informed consent from the competent adult patient. The same applies when patients participate in medical research and the development of healthcare technology.
(g) Informed consent is an ethical and legal requirement when a patient's personal and medical information is being used in technology development.
(h) Where the patients do not have the mental capacity to participate in shared medical decision-making, the decisions would be made by the legal representatives or by the best interest principle [28].

In the area of patient privacy and confidentiality, the following guidelines need to be considered:

(i) Preserving the patients' privacy and confidentiality is key to sustaining the trust and confidence of the patients, their families, the healthcare professionals, and the system.
(j) The use of genetic information, big data, AI, and ML pose greater challenges in the ethical use of patients' information and data to guide decision-making in the clinical and non-clinical context. This is further compounded by the sharing of data for collaborative purposes to drive AI and the vulnerability posed when the systems are breached.
(k) The inappropriate release of patient information has serious implications for healthcare professionals and organizations.
(l) The widespread adoption of digital technology in healthcare threatens privacy, confidentiality, and cybersecurity and should be considered by technology developers as they design systems and infrastructure to address these concerns [29].

9.3.4 Justice

Social justice and distributive justice in bioethics pertain to the fair and equitable distribution of health resources, including consultation, diagnosis and intervention to individuals and the community. The general principles to ensure equitable distribution of healthcare resources include (i) an equal share, (ii) according to need, (iii) according to the effort, (iv) according to the contribution, (v) according to merit, and (vi) according to free-market exchanges [26].

Adhering to these principles can be quite challenging to clinicians and bioethicists and therefore requires sufficient guidelines and structure to help practitioners navigate this complex area to ensure social justice in the execution of healthcare in society. That can be conflicts of interest between all stakeholders in healthcare, and this must be constantly made aware to all. Structures and systems must be incorporated within the delivery of care to ensure unbiased third-party opinions can be obtained on ethical issues. In today's modern-day practice, most healthcare institutions and systems ensure this framework exists in the form of a local ethical committee or board to ensure adherence to the bioethical framework [30].

In terms of social justice and access to Healthcare Technology, healthcare professionals are committed by their professional ethics to promoting justice in the healthcare system, including the fair distribution of healthcare resources. The principle of justice in medical ethics requires healthcare professionals to actively work to eliminate discrimination in healthcare, whether based on race, gender, socioeconomic status, ethnicity, religion, or any other social category. Health equity and access include the burdens of seeking care or using technologies placed on patients, most notably the elderly, disadvantaged, and minorities. People and patients have various skills in using digital technology and face usability, acceptability, and access challenges [5].

9.4 Healthcare technology and ethics

9.4.1 Big data, cloud computing, AI, and ML

The large amount of data produced in healthcare due to the various transactions and interactions in the healthcare systems provides an ideal opportunity for collecting, storing and analysing this data mix. These large and complex data sets originating from the various healthcare point of contact sources (e.g., electronic health records, laboratories, government sources, etc.) stored on computer systems are considered big data. These repositories of data are considered big data by the fact that they are growing in three different dimensions, namely, volume, velocity, and variety. Traditional software is unable to handle and analyse these data. Special analytical software is needed to support a wide range of medical and healthcare functions by harnessing data insights to identify patterns, trends, and associations to guide decision making, disease surveillance, and planning [31]. The specialism of data science provides the knowledge base to understand the disease more comprehensively by integrating our biophysical and clinical knowledge with the socioeconomic impact of disease and the health systems. This is a fundamental component for AI and ML to add value to the healthcare system [8]. To ensure efficient and effective use of these data, there is a requirement for a platform for ease and speed of access. The cloud computing provides this platform. This is described by the National Institutes of Standards and Technology (NIST) as a model for enabling ubiquitous, convenient, on-demand access to a shared pool of configurable computing resources. The essential characteristics of cloud computing include (1) on-demand self-service, (2) broad network access, (3) resource pooling with other tenants, (4) rapid elasticity, and (5) measured services. With the volume and large use of the data by healthcare stakeholders, data safety and security remain challenging [32].

AI is the process of developing an algorithm using a computer system to attempt to reproduce a task that would have otherwise required human intelligence. It can support, facilitate, and enhance healthcare professionals' work and accelerate opportunities to realize the benefits of healthcare. ML is an application of AI that uses technology to learn automatically without a specific programme written by humans to execute it. The combination of AI and big data allows for identifying patterns and predicting future behaviours based on prior behaviour. With the continuous increase in data volume with great speed, ML enables this analysis, responses, and rapid decision-making tasks by the nature of the current hardware with their processing power. These processes of AI are increasingly being used in healthcare, not limited to the areas of diagnosis, monitoring, and managing treatment and research, as shown in Figures 9.5 and 9.6 [8]. AI and ML have also played a significant role in research, drug development, and general administrative applications [33].

The popularity and trends of the impacts of technology in healthcare have not been without challenges. Adoption has not been smooth due to the resistance from the primary stakeholders of healthcare – patients and professionals. For this technology to work, it requires authentic behavioural characteristics of its users who in healthcare have significant biases and aversion for machine-driven decision making, preferring the established models of the professional–patient interaction. This lack of trust in the machines deciding clinically significant issues has resulted in the regulators in healthcare mandating the documentation for the evidentiary and

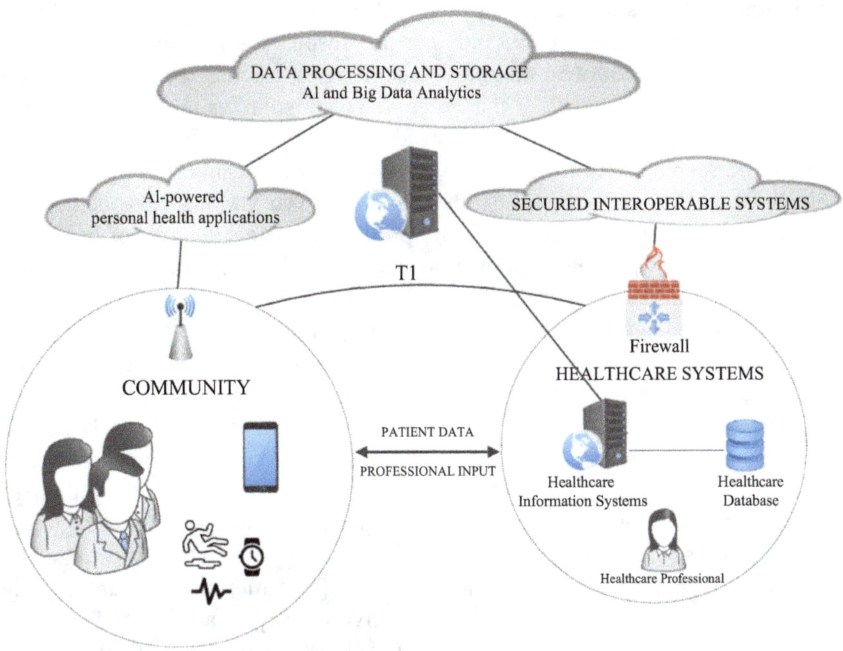

Figure 9.5 Mobile health and AI conceptual guide. Adapted from [8].

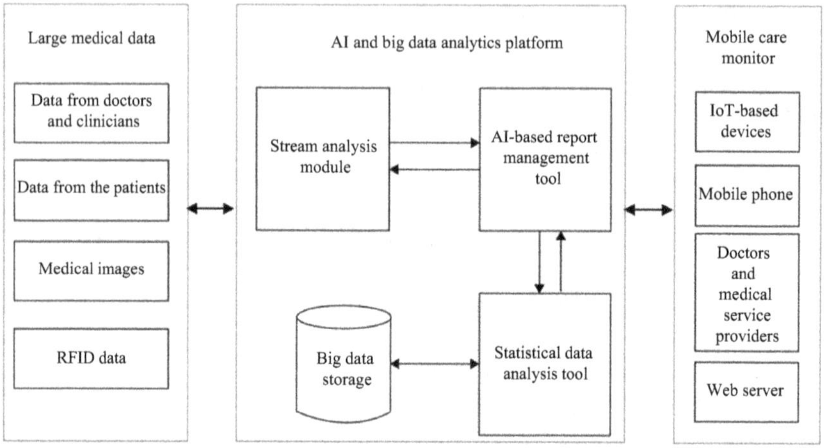

Figure 9.6 Proposed model for AI and big data for mobile health systems [8]

transparent decision-making process with the AI systems. Some have argued that pushing for consensus among primary stakeholders in healthcare to adopt these technologies may not be beneficial for healthcare in general [34].

In their comprehensive report, the United States Government Accountability Office and the National Academy of Medicine summarized that the use of AI has shown promise in healthcare. AI showed that it could improve patient treatment, reduce the burden on providers, and increase resource efficiency at healthcare facilities. They also cautioned that these technologies "... are at varying stages of maturity and adoption, but with the exception of population health management tools, many we described have not achieved widespread use ...." [13].

It can be seen that healthcare professionals face significant challenges in terms of bioethics as they deliver care to their patients. The various advancements in technology that have impacted healthcare produce more challenges for healthcare professionals as they grapple with the impact of the technology and the implication in terms of the bioethics of patient care.

Patients have generally been viewed as being passive recipients of the technology; however, the demand is for healthcare professionals to be more responsible and consider patients' autonomy and ensure that these technology adoptions do not provide harm. Generally, it is accepted that technological advancement in healthcare helps to improve the quality of life of their individuals, giving them an extra hassle-free experience and access to healthcare while simultaneously alleviating the pain and suffering and improving the life span of the individual. On this background, healthcare professionals must ensure that the technology they employ continues to provide beneficence to the patients at all times. They must also ensure that the patient's rights are protected, and confidentiality is always maintained. They must also ensure that adequate information is provided to the patients for their decision-making process. While technology can help in this process, the professionals must also recognize that the technology can fail, and there can be breaches in this technology that will then go against the ethical practice of medicine [35].

When these failures occur within the technological components of the healthcare, errors and untoward events can occur, including and may border onto the areas of negligence with the potential outcomes of litigation. Incorporation of these technologies, therefore, must be carefully weighed by healthcare professionals to ensure that the basic foundations of ethical principles are adhered to in their use in the healthcare systems [36].

The incorporation of a fixed system of values within algorithm design can produce difficulty in ensuring autonomy and shared decision-making which is the accepted practice in most advanced systems of patient care. Rosalind McDougall recommended, "need greater dialogue between bioethicists and A.I. designers and experts to ensure that these technologies are designed in an ethical way in order to ultimately serve patients best." [37, p. 159]. She further argues that while AI is generally designed for and can improve clinical outcomes, patients can be deprived of their value judgments and treatment options if values are fixed within the AI design [37]. Furthermore, the design of AI for healthcare challenges the concept, practice and delivery of empathy, compassion, and trust. These, thus, must be incorporated within the AI design framework for healthcare. Healthcare has been founded on the traditional doctor–patient relationship, and AI can be a source of erosion of this important component of healthcare [38]. Thus, the overarching guiding principle in the design of AI for healthcare should be the appropriate use of data, information sharing, and explanation with shared decision-making. This will then prevent the return to the paternalistic healthcare model, where patients are forced to depend irrationally and without critical judgement on the AI system, the healthcare professional, or both.

9.4.2 Evidence-based medicine, technology, and ethics

Modern healthcare has moved away from anecdotal experiences guiding practice to that based on a high level of evidence guiding today's clinicians' practice. It is an important component of health professional education. It has been defined as decisions about healthcare based on the best available, current, valid, and relevant evidence. These decisions should be made by those receiving care, informed by the tacit and explicit knowledge of those providing care, within the context of available "resources" [39]. Generally, it incorporates the expert clinician's opinion (based on their knowledge and experience) and the evidence from quality data (from the literature and also that unique to the patient and his circumstances). Most importantly, the patients'/caregivers' preferences and context ensure informed and shared decision-making between the clinician and the patient and their caregivers. See Figure 9.7.

Implementing evidence-based medicine requires first the development of a clinical question for which information is required from the body of the knowledge that is already been published in the literature. The evidence is then searched and extracted from the various electronic databases containing the available body of knowledge. Founded on the framework of the clinical questions, once the data has

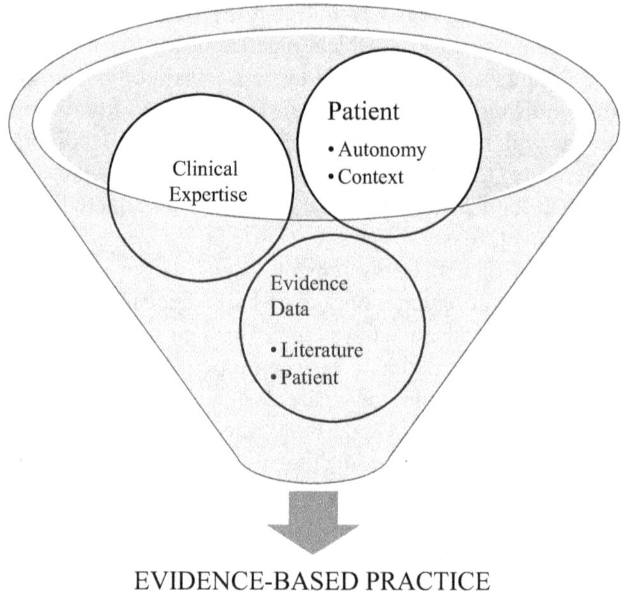

Figure 9.7 Components of evidence-based practice [39]

been located, it is critically appraised for the validity and quality of the evidence that has been published and its applicability in the contacts of the environment in which the evidence is going to be utilized [39].

Once the evidence has been appraised for its quality and validity, it is incorporated into clinical decision-making. This would significantly impact individuals' lives, as the whole purpose of this evidence-based medicine is to improve the quality of care and life of individuals based on sound and reproducible evidence. Following the implementation of an evidence-based change in clinical medicine, it requires an appropriate audit process to ensure that the desired objectives of the changes have been met. And the outcomes are as predicted and expected from the evidence that has been collected from the body of knowledge (Figure 9.8).

When these three components of EBM fall into place, clinicians, patients, their families, and caregivers can make informed, evidence-based decisions. This will ensure meaningful and value-based delivery of services incorporating individuals' interests, values, needs, and choices.

This has been especially important with the current exponential growth of information and data with often contradicting recommendations. In order to overcome these challenges, the Cochrane database was set up as a repository of evidence-based medicine for clinicians to access to search for guidelines to implement in their practice in the 1990s in the United Kingdom [41]. However, it was not without its own challenges. In 2004, a review of drug trials (paediatric antidepressant trials) showed that all trials were negative, the studies were non-existent/biased industry written, and all the data were inaccessible. The positive

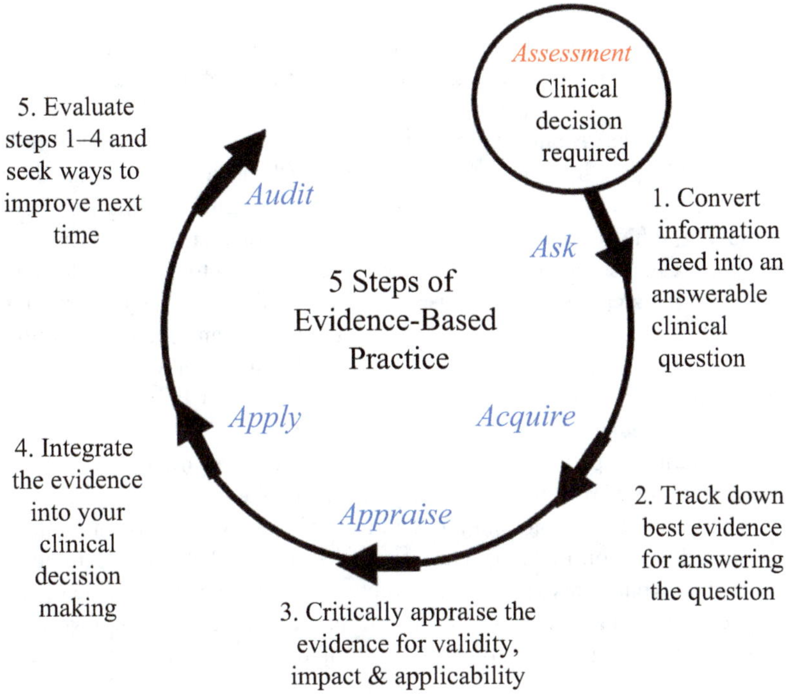

Figure 9.8 Process of evidence-based medicine. Adapted from [40].

published data and the dangers of the drugs were systematically distorted even in reputable medical publications. This occurs even in the leading medical journals. In the same year, the state of New York in the United States filed a fraud action against GlaxoSmithKline (GSK) for false publication when the company's own internal review showed that it did not work and the company selectively published only the favourable results [42].

Such unethical use of data to guide corrupt practices can be overcome using technology to track and validate data collection and analysis. The use of authentic data that is tamper-proof and available for audit to promote transparency and show integrity of collection will ensure the quality of data used for evidence-based research and thereby ensure fraudulent-free analysis and conclusion. The areas that require management are data soundness, data auditability, privacy-preserving, data honesty and data backup. The blockchain approach for data collection and storage has been recommended as a strategy [12].

9.4.3 Blockchain and ethics

Blockchain technology is a distributed database technology using a ledger technology that requires no central authority. In healthcare, it is used for keeping "patients" medical records safe and secure. Entries and transactions are time-stamped "blocks" of data in a chronological sequence and cannot be corrupted retroactively. Each input notifies the nodes that anonymously comprise the distributed, peer-to-peer network, and their replicated copies of the ledger are updated accordingly. It records and stores an audit trail of all transactions. The decentralized nature of the technology makes the ledger highly resistant to fraud and compromise. Also, the integrity of the data is assured based on the immutability of the blockchain. With this comes the replicability of research, adding transparency and removing ethical considerations of research conduct independent of the researchers. It can also be used for the peer review process to disseminate research findings [43]. It also allows for a transparent audit trail of data acquisition and use and thus traceability, preventing retrospective tampering, and securely automating the research process through the Smart Contracts. It allows for a high level of data control, security, and collaboration with all stakeholders, including patients, other researchers and regulators [44].

The modern-day patient journey in the healthcare systems requires the rapid and secure sharing of patient data among the stakeholders. This is crucial for the ethical practice of patient autonomy for the avoidance of maleficence and promoting shared decision-making. The integration of blockchain technology into healthcare data would provide the infrastructure for frictionless, confident, secure, and tamper-proof data sharing for ethical clinical practice. This would also contribute to social justice in that the cost of delivery would be significantly reduced [45].

The implication of this secure, up-to-date, and easily accessible comprehensive repository of individual patient data is the contribution to the personalized patient data for consideration of the evidence-based practice model, as shown in Figure 9.7. In terms of social justice, it will control and prevent fraudulent claims for healthcare interventions and transactions, thereby ensuring the ethical use of public/insurance funding and resources. It will also provide patients open access to their own data for inspection, auditing, and understanding the use of their data in research. They can also contribute to the database with data from their wearables, which could then be stored securely in their records in real-time. This will create a better experience for patients and healthcare providers [46].

The ethical foundation for effective and meaningful decision-making between clinicians and the patients and their families requires an honest, comprehensive evaluation of the patient's needs based on the context as opposed to the benefits and risks of the intervention that will be promoted or prescribed. This is dependent upon trust between the clinician and the patient, the data being used, and the evidence for the decision process. For it to be meaningful, the evaluation of the data has to be comprehensive in terms of considering not only the evidence in the body of the knowledge but contextualized to the patient's environment and circumstances. And these then have to be effectively and meaningfully communicated based on the principle of participation with the engagement of the final decision makers (Figure 9.9).

This is a mandatory requirement of the clinician who has been delegated the responsibility for the health and welfare of the patients, their families, and the community in general.

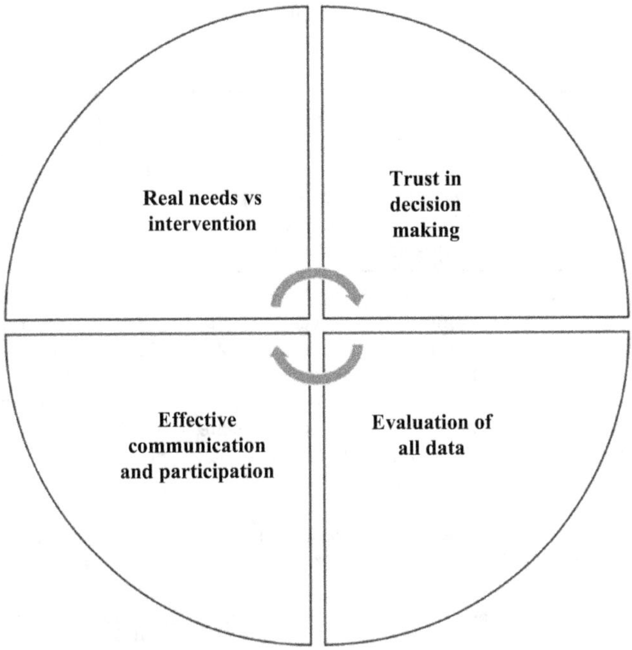

Figure 9.9 Process for shared ethical decision-making in healthcare [47]

Thus, with the implementation of AI systems into healthcare, the infrastructure of the AI systems has to take into consideration these processes to ensure the ethical relationship that will underpin the shared decision-making [47].

Based on this framework, the authors have proposed the following collaborative models for managing the ethical challenges of AI in healthcare (Tables 9.1 and 9.2).

Gundersen and Bærøe [47] suggest that the mere application of the bioethics model to the AI implementation in healthcare may not be ideal as it only looks at the challenges through the monodisciplinary lens of healthcare professionals. This is a comfortable and current approach to the ethical challenges of AI adoption in healthcare but does not address fundamental challenges in the design and development of the algorithm while integrating accountability and transparency while minimizing bias within the AI design.

They refer to the principle that for the implementation of AI and related technology in healthcare, there is a need for the designers and developers of algorithms and coding frameworks to *strictly adhere to the precisely defined guidelines of medical ethics* – privacy and autonomy, maleficence, beneficence, and social justice. This strategy would ensure that the adoption of AI in healthcare would be ethically acceptable to healthcare stakeholders.

Another area of contention with AI in healthcare is algorithmic bias. This is when the algorithm design discriminates against certain groups like gender, ethnicity, and sexual preference. It is thus the responsibility of the AI designers, together with the bioethicist and healthcare professionals, to work together and develop

Table 9.1 Collaborative models components for managing the ethical challenges of AI in healthcare. Adapted from [47].

Short description of the components of shared decision-making	Expanded descriptions of the components of what is required of doctors in shared decision-making. These can be perceived as minimum standards	How AI can undermine the conditions for shared decision-making
(a) Understanding the patient's condition	Doctors must understand the connection between patients' conditions and the need for potential interventions on a general, technical, and normative level and translate them into individual patients' particular contexts	If the clinical outcome of AI is beyond what doctors are able to understand themselves, their clinical competence is undermined, and by that, a crucial presupposition for why the patients have reason to trust them in the first place [38]
(b) Trust in evidence	Doctors must base their decision on sources of evidence they trust to ensure the information is relevant and adequate	If doctors suggest treatments on the basis of AI sources to information they cannot fully account for, they force patients to place blind trust in their recommendations. This is just another version of paternalism
(c) Due assessment of benefits and risks	Doctors must understand all relevant information of benefits and risks and trade-offs between them	If doctors cannot fully understand how and why AI has reached an outcome, say, the classification of an X-ray, uncertainty regarding assessments of risks, benefits and trade-offs will follow. This, in turn, undermines "patients" reasons to have confidence in their judgments as their role as the expert in the relation
(d) Accommodating patient's understanding, communication, and deliberation	Doctors must convey an assessment of risks and benefits to patients in a clear and accessible manner, ensure they have understood the information, and invite them to share their thoughts and deliberate together on the matter	If AI systems make it hard for doctors to understand how and why they reach their outcomes, they cannot facilitate patients' understanding. Instead, they will have to paternalistically require that the patient accept that the AI "knows best"

Table 9.2 Collaborative models for managing the ethical challenges of AI in healthcare. Adapted from [47].

	Transformative and disruptive technology	**Ethical attention**	**Division of labour**	**Benefits**	**Challenges**
Ordinary evidence model	No	Mainly in use, not design	Distinct	Fits well with widely held notions of the professional responsibility	Lacks proper response to challenges pertaining to algorithmic risk, transparency, and accountability
Ethical design model	Yes	Mainly in design, not in use	Distinct	Takes the distinct ethical challenges of medical AI seriously	Technocratic view on ethical choices and the problem of formalizing ethics
Collaborative model	Yes	Both in design and use	Integrated	Alleviates some of the accountability problems and promotes shared decision-making	No proper response to severe ethical risks
Public deliberation model	Yes	Both in design and use and in the public sphere	Partly distinct, partly integrated	Can deal with "meta-ethical risks"	The models need more organizational specification

robust frameworks to guide AI designers and developers in internalizing this fairness in their design [48].

In their collaborative approach, Gundersen and Bærøe recommended a more transdisciplinary and participative approach among healthcare professionals, bioethicists, and AI designers. This allows the AI experts to learn and understand healthcare expertise, incorporate the bioethical framework, and share a joint commitment to ethical product development. For this to succeed, there is a need for a common understanding of the language used by the various stakeholder disciplines of the AI to be used in healthcare. The non-technology members (healthcare professionals and bioethicists) must be actively involved in the design of the AI to be used in healthcare. AI designers must be proactive in engaging healthcare professionals and bioethicists while designing the healthcare AI. This is the process where mutual learning can occur and ensure that the challenges of the end-users are considered in the design phase. Finally, it is also important for this transdisciplinary collaboration to be successful; the outcomes of the collaboration, i.e. the healthcare AI product, are evaluated for its impact on clinical practice. They stated, "The medical literacy of A. I. developers and the A.I. literacy of medical doctors can enable doctors to promote shared decision-making's emphasis on sources of evidence, deemed to be trusted, due harm assessment, and proper communication." [47, p. 12].

As the implication of healthcare is beyond the healthcare professional and the individual and their community, extended stakeholders like healthcare financiers and regulatory bodies have a voice in the ethical implementation, use, and evaluation of technology in healthcare as some of these technologies can be disruptive and transformative and thus cannot be left in the hands of healthcare professionals and AI designers and would require the contributions of policymakers and the public at large.

With the aforementioned ethical challenges of technology use in healthcare, Reddy and co-workers proposed the following model based on the principles of fairness, transparency, trustworthiness, and accountability (Figure 9.10). They emphasized the dynamic nature of the challenges. Thus, the governance framework would need to be ongoing with continuous monitoring and evaluating of the adopted AI. They recommend the integration of these functions into the clinical governance committee incorporating clinicians, managers, patient group representatives, and technical and ethics experts. Their responsibilities would include the monitoring and evaluation of the AI application adopted. They, too, emphasized the importance of creating awareness and educating all stakeholders on the ethical implications of AI in healthcare and recommended the partnership with academic institutions and healthcare providers [14]. This would be in sync with the collaborative model proposed by Gundersen and Bærøe [47].

There must also be full disclosure by healthcare professionals and institutions of the use of these AI applications in the delivery of care to patients and their families. Similarly, the data generators (patients and their families) must be made

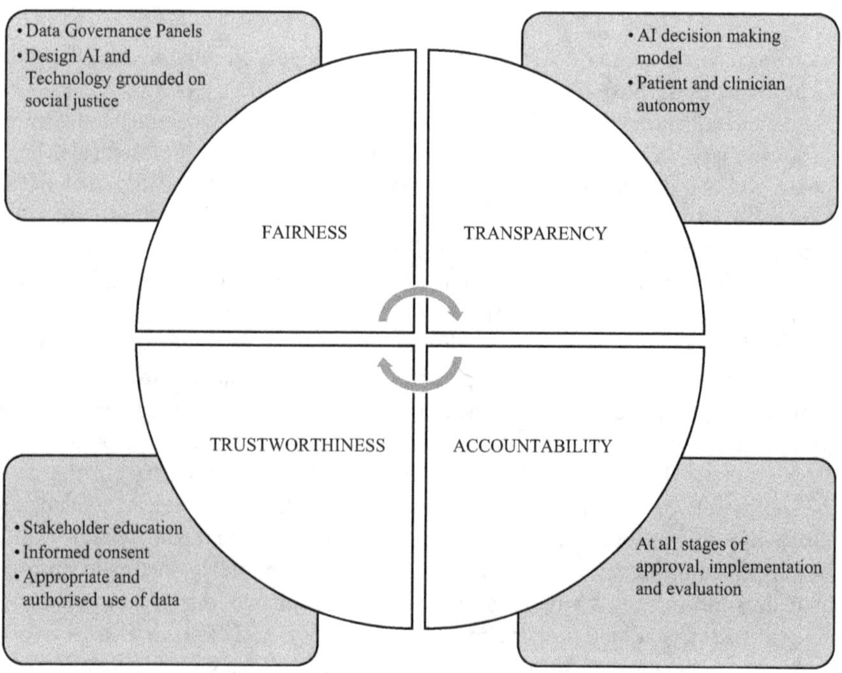

Figure 9.10 Governance model for AI in healthcare. Adapted from [14, p. 493].

aware that their anonymized aggregated data would be integrated within the AI application for ML purposes. The accountability for using the AI in healthcare requires all stakeholders to be engaged in the process of monitoring and evaluating the AI application in healthcare. As with any medical device and intervention, the AI application's safety and effectiveness must be aligned with the ethical framework in healthcare. The authors have recommended the TRIPOD (Transparent Reporting of a Multivariable Prediction Model for Individual Prognosis or Diagnosis) model as guidance for constituting the reporting framework for the AI applications in healthcare. This is a "checklist of 22 items considered important for transparent reporting of predictive models including model specification, performance and validation." [14, p. 5].

9.4.4 Sociotechnical ethics of digital health

In their paper, De Cremer and Kasparov [49] argued that the effectiveness of technology in healthcare depends on the *availability of technology* and thus would be a source of inequality and social maleficence. While technology can be an enabler in healthcare, on the flip side, it can also be a great divider and discriminator, especially to vulnerable members of society. They recommend the use of the following:

- Combine self- and government regulation
  Technology innovators and industry need to collaborate with regulatory and government bodies to create an ethical framework in alignment with the societal and regulatory frameworks.
- Responsible leadership
  These alignments of the industry to ethical principles require strong and moral leadership. Emphasis must not only be on outcomes but also on the processes that lead to the outcomes that must be ensured to be executed in an ethical manner. They also recommend that ethical considerations for developing technology products in healthcare are incentivized when they are incorporated within the structure and systems of the organization, including the leadership and boards. Continuous ethical awareness and education must be promoted within the corporate culture of the organizations.
- Social justice and early access to AI
  The authors note the rapid transformation of AI technology in healthcare but warn of the inequalities, especially the exclusion of certain groups. The industry needs to facilitate inclusivity and timeliness in the roll-out of technology in healthcare ensuring no one is left behind [49].

Shaw and Donia, in their report, proposed a framework based on the available body of knowledge of research studies in the domain of Science and Technology. This interdisciplinary approach aligns well with those recommended by Reddy *et al.* [14] and by Gundersen and Bærøe [47]. The fundamental basis for this framework is that digital health does not just involve the hardware and software but the interactions, engagement, impact, and mutual dependencies between technologies and the social arrangements within healthcare.

On the flip side, these "social arrangements" in healthcare are influenced and impacted by the various digital technologies, not limited to the delivery, monitoring, and evaluation of healthcare.

The sociotechnical framework encompasses the challenges and concerns defined by the technology and the impact and effect of these technology in the social domain of healthcare as the actors interact and use these technologies. This approach, the authors argue, has "the effect of introducing a new series of potential ethical harms that require consideration in ethical analyses of technologies, and in so doing has a higher order impact on our ethical analysis." [5, p. 4]. The main domains considered in this framework are summarized in Table 9.3.

The healthcare digital applications' functionality and requirements for its use can impact the health of individuals from the perspective of their mental health and autonomy. For the development of the hard and software of healthcare technology, the industry needs to ensure the supplies are sourced and utilized ethically without significant ecological impact and ensure there is no exploitation of labour, argued by Shaw and Donia [5].

Consideration must also be given to the universal availability of the infrastructure to deliver healthcare technology to ensure there is no further digital divide, especially among the low-income population they proposed.

The use of wearable devices to track and coerce health behaviour through self-monitoring and evaluation though founded on sound motives; stakeholders, especially healthcare professionals, must be aware of the mental discomfort they can produce, warned by Shaw and Donia [5].

With the seamless ease of communication among stakeholders in healthcare with technology, Shaw and Donia argued that while having all its potential benefits for the delivery and maintenance of health, it also risks misinformation or inappropriate use of these channels and the negative impact that can be produced.

As these technologies transform healthcare processes and systems, they will affect the interactions and roles of healthcare workers and other stakeholders. The availability of aggregated data for health insurers may result in a negative bias towards the availability of coverage for susceptible individuals.

The important role of commercial players in digital health, with the ownership and control of big data, poses significant challenges for regulators and policymakers. There is a potential for the shift of power and control over healthcare systems by profit-centred commercial enterprises, which is another threat to the well-being of individuals and the communities they live in.

Shaw and Donia also explore the role of anticipatory governance for digital healthcare technology. It is a broad-based approach through society that has the ability to monitor and evaluate a variety of inputs in the domain of emerging knowledge based technologies in anticipation of its impact on society rather than reactionary. It requires that regulators and policymakers engage diverse actors, including the lay public, ethicists, and any vulnerable population, to give them a voice on the meaning and desirability of a particular piece of technology. This requires foresight and anticipation of trends and possible outcomes and impacts. This focus will ensure social justice so that everyone has the opportunity for better healthcare.

Table 9.3 Domains of analysis in a sociotechnical approach to digital health ethics. Reprinted, with permission, from [5].

Domain of analysis	Brief description	Example ethical issue
Application Software	The lines of code that constitute a given digital health technology and the health-related practices they compel and discourage	Algorithms that perform with lesser degrees of accuracy for structurally marginalized communities
Material devices and supply chains	The actual material used to build and distribute the devices through which humans interact with digital health technologies	The negative environmental effects of mining for materials to build digital devices
Infrastructures	The infrastructure that is required for digital health to function, including material realities such as the buildings in which health care providers work when delivering virtual care, the cables and wires that enable digital signals to travel over distance, and the corporate structures of the organizations that make digital communication available	Lack of access to the Internet for people living in rural and remote areas
Individual health-related practices	The activities and routines that are compelled by the use of digital health technologies	Adverse mental health implications of continual health-related surveillance
Interpersonal relationships	Digital health technologies have the capacity to impact interpersonal relationships, through shaping the sources of information, expectations, and modes of interaction available to people	Negative impacts on interpersonal relationships as a result of health-related misinformation shared on social media
Organizational policies	The structure, function and routines that characterize organizations, and the ways in which these are formalized in organizational rules and policies	The institution of corporate surveillance on staff
Government policy and regulatory capture	The rules and approaches to governance put in place by state actors, and the influence of digital health stakeholders such as large technology corporations over health-related government policy	The growth in influence of large corporate technology companies over health-related policy

9.5 Conclusion

It is clear that the advancement in technology and its impact on healthcare have brought sufficient ethical challenges. While these may have its awareness in some of the stakeholders and actors who are interested in healthcare technology ethics, they generally remain outside the core understanding and awareness of the healthcare professionals and technology developers who are the principal stakeholders in healthcare technology.

It is important that regulators and policymakers create awareness of the importance of ethical considerations in adopting healthcare technology and have wider public conversations. A transdisciplinary approach should be adopted by all concerned to learn from and about each other's concerns and challenges. This is to ensure that an equitable and inclusive approach is taken to safeguard the adoption and execution of ethical strategies during their implementation.

It is timely that biosocial and technological ethics be included in the curriculum and competencies of health professionals, technology developers, engineers, regulators, and policymakers.

Healthcare technology is too important to be left in the hand of healthcare professionals and technology developers.

References

[1] He, J., Baxter, S.L., Xu, J., Xu, J., Zhou, X., Zhang, K.: 'The practical implementation of artificial intelligence technologies in medicine' *Nat. Med.*, 2019, **25**(1), pp. 30–36.

[2] Nwosu, A.C., Sturgeon, B., McGlinchey, T., *et al.*: 'Robotic technology for palliative and supportive care: strengths, weaknesses, opportunities and threats' *Palliat. Med.*, 2019, **33**(8), pp. 1106–1113.

[3] Reijers, W., Wright, D., Brey, P., *et al.*: 'Methods for practising ethics in research and innovation: a literature review, critical analysis and recommendations' *Sci. Eng. Ethics*, 2018, **24**(5), pp. 1437–1481.

[4] Steerling, E., Houston, R., Gietzen, L.J., Ogilvie, S.J., Ruiter, H.-P. de, Nygren, J.M.: 'Examining how ethics in relation to health technology is described in the research literature: scoping review' *Interact. J. Med. Res.*, 2022, **11**(2), p. e38745.

[5] Shaw, J.A., Donia, J.: 'The sociotechnical ethics of digital health: a critique and extension of approaches from bioethics' *Front. Digit. Health*, 2021, **3**.

[6] Bayramzadeh, S., Aghaei, P.: 'Technology integration in complex healthcare environments: a systematic literature review' *Appl. Ergon.*, 2021, **92**, p. 103351.

[7] Rahman, N.A., Rajaratnam, V.: 'Human-machine interface for healthcare technology manufacturing'. In *Human Machine Collaboration and Interaction For Smart Manufacturing: Automation, robotics, sensing, artificial intelligence, 5G, IoTs and blockchain* (pp. 339–374). Stevenage, UK: IET; 2022.

[8] Khan, Z.F., Alotaibi, S.R.: 'Applications of artificial intelligence and big data analytics in m-health: a healthcare system perspective' *J. Healthc. Eng.*, 2020, **2020**, p. e8894694.

[9] Hermes, S., Riasanow, T., Clemons, E.K., Böhm, M., Krcmar, H.: 'The digital transformation of the healthcare industry: exploring the rise of

emerging platform ecosystems and their influence on the role of patients' *Bus. Res.*, 2020, **13**(3), pp. 1033–1069.
[10] Lu, L., Zhang, J., Xie, Y., *et al.*: 'Wearable health devices in health care: narrative systematic review' *JMIR MHealth UHealth*, 2020, **8**(11), p. e18907.
[11] Marques, I.C.P., Ferreira, J.J.M.: 'Digital transformation in the area of health: systematic review of 45 years of evolution' *Health Technol.*, 2020, **10**(3), pp. 575–586.
[12] Zarour, M., Alenezi, M., Ansari, M.T.J., *et al.*: 'Ensuring data integrity of healthcare information in the era of digital health' *Healthc. Technol. Lett.*, 2021, **8**(3), pp. 66–77.
[13] Aggarwal, N., Ahmed, M., Basu, S., *et al.*: 'Artificial intelligence in health care: benefits and challenges of technologies to augment patient care' *GAO Rep.*, 2020, pp. i–91.
[14] Reddy, S., Allan, S., Coghlan, S., Cooper, P.: 'A governance model for the application of AI in health care' *J. Am. Med. Inform. Assoc.*, 2020, **27**(3), pp. 491–497.
[15] Seh, A.H., Zarour, M., Alenezi, M., *et al.*: 'Healthcare data breaches: insights and implications' *Healthcare*, 2020, **8**(2), p. 133.
[16] Solomon, L.S., Kanter, M.H.: 'Health Care steps up to social determinants of health: current context' *Perm. J.*, 2018, **22**, pp. 18–139.
[17] Sutherland, R.: 'Dying well-informed: the need for better clinical education surrounding facilitating end-of-life conversations' *Yale J. Biol. Med.*, 2019, **92**(4), pp. 757–764.
[18] Golubnitschaja, O., Kinkorova, J., Costigliola, V.: 'Predictive, preventive and personalised medicine as the hardcore of "Horizon 2020": EPMA position paper' *EPMA J.*, 2014, **5**(1), p. 6.
[19] Atkin, C., Crosby, B., Dunn, K., *et al.*: 'Perceptions of anonymised data use and awareness of the NHS data opt-out amongst patients, carers and healthcare staff' *Res. Involv. Engagem.*, 2021, **7**(1), p. 40.
[20] Khan, M., Rahman-Shepherd, A., Bory, S., *et al.*: 'How conflicts of interest hinder effective regulation of healthcare: an analysis of antimicrobial use regulation in Cambodia, Indonesia and Pakistan' *BMJ Glob. Health*, 2022, **7**(5), p. e008596.
[21] Engel, G.L.: 'The need for a new medical model: a challenge for biomedicine' *Science*, 1977, **196**(4286), pp. 129–136.
[22] Abdul Rahman, N., Rajaratnam, V., Burchell, G.L., Peters, R.M., Zweekhorst, M.B.: 'Experiences of living with leprosy: a systematic review and qualitative evidence synthesis' *PLoS Negl. Trop. Dis.*, 2022, **16**(10), p. e0010761.
[23] Bolton, D., Gillett, P.G.: *Biopsychosocial Conditions of Health and Disease*. Palgrave Pivot; 2019.
[24] Tai, M.C.-T.: 'The impact of artificial intelligence on human society and bioethics' *Tzu-Chi Med. J.*, 2020, **32**(4), pp. 339–343.
[25] John, S., Wu, J.: '"First, do no harm"?: non-maleficence, population health, and the ethics of risk' *Soc. Theory Pract.*, 2022.

[26] Varkey, B.: 'Principles of clinical ethics and their application to practice' *Med. Princ. Pract.*, 2021, **30**(1), pp. 17–28.
[27] Blightman, K., Griffiths, S., Danbury, C.: 'Patient confidentiality: when can a breach be justified?' *Contin. Educ. Anaesth. Crit. Care Pain*, 2014, **14**(2), pp. 52–56.
[28] Fernandez Lynch, H., Joffe, S., Feldman, E.A.: 'Informed consent and the role of the treating physician' *N. Engl. J. Med.*, 2018, **378**(25), pp. 2433–2438.
[29] Kayaalp, M.: 'Patient privacy in the era of big data' *Balk. Med. J.*, 2018, **35**(1), pp. 8–17.
[30] McNair, L.: 'Ethical and regulatory oversight of clinical research: the role of the Institutional Review Board' *Exp. Biol. Med.*, 2022, **247**(7), pp. 561–566.
[31] Dash, S., Shakyawar, S.K., Sharma, M., Kaushik, S.: 'Big data in healthcare: management, analysis and future prospects' *J. Big Data*, 2019, **6**(1), p. 54.
[32] Griebel, L., Prokosch, H.-U., Köpcke, F., *et al.*: 'A scoping review of cloud computing in healthcare' *BMC Med. Inform. Decis. Mak.*, 2015, **15**(1), p. 17.
[33] Davenport, T., Kalakota, R.: 'The potential for artificial intelligence in healthcare' *Future Healthc. J.*, 2019, **6**(2), pp. 94–98.
[34] Babic, B., Gerke, S., Evgeniou, T., Cohen, I.G.: 'Beware explanations from AI in health care' *Science*, 2021, **373**(6552), pp. 284–286.
[35] Daskalopoulou, A., Palmer, M.: 'Persistent institutional breaches: technology use in healthcare work' *Soc. Sci. Med.*, 2021, **289**, p. 114399.
[36] Nicolaides, A.: 'Considering medical technology use, ethics and litigation' *J. Med. Lab. Sci. Technol. South Afr.*, 2019, **1**(4), pp. 26–34.
[37] McDougall, R.J.: 'Computer knows best? The need for value-flexibility in medical AI' *J. Med. Ethics*, 2019, **45**(3), pp. 156–160.
[38] Kerasidou, A.: 'Artificial intelligence and the ongoing need for empathy, compassion and trust in healthcare' *Bull. World Health Organ.*, 2020, **98**(4), pp. 245–250.
[39] Dawes, M., Summerskill, W., Glasziou, P., *et al.*: 'Sicily statement on evidence-based practice' *BMC Med. Educ.*, 2005, **5**(1), p. 1.
[40] Sackett, D.L., Straus, S.E., Richardson, W.S., Rosenberg, W., Haynes, R.B.: *Evidence-Based Medicine: How to Practice and Teach EBM* (2nd ed.). Churchill Livingstone; 2000.
[41] Rosenbaum, S.E., Glenton, C., Cracknell, J.: 'User experiences of evidence based online resources for health professionals: user testing of The Cochrane Library' *BMC Med. Inform. Decis. Mak.*, 2008, **8**(1), p. 34.
[42] Lancet, T.: 'Depressing research' *The Lancet*, 2004, **363**(9418), p. 1335.
[43] Agbo, C.C., Mahmoud, Q.H.: 'Blockchain in healthcare: opportunities, challenges, and possible solutions' *Int. J. Healthc. Inf. Syst. Inform. IJHISI*, 2020, **15**(3), pp. 82–97.
[44] Benchoufi, M., Ravaud, P.: 'Blockchain technology for improving clinical research quality' *Trials*, 2017, **18**(1), p. 335.
[45] Stafford, T.F., Treiblmaier, H.: 'Characteristics of a blockchain ecosystem for secure and sharable electronic medical records' *IEEE Trans. Eng. Manag.*, 2020, **67**(4), pp. 1340–1362.

[46] Gordon, W., Wright, A., Landman, A.: 'Blockchain in health care: decoding the hype' *NEJM Catal.*, 2017, **3**(1), doi:10.1056/CAT.17.0523.

[47] Gundersen, T., Bærøe, K.: 'The future ethics of artificial intelligence in medicine: making sense of collaborative models' *Sci. Eng. Ethics*, 2022, **28**(2), p. 17.

[48] Suresh, H., Guttag, J.: 'A framework for understanding sources of harm throughout the machine learning life cycle'. In *Equity and Access in Algorithms, Mechanisms, and Optimization (EAAMO '21)*. Equity and Access in Algorithms, Mechanisms, and Optimization (pp. 1-9). ACM; 2021.

[49] De Cremer, D., Kasparov, G.: 'The ethics of technology innovation: a double-edged sword?' *AI Ethics*, 2022, **2**(3), pp. 533–537.

Chapter 10

Medical equipment engineering and manufacturing standard and policies

Soon Cheng Yap[1] and Wai Yie Leong[1]

The manufacture of medical devices has included the design of the hardware and software which is required to comply with the standards that have been set by the international authorities such as FDA or IEC standards. This is to ensure that the final product that is manufactured by the medical equipment manufacturer, in making a safe and effective use of the devices to the end user. Throughout the manufacturing process, the risk assessment is one of the important keys to the success of launching medical products [1]. This is because those related assessments or testing that have been done during the manufacturing process will act as a valid proof to verify the performance of the device so that it is safe to be used by fulfilling safety requirements such as the electrical safety test, electromagnetic compatibility (EMC) or GUI testing.

10.1 Introduction on medical equipment engineering

Engineering on medical equipment is a field that applies the knowledge of engineering principles and medical related that infused both, and to develop the innovative medical devices through new and advanced technology, in improving the healthcare quality for the society. The manufacture of the medical equipment and system could be served with the purpose of diagnostic, therapeutics, and monitoring, with the design interface and development of workflow such as the innovation of Internet of Things (IoT), cloud computing, and big data that integrates into the existing healthcare system, health information system (HIS), that transforms the traditional medical systems into more intelligent, digitized and informative systems [2]. The current development of medical equipment and devices, the invention of its design could be simpler, user friendly, and reduce operation time by giving more precise diagnoses and safer treatments to the patients. However, the doubts on new digitized medical equipment are always getting suspicious on how the new design or methodologies can deliver better performance in terms of efficiency,

[1]Graduate School of Medicine, Perdana University, Malaysia

consistency, and reliability, by comparing with the same functionality of existing medical devices. Meanwhile, the challenges of new medical technologies might conflict with the ethical implications that relate to its treatment and complications on human–machine interactions [3]. Example of the use of non-invasive blood pressure (NIBP) device is operated by the inflation and deflation of the cuff, in getting the patient's blood pressure (BP). In current development of NIBP, it is operated automatically and triggered the measuring by pressing a measure button, in completing the measurement of patient's BP within 15–20 s, instead of the manual pumping by using the mercury sphygmomanometer with a stethoscope, where that is not required in use on automated NIBP device. The measurement of NIBP usually integrates on the monitoring type medical devices such as vital sign monitor, patient monitor, and defibrillator. Hence, Figure 10.1 shows the example of a vital sign monitor that has integrated the parameters of BP, saturation of oxygen (SpO_2), and pulse rate (PR). Unfortunately, the feature of automated NIBP device could have negative impacts as well, where tragedies might happen during the medical procedures. That was a case study of medical negligence filed in year 2011, regarding the automated NIBP with the use of a malfunctioned cuff which this NIBP device itself had inflated for more than 5 h during the surgery. During the surgery, the mean arterial pressure (MAP) of the patient was supposed showing "60" in mmHg reading of inflation that indicates the venipuncture mode in order to facilitate the operation of intravenous catheter [4]. However, the false error had occurred between the communication of software and hardware display without any alarm triggered or error message on monitor, resulting in an anesthesia patient that was under the dilemma of 'venous stasis' and the patient's arm amputated during the surgery.

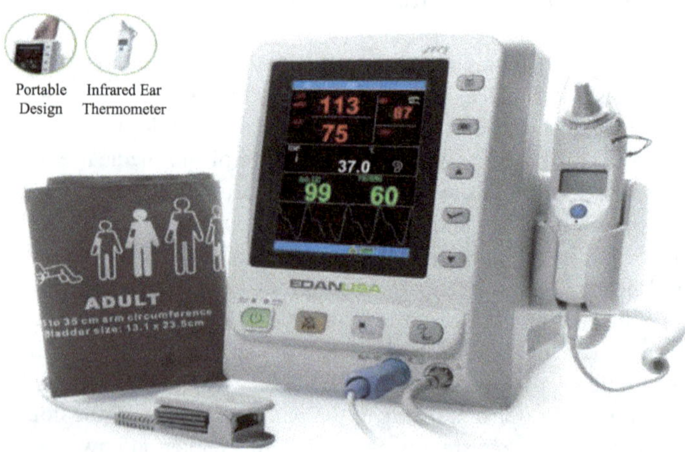

Figure 10.1 Example of M3 vital signs monitor, company of Edan USA that integrated the features of NIBP, SPO_2, and PR with portable design for the users

Before the large-scale production of a medical equipment, the manufacturer is required to undergo the process of getting approval by the authorities before the launching and marketing that comply with these medical device standards and regulations accordingly to the regulatory bodies of different countries [5–7]. Furthermore, the safety and effectiveness on new designed medical equipment is a massive challenge for the manufacturers that ensure that their devices are reliable and safe to be used in order to get approval. From the review on the regulation of medical equipment, one of the requirements after post sales activity is to maintain the safeness and useable of medical devices by performing the planned preventative maintenance service (PPM) [8]. In Japan, the coordination and management of maintenance services are the responsibility for the medical equipment safety manager (MESM) in Japan's hospital. For example, the medical devices that should be maintained including ventilators, artificial heart or lung apparatus, biventricular assisting devices, hemodialysis apparatus, infant incubators, defibrillators, radiation medical equipment which has been stated under the revision of their medical law. However, due to shortage of staff, the position of MESMs is usually handled by the physician or clinical engineer technologist of the hospital, who might not have adequate skills and experience in handling on coordination of maintenance service, that could affect the levels of safety and effectiveness of medical devices and induce the seriousness of medical adverse events and lawsuit against them. This is required to clarify and emphasize the importance of responsibility and authority of MESMs and resolve the shortage of manpower for handling on maintenance services [9]. This situation is indicating the high possibility of human induced error could happen rather than the issues on manufacturing or design interface of medical equipment. Hence, the PPM schedule should be more alert by the correct candidate of MESMs, in order to monitor and control the progression of maintenance of the medical devices, and he or she should be handling more professionally if machine failure occurs.

Clinical testing such as *in vivo* testing is required to be performed from the medical device, whereby it is to collect the clinical data and review before the launching of the market. Meanwhile, the post-surveillance is controlled by the international authorities such as United States Food and Drug Administration (FDA) and European Union (EU) to investigate and approve the reliability of medical devices in terms of mechanical, physical and clinical performance. The classification of the medical devices is based on the degree of risk and can be classified as significant, non-significant and lowest level of risks with different submissions of the document to those authorities. The occurrence of adverse events cannot be fully evitable but can try to reduce the formation of unwanted errors and unnecessary hazardous risks through implementing standards and design requirements. Figure 10.2 shows the incidence of adverse events that happened in several countries' hospitals, such as the formation of injuries, hospitalization or death, whereby the percentage lies between 4% and 17% of the occurrences of adverse events, including the operation or drug-related factors [10]. Nevertheless, this figure does not fully represent the quality of the overall healthcare system globally. Medical failure and unfortunate adverse events that happened in the past lead to the

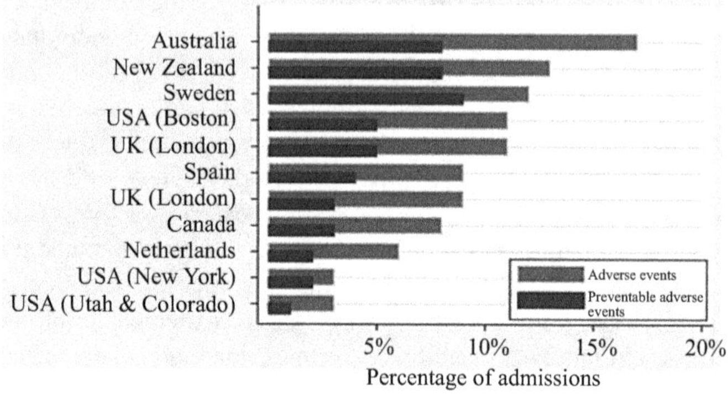

Figure 10.2 Statistics on incidence of hospital adverse events happened in several countries [10]

advancement of healthcare and medicine systems towards a brighter future whereby the technology that integrates into the healthcare system can be improved on its design and giving better experience and treatments for the patients.

10.2 Manufacturing failure on medical devices

Innovation on medical devices with latest technologies can transform the existing healthcare system into more advanced and modern healthcare system such as the current trend on medical graded of wearable monitoring devices whereby it can access and monitor the heart-related bioactivity such as arrhythmia on the heart disease patients with the analysis of Electrocardiogram (ECG) and BP by using artificial intelligent (AI) for the prediction of abnormal activity or disease-related factors. However, the failures on medical devices will bring along the negative impacts to the patients, hospitals, and manufacturers. It could be happening in the lawsuit against the manufacturers due to the failure or malfunction of the medical devices. This is because the losses on patients from such adverse events would be permanently affecting the patients in lifetime. Hence, the procedure of the good manufacturing practice (GMP) is the quality guidance for the manufacturers on manufacturing their medical devices before the launch to the market, with the compliance of the recognized standards. The standards of ISO13485 from EU and 21 CFR Part 820 from FDA are one of the harmonized standards for the manufacturer to ensure the quality of the devices and reduce the potential risk with a proper and good management for quality control on their medical products and services. Table 10.1 shows the 15 subsections under 21 CFR Part 820 of the FDA regulation that required the management to inspect, validate, and verify the quality of the medical devices with assessment from time to time during the entire manufacturing process. Recall process might be implemented when that is a confirmed defective medical device that has the risks of endangering people's lives and

Table 10.1 Management responsibility on the quality control under FDA regulation of Title 21 CFR Part 820 [11]

FDA 21 CFR Part 820:
+ General provisions + Quality systems requirements + Design controls + Documents controls + Purchasing controls + Identification and traceability + Production and process controls + Acceptance activities + Nonconforming product + Corrective and preventive actions + Labeling and packaging control + Handling, storage, distribution, and installation + Records + Servicing + Statistical techniques

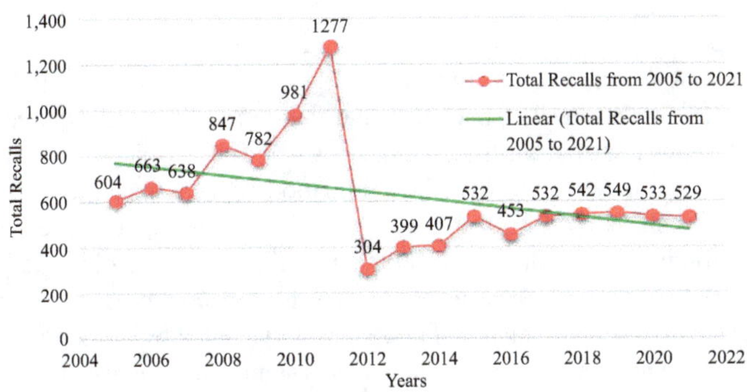

Figure 10.3 Total number of recalls on medical device from FDA Year 2005 till 2021 [12]

required to collect from the market and for redesign and remanufacturing purposes. The factors on low-quality raw materials, counterfeit medical devices, software glitches, ineffective technical performance, or off label medical devices are the failure of the manufacturers, where they fail to implement a more effective quality control on the products, in leading the threats to the patients [12]. Figure 10.3 shows the total number of recalls on medical devices from year 2006 till 2011, with the highest records of 1,277 cases in 2011 whereas it dropped to 304 cases in the next year.

Table 10.2 Indication of the level of severity, occurrence and detectability [14]

Score	Severity	Occurrence	Detectability
1	None	Extremely remote	Almost certain
2	Very minor	Remote, very unlikely	Very high
3	Minor	Very slight chance	High
4	Very low	Slight chance	Moderately high
5	Low	Occasion	Moderate
6	Moderate	Moderate	Low
7	High	Frequent	Very low
8	Very high	High	Remote
9	Hazardous with warning	Very high	Very remote
10	Hazardous without warning	Extremely high	Absolutely uncertainty

10.3 Methodologies on existing analysis on medical equipment management

Failure Modes and Effect Analysis (FMEA), one of the methodologies to identify the potential failure modes, evaluate and mitigate the risks which are applicable to implement on the medical devices manufacturing. The identification of the potential failures was determined through the indication of severity (S), occurrence (O), and detectability (D) on the risk analysis of the medical devices. The risk priority number (RPN) is the product of the severity, occurrence, and detectability, which gives an overall value to evaluate the potential failure of the medical products and correct the failure with the respective actions required to be implemented [13]. Meanwhile, the RPN value also indicates the seriousness level of that particular failure mode and is required to control and reduce the potential risk in the corrective ways. The definition of severity is the effect of seriousness in reflecting from the failure modes, occurrence is the probability of frequency that might happen on that particular failure modes and whereas the detectability is the ability of difficulty that can be detected as the cause of the failure modes [14]. Table 10.2 demonstrates the levels of severity, occurrence and detectability by respecting the seriousness of potential failure that is evaluated by the scoring of 1 to 10. Higher the RPN value indicates the potential risk is significant whereas the low RPN is a low-risk process and it could be eliminated or exempted based on the scenario that was justified by the manufacturer or medical equipment designer [14,15]. The final scoring of this FMEA analysis is comparatively subjective and dependent on the experience from the previous incidents or cases that has been experienced by the manufacturers. Meanwhile, some of the researches have modified the FMEA into healthcare failure mode and effect analysis (HFMEA) that is implemented into the healthcare process, instead of the process of design or manufacturing of the medical devices.

10.4 Impact on medical equipment management

Human factor engineering (HFE) is one important consideration on the design interface of the medical equipment whereby its methodologies apply the factor of ergonomics that identify all the possible points of interface between the user and the medical equipment, leading the user to satisfy the use of the equipment. The factors include the user might have a limited knowledge, unfamiliar on the machine interface of the medical equipment or the limitation of the software and hardware elements. The standard of IEC 62366 or HE75: 2009, is to minimize the human error which could be lacking on training, inattentive, or not reading the instructions. Even though the device itself might not have any technical or clinical aspect of error but the formation of human pattern on their work practice. Thus, the concept of the HFE standard is applied for creating the working environment that is mainly on the user's consideration for easy and safer operation of the medical equipment. For example, the design interface of clinical guidelines that embedded into the medical equipment system is giving a warning or error message to the users that might indicates the abnormal activity in real-time monitoring such as the limits of overdose on drug devices. Hence, the development cycle of medical devices is required to integrate with the consideration of safety related usability that evaluate and mitigate the usability-induced use errors from the interface of the medical devices such as the reliance on memory-based medical system, invisible of devices' interfaces, and poor design of user interface.

Recall is one of the remanufacturing processes in order to redesign on those defects and failure modes of the medical devices, whereby the manufacturers should be more alert on their quality control processes by validating and verifying the performances through various risk assessments in gaining the confidence from the market and their customers [16]. Root cause analysis (RCA) is one of the methodologies on the investigational of the incident event with a causal chain of events presented [17]. Before the development of new medical devices, the engineer may look at functionality, components of the devices with their justification based on the scientific experiment and compliance with the regulatory [18]. This is because the occurrence of death or losses on patients might happen during a surgery or a misdiagnosis, in causing the adverse event in hospitals. Figure 10.4 shows the

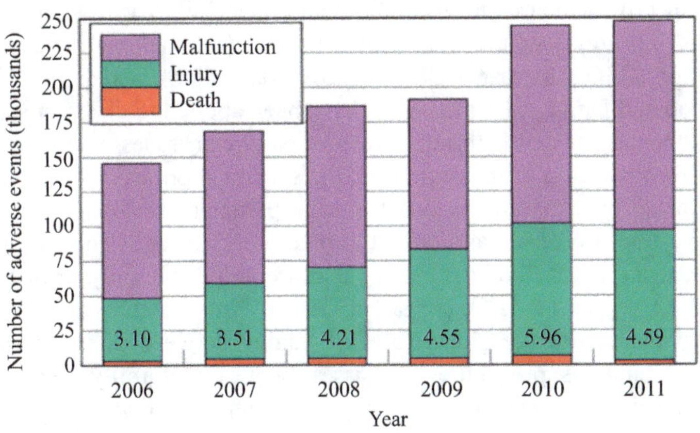

Figure 10.4 Number of adverse events in hospital including the injuries, death, and malfunction of electronic or software based medical devices [19]

number of adverse events that happen on the failure of the medical devices, in causing the malfunction of the devices, formation of injuries and death to the patients. Based on the FDA database, the highest number of adverse events is about 250,000 cases that happened in year 2011 whereas the effect of malfunction is the highest portion that causes the failure mode of the medical devices.

10.5 Introduction on manufacturing standard and policies

Manufacturing on medical devices: one of the concerns is the measurement that applies differently to adult, pediatric, and neonatal because of different body sizes, body shape, and anatomical structure, resulting in the standard on measurement and design perspective being varying to each other. For example, the use of NIBP measurement, the particular design of the cuff width is depending on the measure of arm circumference. Based on the recommendation of British Hypertension Society, the cuff size should be 12 × 26 cm for adult arms, 12 × 40 cm for obese arms, whereas for lean adults' arm and children, the cuff is about the size of 12 × 18 cm [20]. The respective specific standard of IEC 80601-2-30 describes the electrical requirement of safety use and its performance on automated non-invasive sphygmomanometers. Moreover, the design of the cuff is also capable of being used for lower limb measurements for those patients, who lost their arms from an accident or due to birth defects. Those published standards are to ensure the safety and effectiveness of medical equipment, in order to reduce the potential risks that could be avoided accordingly with the guidelines provided. Meanwhile, it is to ensure the quality of these manufactured medical equipment that comply with the requirement settings from the regulatory bodies. For IEC standards, it is a wide range of safety requirement from general to specific standards, including the electromagnetic emission (IEC 61000), human factor engineering (IEC 62366), and electrical safety requirement (IEC 60601) that can be further breakdown into a series of specific standards for each different medical electrical equipment.

From this review, the standards of IEC (International Electrotechnical Commission), ISO (International Standard Organization), and FDA (The United States Food and Drugs Administration) have been applied to different sectors from the global consensus that is trying to resolve particular issues with the appropriate solution. By providing those guidelines, the specification and requirements are to share with the public policymakers from the particular sectors. From the global perspective, the use of a standardized regulation is easier to follow and inspect, instead of using the different standards that are applicable only in that particular country. The World Trade Organization (WTO) is the intergovernmental organization that deals with the global rules of trading between different nations and ensures the standards, procedures, and assessment of conformity used to eliminate the inefficiencies as a trade barrier and monitor the trade policies. IEC publishes the information on electrical, electronic, and related technologies that comply with regulation, and has been recognized by WTO in order to resolve the technical barriers on the trade agreement between the national and regional organizations.

10.6 Standards on quality management system (QMS)

International Organization for Standardization (ISO) develops the standards of the management system that the regulation is released according to different sectors of manufacturing and working practice, in giving of the framework of safety and effectiveness from the organizations and to the public. The organizations are required to comply with those sets of various regulations, in order to get the certification from ISO as the proof of regulatory compliance that the manufactured products or system that is recognized and certified by those power and prestige authorities, in gaining the confidence of the consumer. ISO 9001 standard is one of general quality management systems that use the procedures, policies, and processes in maintaining and assuring the quality of the products and services during production, servicing, and development, whereby it could meet the customers' requirement and enhance their satisfaction in leading the cooperative and growth on business [21]. Table 10.3 lists the standard of ISO 9001: 2015 that has different aspects on this quality management system where the requirements are applied within an organization internally from the objectives of organizations, board of management, and the performance employees. In common, the implementation of QMS is using the concept of Plan-Do-Check-Act (PDCA) cycle for improving their products and services, with the execution on design & build, deploy, control & measure, review, and improvement [22].

10.6.1 ISO 13485

The regulation of ISO 13485 is the framework of the quality management system for the sector of medical devices and is required to be followed by the manufacturer according to the compliance of its regulatory and legal. The working principle is similar to ISO 9001 where the responsibility of management of an organization is to plan and execute the settings on quality objectives and targets on the QMS system that are beneficial to their own medical devices and services. This requires demonstrating the manufacture of medical devices that meet the customer requirement and satisfaction and deliver the system with minimal risks. Furthermore, the supplier corrective action request (SCAR), which is under the section of corrective and

Table 10.3 Aspect of the QMS on ISO 9001: 2015 standard [21]

Clause 0–3	**Introduction and scope of the standard**
Clause 4	Context of the organization
Clause 5	Leadership
Clause 6	Planning
Clause 7	Support
Clause 8	Operation
Clause 9	Performance evaluation
Clause 10	Improvement

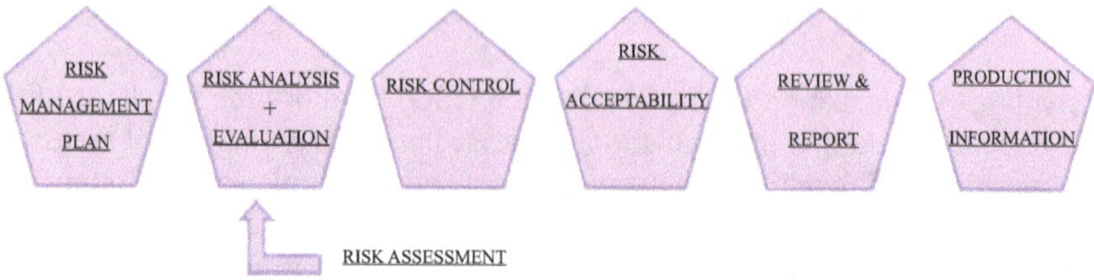

Figure 10.5 Process of risk management on the manufacturing of medical devices [1]

prevention action (CAPA) in this standard [23]. The challenges of CAPA are to solve the recurring quality problems that existed on medical devices, whereby the process is required to collect and analyze on those problems with the appropriate methodology. These existing and potential quality issues should be identified and investigated by related authorities, and the medical devices might be required to undergo the recall process from the market for its correction of the faults or defects. The update of ISO 13485 includes the focus on requirement of software, packaging and distribution, feedback handling and the measures of post-market surveillance, to ensure the products that manufacture and deliver to the highest quality to the customers.

10.6.2 ISO 14971

Standard of ISO 14971 is to provide the framework on the risk management for the lifecycle of the medical product by following its techniques on this effective management, in order to reduce uncertainty that related on the safety issues and deliver the solution to the error of medical products that try to mitigate the error and failure [1]. The process of the risk management includes the planning of risk management, risk analysis, risk control, risk acceptability, review and report with the detailed information of the product. Meanwhile, in between the process, the requirement of the product design has to be set when that is a use on implementation of the risk assessment during the phase of analysis and evaluation. Figure 10.5 shows the total workflow on the process of risk management during the design and manufacture of the medical devices. The methodology on this risk assessment usually is implementing the RPN value which has been discussed on Section 10.1.3 with indication level of severity, occurrence, and detectability, by evaluating the potential risk, and the seriousness of the failure mode.

10.7 Technical standard for safety measurement

10.7.1 Electromagnetic compatibility

Electromagnetic compatibility (EMC) provides the proper immunity standards for the power supplies that require to testify the electronic equipment including the sector of medical devices, under certain specific tests and comply with the performance and its acceptance criteria with the standards given. Table 10.4 shows the

Table 10.4 Standard on EMC

Immunity standard of EMC	Reference standards
Limit for harmonic current	IEC/EN 61000-3-2
Limitation voltage fluctuation/flicker	IEC/EN 61000-3-3
Electrostatic discharge test	IEC/EN 61000-4-2
Radiated RFI immunity	IEC/EN 61000-4-3
Electrical fast transients	IEC/EN 61000-4-4
Mains surges	IEC/EN 61000-4-5
Conducted RFI	IEC/EN 61000-4-6
Mains frequency magnetic field	IEC/EN 61000-4-8
Pulsed magnetic field	IEC/EN 61000-4-9
Damped oscillatory magnetic field	IEC/EN 61000-4-10
Supply voltage dips and interruptions	IEC/EN 61000-4-11

list of immunity tests of the EMC standard which comply with IEC/EN 61000 and its reference number represents the specific tests accordingly. However, the IEC/EN 61000 does not cover only the standard for immunity limits but it does include the measurement techniques, installation guidelines or functional safety on different subsections of the standards. During the design phase of the medical equipment, the design engineers are required to follow and comply with the standards with the testing and evaluate the effectiveness of the supply on the equipment. For IEC/EN 61000-3-2, the testing of harmonic currents is to supply the mains networks with the voltage of 220 V and phase current is about 16 A, in order to examine and limit the harmonic distortion and current over the AC line. This is because the higher distortion of the harmonic will cause the increase of harmonic current on the AC power system, leading the temperature increases on electronic components such as the distribution transformer until it overheats and fails to operate permanently. Usually, the harmonic current over the AC power line is required to be kept as low as possible, thereby decreasing the effect of the distortion.

IEC/EN 61000-3-3 is the standard given that analyze and limit the voltage fluctuations and flicker in low-voltage application with the rated current of equal or less than 16 A per phase on the equipment. This is to ensure that the effects of the fluctuations are not affecting the system of the equipment during the normal operation. Hence, the occurrence of voltage fluctuation over the power system network is due to sudden rapid change on the real and reactive power of the output loads, resulting in the phenomena of lamp flicker, whereby the intensity of lamp is varying on the changes of the supply voltage when it is overloaded. Therefore, it is important that the design circuit of the equipment is not designed with the feature of high output impedance, where the current could be drawn significantly and causing the output voltage drops drastically that prevent the equipment to operate properly. Figure 10.6 indicates the limits of the flicker and voltage changes within the variation of the parameter and its specific condition. IEC/EN 61000-3-5 and IEC/EN 61000-3-7 are the standards for low-voltage equipment that deals with rated current greater than 16 A and for fluctuating loads on the middle voltage and high voltage systems respectively.

Parameter	Limit		Conditions
Short-term flicker indicator	Pst	1.0	
Long-term flicker indicator	Plt	0.65	
Relative voltage change	d(t)	3,3%	For more than 500ms
Relative steady-state voltage change	dc	3,3%	
Maximum relative voltage change	dmax	4%	Without additional conditions
		6%	For equipment which is switched manually or switched automatically more frequently than twice per day
		7%	For equipment which is attended while in use (hair dryers, vacuum cleaners, mixers, lawn mowers, electric drills), or switched on automatically, or is intended to be switched on manually, no more than twice per day

Figure 10.6 Requirement on the limits in short and long terms of flicker, relative voltage change on steady state, and maximum limit

Meanwhile, the electromagnetic harmonic is one of the distortions that affect the performance of medical devices including the hardware application and software as well. The reason for malfunction on medical devices could be the existence of electrostatic discharge (ESD) that is characterized as the peak discharge current with the produce of transient electromagnetic fields [24]. High amount of accumulated ESD, it might cause injuries or death to the human body and damage the medical devices during the duration of operating. Hence, for such IEC standard of 61000-4-2, is to testify the immunity of ESD and robustness of medical electronic equipment by injecting an ESD pulse from ESD gun into the subject equipment, with the methodology of contact discharge [24]. Otherwise, the air discharge method is getting the ESD gun brought closer to the equipment until a discharge happens. The most severe ESD threat (level 4) has been considered in testing of 8 kV and 15 kV with the contact discharge and air discharge, respectively.

10.7.2 IEC 60601-1 and IEC 60601-2

IEC 60601-1 is the general standard of electrical safety and essential requirement on the medical electrical equipment to ensure the safety use of medical devices where that is a concern on the dangers of the electricity and power supplies that supplied to the medical system, whereby the IEC 60601-2 is for the safety measurement on different types of specific medical equipment. This is to control the design of the medical system to prevent any form of hazards to the operators or patients during the medical treatment. For example, the standard of IEC 60601-2-5 or IEC 60601-2-16 is the safety use of ultrasonic physiotherapy equipment and hemodialysis or hemofiltration equipment, respectively. For IEC 60601-1-8, it is the usage of the audible alarm that is required to integrate into the medical system for the error detection of the medical equipment or treatment and act as the warning to alert the operators. In third edition of IEC 60601-1, that defining the electrical performance for safe operation in terms of relevant to the concept of mean of protection (MOP) which has divided into two different protections, known as "means of operator protection" (MOOP) and "means of patient protection"

(MOPP) that concern on the safety from the perspective of patients and operators, that the physical contact is connected via probes, however, by comparing to the second edition, it is more focusing on the vicinity of the patient with the risk guideline of the medical equipment is within 6-foot radius from the patients. In this edition, three different classifications of medical devices are named as Type B (body), Type BF (body floating), and Type CF (cardiac floating). Each of the classification of equipment is equipped with a different value on its parameter. Table 10.5 shows the second edition of the IEC 60601 standards on the various parameters with three different classes of the medical devices in terms of isolation, creepage and insulation. Meanwhile, Table 10.6 shows the third edition of the requirement that was revised with the reference point in terms of "Protection." For type B devices, they could have two isolation barriers and be divided into One MOOP and One MOPP that have the different requirements on the isolation and creepage. The fourth edition of IEC 60601 standard tries to emphasize the managing and analyzing the risks that present on the disturbances of EMC. Furthermore, the use of symbols and markings are required to specify the identification of the equipment such as the electrical requirement, model number and serial number, and in usual as the safety information of the equipment. Figure 10.7 shows the example of the labeling on the defibrillator that indicates the classification of medical devices, CE marking and the icons that represents the device type with or without physical contact on patients

Table 10.5 Second edition of IEC 60601 requirement that indicate the levels of isolation, insulation and their creepage of an isolation transformer or DC–DC converter

Classification	Type B	Type BF	Type CF
Description	Equipment operates within vicinity, without patient contact	Physical contact with patient contact	Physical contact with the heart
Isolation	1,500 Vac	3,000 Vac	4,000 Vac
Creepage	2.5 mm	5.0 mm	8.0 mm
Insulation	Basic	Double	Double
Example of medical devices	X-ray, MRI imaging	Blood pressure monitoring	Defibrillator

Table 10.6 Third edition of IEC 60601 requirement

Classification	One MOOP	Two MOOP	One MOPP	Two MOPP
Isolation	1,500 Vac	3,000 Vac	1,500 Vac	4,000 Vac
Creepage	2.5 mm	5.0 mm	4.0 mm	8.0 mm
Insulation	Basic	Double	Basic	Double

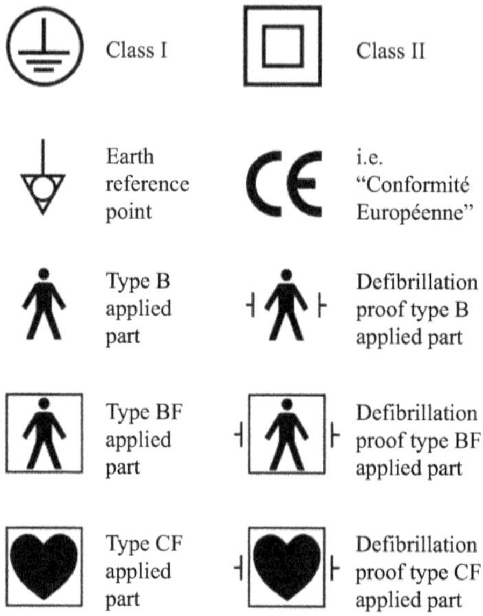

Figure 10.7 Example of the marking on the medical equipment of defibrillator

10.8 Standard of human factors engineering

10.8.1 IEC 62366/AAMI TIR59: 2017

The European Union's regulation of IEC 62366 is the standard for the human factors engineering (HFE) that is applicable to all manufacturers of medical devices, whereby this standard is harmonized, in order to promote the safety in use with the reduce of the unaccepted error and avoid the adverse events after the users are in use of the devices. Moreover, in FDA, the term of HFE is known as the guidance of "Applying Human Factors and Usability Engineering to Medical Devices" that was finalized in the year 2016, with the efforts from the Association for the Advancement of Medical Instrumentation (AAMI) that conceptualized the HFE to a part of design on the medical devices, AAMI/IEC TIR62366-2016, that the standards for the analysis, design, verify, and validate of safety-related usability through the development cycle of medical devices [25]. Figure 10.8 shows the timeline of the harmonized HFE regulation between the EU and FDA for the usability of medical devices that complies with the regulatory requirements. By implementing the HFE standard, it is to reduce the use error with the safe innovation and the proven clinical benefit. It has included the software interface and hardware design that matches with the user specification and requirement in order to reduce the use error and the safety concern when that is a use of a medical device. The process is required to explore on the user interface specification, evaluation plan, and interface design, according to the predictive hazards-related use scenarios and avoid the known or foreseeable hazards. From the review on HFE

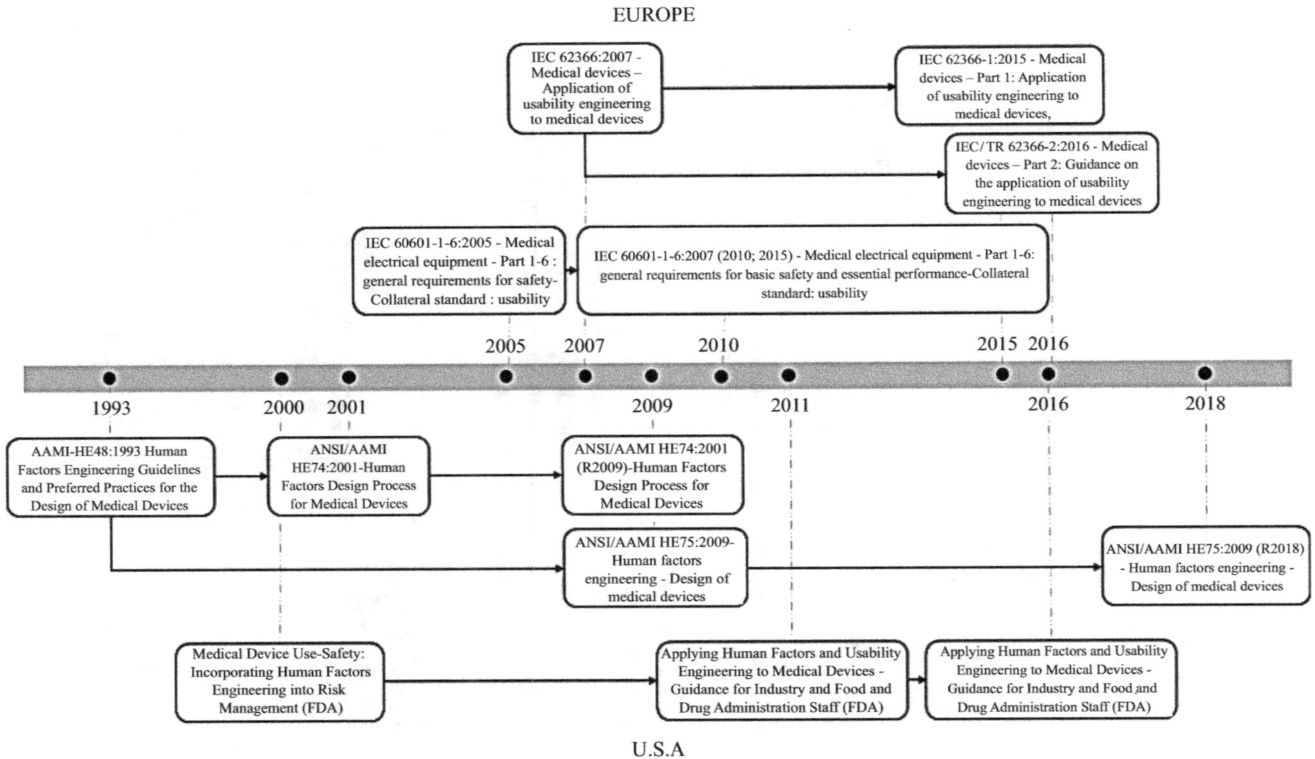

Figure 10.8 Timeline of IEC 62366 that harmonized between the EU and FDA [25]

regulation, the failure of medical devices that induced the recall process between year 1985 and 1989 was up to 50% because of this the user interface design was poor and the FDA has been moved in and controlled over the manufacturers to the development of device products due to the occurrence of adverse events [26].

10.9 Medical device software

10.9.1 ANSI/AAMI/IEC 62304

Embedded software on the medical devices is an inclusive component that had been built into the medical devices, whereby the integration of human–machine interaction is an important console that helps and assists the healthcare professional on measuring, giving the diagnostics, and treatments that are beneficial to them instead of performing the tasks manually and longer time required. However be the defects of the software on medical devices, it would affect the performance of the devices, endanger the patients and healthcare professionals. Figure 10.9 shows the number of recalls of the computer-related failure that occurred within the year 2006 till 2011, whereby the highest number of 319 recalls has been performed in the year of 2011. In overall, the number of recalls is increasing regardless of non-computer or computer-related factors throughout the years. The software glitches as the bugs on the medical device might be giving the wrong dose to the patients, or undesirable impacts such as skin burning cases, wrong dose of drug to the patients [12]. Recall process might be induced by the software failure of the medical devices, on the quality improvement [27]. Thus, the standard of IEC 62304 for compliance with the development of software that tries to reduce the failures on the interface, and provide framework of medical device software life cycle process with good software engineering [28]. One of the important features on the IEC 62304 is using the concept of road mapping in

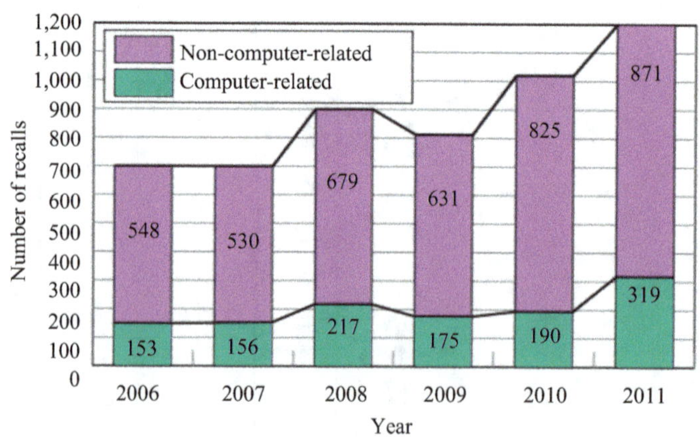

Figure 10.9 Number of recalls on failure of non-computer and computer related on medical device from year 2006 to year 2011 [19]

Table 10.7 *Process of software life cycle of healthcare software that comply to the standard of IEC 62304 [28]*

1.	Software risk management process
2.	Software development planning
3.	Software requirement analysis
4.	Software architectural design
5.	Software detailed design
6.	Software unit implementation
7.	Software integration and integration testing
8.	Software system testing
9.	Software release
10.	Software configuration management
11.	Software problem resolution

tracing the failure of the medical software to standardize and visualize the software life cycle is not a standalone standard and requires to comply with other related standards, such as the quality management standard of ISO 13485, RMS of ISO 14971 and the usability standard of IEC 62366 to ensure the conformity of the medical devices [21,22,29]. To develop the software of the medical devices with the classification of three classes as Class A, Class B, and Class C which depending on the risks of the seriousness of software, software as medical device (SaMD) such as the program of Electroencephalograph (EEG) that acquisition and review the waveform of seizure, sleep study for the patients [30]. Meanwhile, the revolution of the medical device could be the current trend of mobile health apps in monitoring health. New version of IEC 62304 includes the cybersecurity requirements on the medical devices. Table 10.7 lists the process of the software life cycle under the standard of IEC 62304 in designing healthcare software [31–45].

References

[1] S. Mishra and V. K. Shukla, "Latest risk management guideline (ISO 14971:2019) & environmental aspects of medical device," *International Journal of Drug Regulatory Affairs*, vol. 8, no. 2, pp. 15–24, 2020.

[2] S. Tian, W. B. Yang, J. M. L. Grange, P. Wang, W. Huang, and Z. W. Ye, "Smart healthcare: making medical care more intelligent," *Global Health Journal*, vol. 3, no. 3, pp. 62–65, 2019.

[3] V. Rampton, M. Bohmer, and A. Winkler, "Medical technologies past and present: how history helps to understand the digital era," *Journal of Medical Humanities*, vol. 43, pp. 343–364, 2021.

[4] S. M. Shulman, Y. Namn, S. Lando, and P. Discepola, "Forearm loss caused by automated non-invasive blood pressure cuff malfunction: a hearsay report," *Open Journal of Anaesthesiology*, vol. 5, no. 11, pp. 227–232, 2015.

[5] S. K. Gupta, "Medical device regulations: a current perspective," *Journal of Young Pharmacists*, vol. 8, no. 1, pp. 6–11, 2016.

[6] T. W. Li, P. W. Tu, L. L. Liu, and S. I. Wu, "Assurance of medical device quality with quality management system: an analysis of good manufacturing practice implementation in Taiwan," *Biomed Research International*, vol.2015, pp. 1–7, 2015.

[7] R. M. G. Bretana and A. L. F. Rendon, "Impact of regulations on innovation in the field of medical devices," *Research on Biomedical Engineering*, vol. 34, no.2, pp. 356–367, 2018.

[8] E. Iadanza, V. Gonnelli, F. Satta, and M. Gherardelli, "Evidence-based medical equipment management: a convenient implementation," *Medical & Biological Engineering & Computing*, vol. 57, pp. 2215–2230, 2019.

[9] K. Ishida, M. Hirose, K. Fujiwara, H. Tsuruta, and N. Ikeda, "Analysis of medical equipment management in relation to the mandatory medical equipment safety manager (MESM) in Japan," *Journal of Healthcare Engineering*, vol. 5, no. 3 pp. 329–346, 2014.

[10] N. Rafter, A. Hickey, S. Condell, *et al.*, "Adverse events in healthcare: learning from mistakes," *QJM: An International Journal of Medicine*, vol. 108, no. 4, pp. 273–277, 2015.

[11] K. M. Rojas, L. Cosler, and D. L. Santos, "A narrative review of FDA human factors validation requirement: the needs of key stakeholders and proposal of an industry (human factors service providers) maturity assessment tool," in *Proceedings of the International Symposium on Human Factors and Ergonomics in Health Care*, 2019, p. 222.

[12] S. V. Singan, "Medical device failures – impact on medical device & healthcare industry," *International Research Journal of Modernization in Engineering Technology and Science*, vol. 3, no. 7, pp. 741–748, 2021.

[13] E. Ullah, M. M. Baig, H. GholamHosseini, and J. Lu, "Failure mode and effect analysis (FMEA) to identify and mitigate failures in a hospital rapid response system (RRS)," *Heliyon*, vol. 8, no. 2, p. e08944, 2022, doi: https://doi.org/10.1016/j.heliyon.2022.e08944

[14] J. E. Rah, R. P. Manger, A. D. Yock, and G. Y. Kim, "A comparison of two prospective risk analysis methods: traditional FMEA and a modified healthcare FMEA," *Medical Physics*, vol. 43, no. 12, pp. 6347–6353, 2016.

[15] R. Onofrio, F. Piccagli, and F. Segato, "Failure mode, effects and criticality analysis (FMECA) for medical devices: does standardization foster improvements in the practice?" *Procedia Manufacturing*, vol. 3, pp. 43–50, 2015.

[16] S. Eze, W. Ijomah, and T. C. Wong, "Accessing medical equipment in developing countries through remanufacturing," *Journal of Remanufacturing*, vol. 9, no.2, pp. 207–233, 2019.

[17] A. Tase, P. Buckle, M. Z. Ni, and G. B. Hanna, "Medical device error and failure reporting: learning from the car industry," *Journal of Patient Safety and Risk Management*, vol. 26, no. 3, pp. 135–141, 2021.

[18] M. Tamsin and C. Bach, "The design of medical devices," *International Journal of Innovation and Scientific Research*, vol. 1, no. 2, pp. 127–134, 2014.

[19] H. Alemzadeh, E. K. Lyer, and Z. Kalbarczyk, "Analysis of safety critical computer failures in medical devices," *IEEE Security and Privacy Magazine*, vol. 11, pp. 14–26, 2013, doi:10.1109/MSP.2013.49

[20] P. Palatini and R. Asmar, "Cuff challenges in blood pressure measurement," *Journal of Clinical Hypertension,* vol. 20, pp. 1100–1103, 2018, doi: 10.1111/jch.13301.

[21] S. Mourougan and K. Sethuraman, "Understanding and implementing quality management system," *IOSR Journal of Business and Management (IOSR-JBM)*, vol. 19, no. 5, pp. 41–51, 2017.

[22] S. I. Ali and S. Khatoon, "Implementation of total quality management," *International Journal of Emerging Trends in Engineering and Development*, vol. 6, pp. 114–119, 2016, doi: 10.13140/RG.2.2.32353.61283

[23] S. Aggarwal and S. Aggarwal, "Maintaining regulatory compliance in medical devices through ISO 13485 and 14971," *Cancer Therapy & Oncology International Journal*, vol. 2, no.3, p. 555589, 2016.

[24] M. Kohani, A. Bhandare, L. Guan, and D. Pommerenke, "Evaluating characteristics of electrostatic discharge (ESD) events in wearable medical devices: comparison with IEC 61000-4-2 Standard), *IEEE Transactions on Electromagnetic Compatibility*, vol. 60, pp. 1–9, 2017, doi:10.1109/TEMC.2017.2773271.

[25] S. Pelayo, R. Marcilly, and T. Belland, "Human factors engineering for medical devices: European regulation and current issues," *International Journal of Quality in Health Care*, vol. 33, no. 1, pp. 31–36, 2020.

[26] K. M. Rojas, L. Cosler, and D. L. Santos, "A narrative review of FDA human factors validation requirement: the needs of key stakeholders and proposal of an industry (human factors service providers) maturity assessment tool," in *Proceedings of the International Symposium on Human Factors and Ergonomics in Health Care*, vol. 8, pp. 222–233, 2019, doi:10.1177/2327857919081056.

[27] P. Rust, D. Flood, and F. McCaffery, "Creation of an IEC 62304 compliant software development plan," *Journal of Software: Evolution of Process*, vol. 28, no. 11, pp. 1005–1010, 2016.

[28] A. Varri, P. K. Zuppan, and R. D. L. Cruz, "IEC 62304 Ed. 2: software life cycle standard for health software," in *2019 International Medical Informatics Association (IMIA) and IOS Press*, vol. 264, pp. 868–872, 2019.

[29] A. Jain, N. Ganesh, and M. P. Venkatesh, "Quality standards for medical devices," *International Journal of Drug Regulatory Affairs*, vol. 2, no. 4, pp. 19–24, 2014.

[30] M. N. Teferra, "ISO 14971-medical device risk management standard," *International Journal of Latest Research in Engineering and Technology (IJLRET)*, vol. 3, no. 3, pp. 83–87, 2017.

[31] W. Y. Leong, "Implementing blind source separation in signal processing and telecommunications," Thesis, The University of Queensland, Australia, 2005.

[32] W. Y. Leong and D. P. Mandic, "Towards adaptive blind extraction of post-nonlinearly mixed signals," in *16th IEEE Signal Processing Society Workshop on Machine Learning for Signal Processing*, pp. 91–96, 2006, doi: 10.1109/MLSP.2006.275528.

[33] W. Y. Leong, J. Homer, and D. P. Mandic, "An implementation of nonlinear multiuser detection in Rayleigh fading channel," *EURASIP Journal on Wireless Communications and Networking*, pp. 1–9, 2006.

[34] W. Y. Leong, J. H. Chuah, and T. B. Tuan (eds.), *The Nine Pillars of Technologies for Industry 4.0.* Stevenage, UK: Institution of Engineering and Technology, 2020.

[35] M. Palaniswamy and W. Y. Leong, "Mechanical properties of the human vertebrae between normal, post corrective and post operative," in *2014 IEEE International Symposium on Robotics and Manufacturing Automation (ROMA)*, Kuala Lumpur, pp. 188–193, 2014, doi: 10.1109/ROMA.2014.7295886.

[36] W. Y. Leong, *Human Machine Collaboration and Interaction for Smart Manufacturing: Automation, robotics, sensing, artificial intelligence, 5G, IoTs and Blockchain.* Stevenage, UK: Institution of Engineering and Technology, 2022.

[37] W. Y. Leong, *Medical Equipment Engineering: Design, manufacture and applications.* Stevenage, UK: The Institution of Engineering and Technology, 2023.

[38] W. Y. Leong and J. Homer, "Blind multiuser receiver in Rayleigh fading channel," in *2005 Australian Communications Theory Workshop*, pp. 155–161, 2005.

[39] W. Xiaofan, P. H. J. Chong and W. Y. Leong, "Performance comparison of CSMA/CD, CSMA/CA, CSMA/RI, CSMA/PRI and CSMA/PR with BEB," in *5th IEEE Conference on Industrial Electronics and Applications*, Taichung, pp. 1843–1848, 2010, doi: 10.1109/ICIEA.2010.5515401.

[40] H. F. Min, W. Y. Leong, "Investigating target detection and localization in wireless sensor network," *Procedia Engineering*, vol. 41, pp. 75–81, 2012.

[41] U. Mehrotra and W. Y. Leong, "NSEEAR: A energy adaptive routing protocol for heterogeneous wireless sensor networks," in *35th Annual Conference of IEEE Industrial Electronics*, Porto, Portugal, pp. 2647–2652, 2009, doi: 10.1109/IECON.2009.5415255.

[42] W. Xiaofan, P. H. J. Chong and W. Y. Leong, "Evaluation of performance on random back-off interval and multi-channel CSMA/CA protocols," in *TENCON 2009–2009 IEEE Region 10 Conference*, Singapore, pp. 1–5, 2009, doi: 10.1109/TENCON.2009.5396103.

[43] W. Y. Leong and J. Homer, "EKENS: A learning on nonlinear blindly mixed signals," in *IEEE International Conference on Acoustics, Speech and Signal Processing (ICASSP 2005)*, Philadelphia, PA, USA, vol. 4, pp. 81–84, 2005.

[44] M. Palaniswamy and W. Y. Leong, "Head and neck posture in young adults with chronic neck pain," *International Journal of Recent Advances in Multidisciplinary Research*, vol. 4, no. 11, pp. 2946–2951, 2017.

[45] C. R. Andrew Ng, W. Y. Leong, "An EEG-based approach for left-handedness detection," *Biomedical Signal Processing and Control*, vol. 10, pp. 92–101, 2014.

Chapter 11

Reimagining medical equipment engineering education: does industry 4.0 need education 4.0?

Randeep Singh Sidhu Jeswant Singh[1]

In this particular chapter that there has been a discussion on the medical equipment Engineering education and its effect on the industry 4.0 has been spoken. Further there has been the shedding of the light on the concept and current scenario of industry 4.0 and education 4.0 has been viewed. In the research methods, the effective tools have been discussed along with the inclusion and exclusion criteria and Boolean search strategy. The data types and database have also been included in this section. In this research paper, it is discussed how education 4.0 in industry 4.0 enabled personalized learning in engineering education. It also helps in the development of the medical equipment that provides technical solution to the education. It also helps in the discussion on these points that help to understand the condition of the industry 4.0.

11.1 Introduction

The primary focus of this chapter is progress on reimagining medical equipment in the field of engineering education. In this context, it is going to explain the future of medical engineering which is set up with advanced digital medical technologies such as artificial bits of intelligence, robotics, additive manufacturing, and cloud computing. The future of medical equipment in engineering education depends on advanced technologies and healthcare workers are forced to increase healthcare technologies in order to keep their importance in the future. The study is also focused on the main objectives and purpose of medical equipment in the field of education and industry sector. The background of this study is focused on education 4.0 which refers to the purposeful concept of learning which is connected with the fourth industrial revolution and concerned with changing the next education with advanced technologies.

Figure 11.1 depicts the ultrasonic molding device that is extensively used in medical industry. The use of this device is important regarding making medicine compressed pellets or pellets of other materials [1]. It is only an expel of device; however, several other devices are used in medical industry and different technologies from industry 4.0 can help to improve them, such as Internet of Things (IoT) and

[1]PEOPLElogy Group, Malaysia

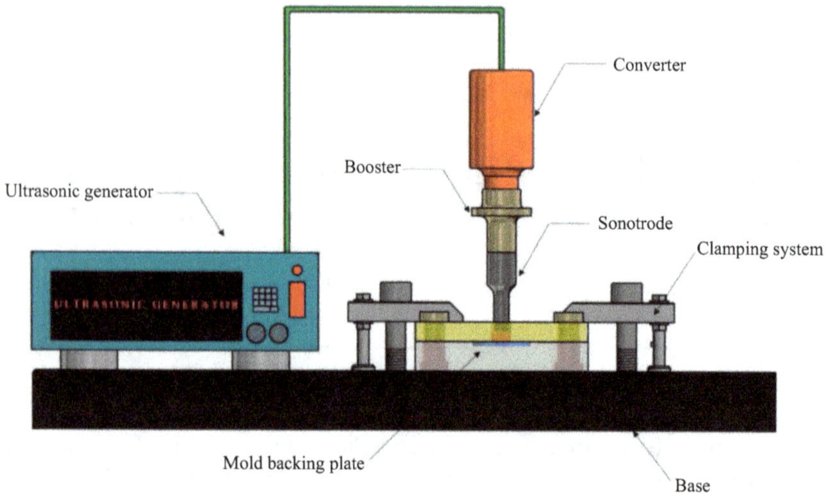

Figure 11.1 Ultrasonic compression molding platform. Source: Heredia-Rivera et al. [1].

Artificial Intelligence (AI). The study will discuss medical equipment in engineering education and in industry sectors which are analyzed by the concept of education 4.0, its present situation, and the needs of industries 4.0. The education system is directly connected with industry development so that as the industries get developed, the education system also gets developed and vice versa. Digital technologies are playing a major role in the development process so this study mainly analyses how it is affected. Furthermore, digital innovation focuses on the developed training models which results in the overall development of the educational processes and knowledge of an individual. Therefore, it can be stated that the major development process is mainly focused on digital technologies that are working in the education system.

Industry 4.0 aims to change the engineering and manufacturing sector by identifying the various factories where cyber processing systems are connected with digital technologies such as the IoT, assisting machinery, and workers to operate their tasks within time. Furthermore, Figure 11.2 depicts that different disruptive technologies have being integrated in the healthcare sector, which helps to make them more efficient in treating patients [2]. Education 4.0 has changed which is important for industry 4.0 and it helps students to get better employability and help to prepare for their future with better return expectations through education. Creativity is the main factor in industrial revolution 4.0 where trained or creative workers can control the changes or innovation in the education system. Education 4.0, it helps students to get employability with proper training.

11.1.1 Aims

The aim of the study is "*to identify the needs of Education 4.0 in Industry 4.0 for remaining Medical Equipment Engineering Education*."

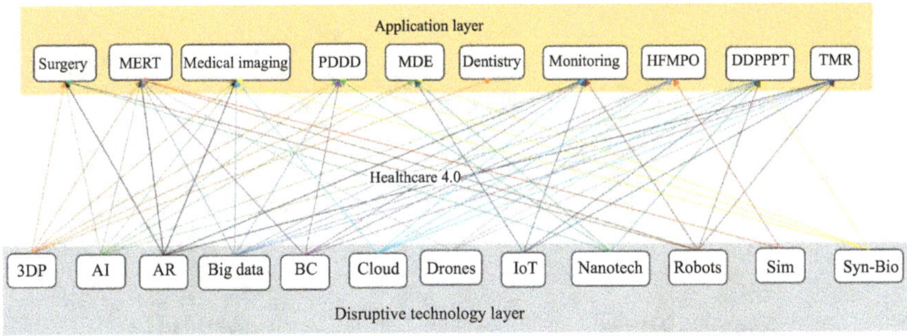

Figure 11.2 Disruptive technologies converging in healthcare. Source: Bongomin et al. [2].

11.1.2 Objective

- To identify the need for education 4.0 in industry 4.0 for reimagining medical equipment engineering education
- To evaluate the current system of education in industry 4.0 for reimagining medical equipment engineering education
- To assess the impact of digital technologies in education that needs for industry 4.0 in engineering education
- To investigate new models of education 4.0 in industry 4.0 for remaining medical equipment engineering education

11.2 Background

11.2.1 Education 4.0 looks like

Education 4.0 is a technique of learning that is connected with the fourth industrial revolution and also focuses on changes in the future of the education sector through advanced automation and technology. It is purposeful concepts that help to learn that connect with the fourth industrial revolution and also help to transform the future in the sector of education by using advanced technologies [3]. Education 4.0 mainly focuses on the knowledge development processes of through implementation and inclusion of modern technologies. The main focus is to develop knowledge among the people regarding the basic areas through a refined pragmatic and practical approach. It includes usages of technologies such as Virtual Reality, Augmented Reality and even Artificial Intelligence. The focus is given on areas of knowledge that are important and contents that might be harmful are often filtered through implementation of Education 4.0.

In Figure 11.3, it has been seen that education 4.0 encourages digital education which helps in the modernization which helps in development of industry 4.0 [5]. It has enhanced its branches to use digital technologies in an innovative way. Education 4.0 involves various sectors where educational activities can grow rapidly [6]. Education 4.0 involves AI, machine learning, business analytics, digital marketing, investor markets, MIS, SAP family business management, and hospitality management.

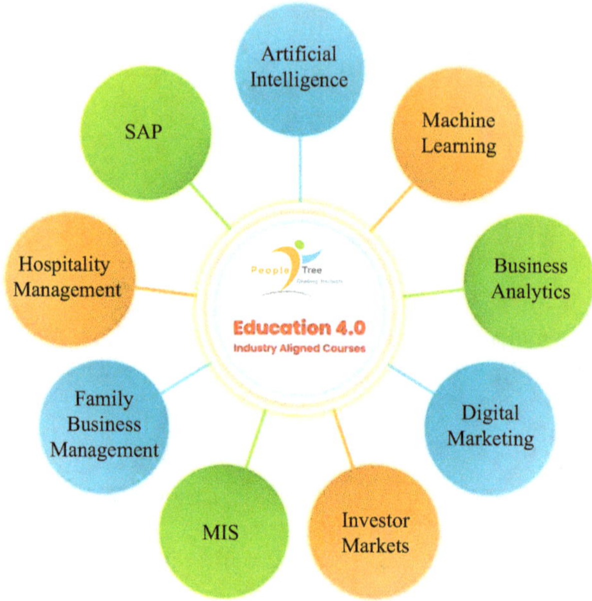

Figure 11.3 Education 4.0. Source: PTeS.edu.in [4].

These fields of study help in the growth of the educational field in an innovative way. These sources are interconnected with each other and flourished globally.

Education is an integral part of human development and through this education, humans can develop their wealth and can employability easily. Education 4.0 will use technologies that do not exist at present, and it will focus on creative thinking rather than rote learning [7]. On the other hand, it is also said that creativity is also a key feature of industrial revolution 4.0. Only trained and skilled workers can control the innovative changes and the concepts of mechanisms in the education system. According to education 4.0, it helps students to get employability which is the purpose to take any challenges.

There are major trends of education 4.0 that includes personalized learning, remote learning opportunities, a plethora of education tools, project-based learning, easy and accurate assessment, and data at the fingertips. The education system assists the students to develop self-confidence and knowledge to provide better work. In addition to this, it also focuses to increase learning surrounding to develop the abilities of all students that are near them. The education 4.0 system assists to grow the industry revolution 4.0 that can immediately affect the country's development. Moreover, the learning process when complete in a fun or interesting way the understanding of students gets also enhanced. It provides theoretical knowledge to students that they can learn about time management skills, collaborative skills, organizational skills, and leadership skills that are needed for their employees for future success.

Education 4.0 is the key factor for future circumstances; it is all about involving in the times and for higher education systems and helps to understand major requirements of their future success [8]. The method to connect industry requirements with education such as *remodeling of curriculum, building digital skills, opting for digital tools for virtual learning, tweaking course delivery, and technology-building classrooms* are most useful. These are some methods that can prepare students with education 4.0 to attempt their future challenges. Some of the top digital skills and requirements that education 4.0 has to demand the students are such as complex problem solving, cognitive flexibility, negotiation, coordinating with others, emotional bits of intelligence, judgment and decision making, critical thinking creativity, and services orientation. Such types of skills are demandable for education 4.0 for preparing the student with good training and controlling the change in the education system.

11.3 Medical equipment engineering education in industry 4.0

11.3.1 Concept of education 4.0

"***Engineering Education 4.0***" is the education and its approaches that have shown a lot of inspiration from the industry 4.0 revolution. It has shown a lot of flawlessness and satisfaction for making a lot of time-saving in engineering education [9]. It helps in doing a lot of the skill development and the efficiency in the overpowering study of the education of engineering. Industry 4.0 is a type of the current trend of automation and the exchanging of data in the manufacturing technology as the major part has included cyber-physical systems. Cognitive learning and the techniques given to the facilities are available of the content of the understanding. The information processing is enabled for problem-solving skills and the enhancement of the learning.

There has been a need for a huge education 4.0 of biomedical engineering in industry 4.0 and because of this, a few of the industries still need the eventual shifting of the computerization of the manufacturing of and the designing of medical equipment. There has been a need for education 4.0 so that engineers can bring a lot of rapid innovation in the industrial revolution for getting more of the data. Modern medical equipment is evolving fast but there has been a lack of education and it needs a lot of developed engineering education. The following is the education innovation that was oriented in biomedical engineering. In engineering of the education 4.0, the engineers are taught about the technology with the use of the IoT, additive manufacturing, and many more other things [2].

In fact, it has been seen that the current medical technology engineering courses have been designed for showing the impact of the different knowledge from the natural sciences in medical equipment education [10]. There has been training on systems such as the IoT that have a connection with the machine–human and other machines. Figure 11.4 shows the blueprint of a medical manufacturing device uses computer-aided design (CAD). Moreover, it is a reconfigurable manufacturing

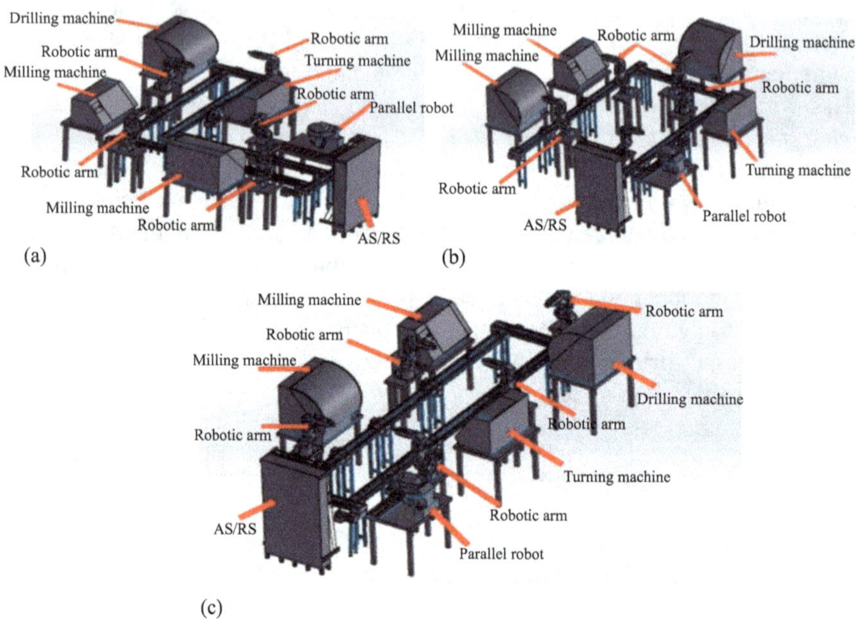

Figure 11.4 CAD modeling of L-shaped RMS system. Source: Salah et al. [11].

system (RMS) device and VR technology had been incorporated to teach students to operate this machine [11]. Education 4.0 has been giving a lot of catering to the needs of the society in the era of innovation in medical equipment engineering education which has been very much helpful for industry 4.0 [12].

11.3.2 Current scenario of industry 4.0 in education

Today many of the medical equipment-making industry has been trying to make a lot of the adoption in digital technology very aggressively. However, it has been said that this adoption of the new technology in the industry has been possible due to the reason of providing education 4.0 to the engineering student or the engineers [13]. Due to the effect or the outbursts of the Corona virus, all the industry has been trying to focus on the creation of the operation across the making of medical equipment in a more advanced way. The prime focus in the current scenario is the accumulation of the transformation of the biomedical industry into industry 4.0 through education 4.0. Technologies are mainly based on machinery because when machinery is not developed, the technologies cannot be adapted. In Education 4.0, machinery is mainly dependent on education because as the education system grows, the technologies play a major role. IoT is a major factor in changing the education system as in the education system internet plays a major role.

This figure has shown the current scenario of industry 4.0 in education. United States is the leading country in industry 4.0 where it receives 28% of the population all over the world due to the modern technologies and skills of the population [14].

Various technologies are adapted for the development of better educational facilities. On the other hand, it is also that Germany receives moderate education where the population rises only 25%. Besides, there are many countries like France, China, and the Netherlands that receive the lowest population for education 4.0.

It has been seen that education 4.0 has given a lot of fundamental changes in the business of the industry revolution [15]. Moreover, it has been said that education has brought a lot of the shifting from traditional manufacturing to industry 4.0. Engineers in biomedical technology have been enabling the setting of the technology that includes the automatic robot, simulation of the technology, cloud computing, and big data. It has been noted that through education 4.0, there has been the possibility of getting the Revolution of Forth Industry in the intelligence with the value chains and the product life cycles. The industry growth is happening a lot so that there have been many difficulties facing the manufacturing of medical devices [16]. There have been a lot of problems that have been faced due to the effect of the quality control in all the devices. There are many ways education 4.0 and changing the medical devices of the future will improve the industry. It has been seen that the application of smart technology has enabled unwieldy devices to be portable. The industry is trying to build up an upgraded version of the glucose monitoring systems through the hands of modern engineers. Some of the medical equipment industry is trying hard to build up automation in insulin pumping. The reason is so that through which the pumps or the system can be taken and transported easily.

11.3.3 Effect of digital technology on education

Emerging technology has been fundamental, and its transformation has created a lot of interaction with medical devices. In the past decade, technology has been going through contributions contributing interesting features to the product and its standards. The infant industry has realized that consistency and efficiency have been included in the introduction of medical devices. It is trying to create a lot of innovation in the mind for working in the industry for mitigating the needs of the customer. On the other hand, the application of digital technology used as AI is one of the most important technologies that have been released in industry 4.0 [17]. AI-powered technology helps in the development of natural language processing along with audio recognition for getting interacted and consumed with the media. This also helps the people to access the organizational data which is needed by the people. In the context of the medical education, the use of AI is too useful as it helps in improving the diagnosis accuracy and in streaming medical training programs. Moreover, the use of artificial technologies also helps in establishing a proper relationship with the healthcare givers and healthcare professionals. Thereafter, it develops the learning experiences in the educational development in the current situation. It helps the medical education about the content of keeping up to date about the inclusion of the education and its environment. There have been a lot of problems that have been faced due to the effect of the quality control in all the devices.

The improvement in education sectors depends on the integration of digital technologies. However, this also helps to keep a continuous improvement of the overall education sector for contributing to career growth. On the other hand, the implementation of different advanced technologies within the education sector helps to cover the annual course for the students. Moreover, the analysis of *AI, the IoT*, and *machine learning* improves the overall infrastructure of education as most students are able to encourage their bright future. The implementation of different educational platforms also depends on the use of digital technologies while dealing with more improvement in personal and professional growth. The implementation of a daily routine based on the use of innovative techniques is also useful for most students to deal with innovative digital techniques within the course structure. Moreover, the level of intelligence among the students has been increased through the use of different digital tools within the course curriculum.

11.3.4 Need for industry 4.0 in education

It has been observed in the last few decades about witnessing the birth of technological advancement in the industry. It includes the IoT, AI with a lot of machine learning. This technology and its education have brought up a lot of the transition in industry 4.0 for getting the digitalization of manufacturing and gaining a lot of profit. It has been said that this has given a lot of the new hybrid and its concepts that have been leading to the management of the different types of efficiency in the use of the IoT in the new technologies [18]. It can be said that the advancement of digital technology has been bringing up a lot of jobs that will help in making medical equipment.

Digital technology has revolutionized medical equipment engineering and its education [19]. There is a huge demand for industry 4.0 in education due to the demand for technology which is present in innovative ways. The innovative strategies are developed and adopted for the development of the industry 4.0 which are required for the development of the industry 4.0. Artificial technology, robotics, and IoT are required for the development of industry 4.0. In the advanced world, the techniques have to be innovative, and skill based which when applied to give better outcomes in education. Education is such a platform that requires a huge demand for technologies for better application which help in the growth of the technologies. Amidst of COVID-19 various strategies are applied for the development of education. Various innovative strategies are adopted for the development of education. The digital apps although help in education, it also makes the communication strong between the people.

It can be said that the future of education and its system will help the preparation of the student for the demands of the future in the manufacturing industry 4.0. In some advanced countries, the education system of the engineer has been taking up a step ahead for the reorientation of the education system for betterment in the suiting of the industry with a lot of the modern ideas [20]. It will help the fourth industry for manufacturing many of the advanced medical products and it will help in better work in life. It will help in the creation of data science and advancement with a lot of technology awareness and the understanding of the impact of the technology.

11.3.5 Analysis of engineering education

The new model of Engineering Education is mainly focused to develop scientific subjects such as Math and Science group subjects. The subject mainly assists to enhance the effectiveness of engineers and expects better work from them. It will help in designing the pairing of the broad set of soft skills that are essential for success. It will help in bringing up a lot of creativity while working in the industry globally [21]. In today's fourth revolution industry, there has been a possibility that the application of the T model will give the definition and light towards the future of the successful and its engineering.

It will give the idea about the engineer to become a clear innovation with a lot of ethics and humanistic for clearly communicating with each other. The demand for engineering and its education among graduates is increasing daily due to the current services and the technology for meeting the different types of needs of society and the increase of work in the future [22]. This type of education has to lead to the proper education for which industry 4.0 will get a lot of the effect and the technological development of the industry will get a lot of the enhancement [23].

11.3.6 Evaluation of current system of medical equipment engineering education

The evaluation of the current system of medical equipment in engineering education considers the following engineers who make medical equipment. There is a particularly strong demand for medical equipment engineering education for the industry by using digital technologies where it can be shown that almost 20% of all biomedical engineers are employed [24].

11.3.6.1 Robotics engineer

Robotics engineering is very complex which shows the engineer working in a robotics position and is responsible for programming, analyzing, testing, and designing the robot system that can work in replacing humans. It is one of the digital technologies in engineering education for industry 4.0 [25]. A robotics engineer designs robotics software that is used for developing vital robotics systems to save lives in the medical field.

11.3.6.2 Medical device design engineer

Medical device designers are highly responsible for designing, envisioning, and producing modern tools and equipment which can be used for diverse surgical processes. These devices can be used in clinics or other medical elements [26].

11.3.6.3 Imaging engineer

The role of an imaging engineer involves the installation, maintenance, and inspection of medical imaging equipment. These specific types of imagine engineers have a duty to install, repair, and perform to manage medical equipment such as CT equipment, arthroscopic equipment, and so on.

11.3.6.4 Biomedical engineer

Biomedical engineers have greatly contributed to the advancement of medical equipment and technologies. Biomedical engineers develop digital technologies such as medical diagnostic machines, artificial organs, and prosthetic devices [27].

11.3.7 Relation between industry 4.0 and education 4.0 in medical equipment engineering education

The strong relationship between Industry 4.0 and Education 4.0 acts as one of the major and significant ineffective factors in the education system, the focus of education changes to more practical and experience based concepts that are trying to connect industry, and this is what created the educational revolution is called education 4.0. It is a conceptual method for the future of education that responds to the need of the industrial revolution. On the other hand, the main objective of industry 4.0 is to make the manufacturing process easy and faster, and customer-centric beyond automation and optimization to search for new business opportunities and theories. The impact of industry 4.0 is in many fields such as business, government, and medical.

In Figure 11.5, industry revenue for medical equipment is shown from the year 2016 to 2027. It has been shown that the years 2012, 2013, 2014, 2015, 2016, and 2017 have high industry revenue for medical equipment sector [28]. It has also shown that from the year 2020 onwards due to the pandemic situation, the economic condition gets hampered which lowers the industrial revenue. It is also shown that in the middle of 2019, the industrial revenue was lowered down.

The development of the computer into a cyber-physical system led to the growth of advances and modern technology systems such as *cloud computing, machine learning, augmented, data sciences, the IoT, and virtual reality are some of the successful achievements of the industrial revolution* [29]. Some of the major value points related to aligning the industry and education system such as building a flexible learning path, continuous teacher training, more divergences, and pluralism, education must be a goal target.

11.3.8 Concept gap

In this particular chapter, the main issue that has been faced is the sign in the problem by the analyzer or the investigator. The main issue is that there has been a huge issue

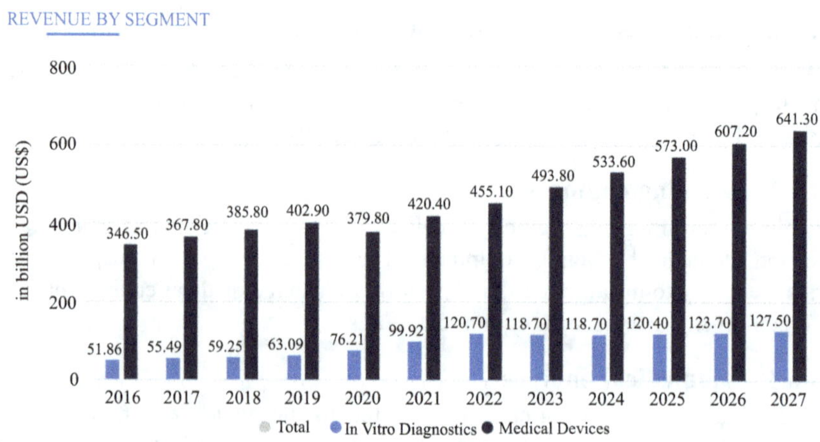

Figure 11.5 Industry revenue of medical equipment. Source: Statista [28].

relating to the gathering of the information on the current study of the making of the article. There have been a very few limitations in the information for the accumulation of the creation of the conclusion at the end [30]. Moreover, it has been seen that as a part of the comparison, it has been noted that secondary data has provided a lot of information or knowledge about the study topic. However, this has created a lot of issues regarding the collection of a huge amount of information from secondary sources. There has been a lack of data authentication of the source as there have been no proper sources for cross-checking the data. This led the investigator to take into consideration the adequate number of theories and models for getting any type of relation to the research topic. In the end, it can be said that the concept of the topic is not very clear to the investigators [31]. Hence, still, there has been the presence of a conclusion at the end but it has been very much vague for the chapter.

11.4 Methods

11.4.1 Data collection strategy

Data collection is a crucial factor in industry 4.0 as it helps to generate raw and unbiased information, which can be used to reduce several issues. In medical engineering and education industry, this aspect is important as several technologies generating data and transforming them helps to have a better understanding of any situation and process. Moreover, in many cases, it can be beneficial to reduce the expense of resources and maintaining safety. The use of AR and VR technology is one such example where the trainee or student uses virtual interaction to understand the process of different tools and techniques. Therefore, in other cases, these techniques can be modified to get necessary data out of different processes and techniques and this is the primary aspect of implementation of technology in medical engineering and education.

11.4.2 Data types

In a research process, data types are divided into two types: primary data types and secondary data types. The primary data types are interviews (face-to-face or telephone), surveys (mail or online), questionnaires (paper or online), focus groups, and locations of competitors. The secondary data types are usually books, journals, articles, and websites.

Industry 4.0 is all about data and using them efficiently to resolve issue, which is similar in the case of medical industry. Here, data comes in different forms such as visual, nominal, audio, and other means; however, the primary goals stay the same to use these data to generate relevant knowledge that can help to improve the bigger issues in medical sector.

11.4.3 Data collection method

In the research study, the data collection method is an essential tool as it helps in collecting relevant information in an effective way which is more necessary to the respective research [32]. There are usually two types of data collection methods used in most research processes and those are the primary method. The methods are further classified into two subdivisions: quantitative and qualitative. The primary data collection method deals with the process of collecting relevant information from direct sources through the process of interviews or surveys.

Data collecting in industry 4.0 is primarily based on through different technologies such as IoT, data collection devices, or through manual process. Then, they are managed properly to get relevant information out of them. This information then can be implemented in personalized treatment for each patient to improve their treatment process. Other than that, these data, in some cases, may help to identify and mitigate rare issues and diseases. However, data collection in the medical industry can be used in many cases, such as example would be automating different medical devices through the implementation of IoT or the automation of Robots. In addition, AI (artificial technologies) is used to make different digital processes smart.

In this research process, the data has been collected from secondary sources maintaining the secondary data collection method [33]. The effective data has been collected from the relevant articles and journals without diverging from the main topic of the research in terms of the impact or requirement of education 4.0 for the purpose of industry 4.0. Along with this, the secondary method has been chosen as it can help in compiling, gathering, and analyzing the information which has been gained from the previous research [34].

11.4.4 Inclusion and exclusion criteria

Table 11.1 Inclusive and exclusive criteria

Parameters	Inclusion criteria	Exclusion criteria
Study topic: "*Reimagining Medical Equipment Engineering Education: Does Industry 4.0 Need Education 4.0*"	• Reimagining the future scope of the medical industry through advanced technologies regarding the fourth industrial revolution • Industry 4.0 and its requirement of education 4.0 in terms of medical equipment engineering purposes	• Diverged from the fourth revolution of industry and educational purposes regarding engineering studies and medical equipment • Unclear or insufficiency in the discussion of the research topic of industry 4.0 and education 4.0.
Study type	Empirical research and academic theoretical aspects such as chapters from books, journal papers, professional reports, web pages, press articles, thesis, research notes, and abstracts	Ambiguous research process and methodology
Study language	Written in the English language	Written in another language or in a mixed language
Study frame-time	Published from 2017 onwards with extra concentration on studies of the research topic	Published before 2017

Source: Self-made.

11.4.5 Database

This research has been based on some effective points or keywords such as industry 4.0, education 4.0, current education system, digital technologies, the new model of engineering education, AI, cloud computing, and medical equipment. The research process is associated with the main topic of the research in terms of the requirement of education 4.0 for the industrial revolution and development [35]. From the entire research, it has been extracted that the need of understanding the main purpose of the industrial revolution is essential in order to align the education 4.0 revolution in terms of engineering education and digital technologies [36]. The information about the advanced model of the engineering education system has also been known from the research study along with the current education systems. The research keywords can help the users in getting relevant records by searching with those terms [37].

11.4.6 Database search strategy

The Boolean strategy in a research method allows the researcher to combine or limit the searched variables of a research study. Utilizing Boolean terms such as AND, OR, and NOT, the searcher can define the interrelation among the relevant concepts. The OR term is used to broaden the results as this can expand the search in order to incorporate all records or data containing either concept. The AND term is used to narrow the results of the search and this only instructs the user regarding the resource in retrieving only those records or documents having both the phrase and words. On the other hand, the term NOT is used to narrow the results by removing specific words from the search.

In Figure 11.6, the OR Boolean term has been shown to be based on the research topic [38]. This search strategy is effective for this particular research as this has helped the user in getting all the necessary documents and records as this can increase the possibility of removing relevancy while the best keywords have not been searched or selected.

11.4.7 Big data

Big data is an important factor to consider in the case of industry 4.0. Relevancy of big data is important as it has vast historical data that comprises of human interaction, behavior, choices, and their change overtime. It is crucial to consider these factors in the healthcare and medical sectors as it helps to design effective medicines, treatments, and devices, which resolve the critical, rare and chronic diseases. Managing big data was troublesome in past as it needed proper computation, processing power to untangle unstructured and irrelevant data [39]. However, industry 4.0 has enabled different industries including medical industries to manage these data and generate proper structure data for future that can be utilized in future with more efficiency. Therefore, it can be considered that big data has a crucial role in upcoming medical revolution.

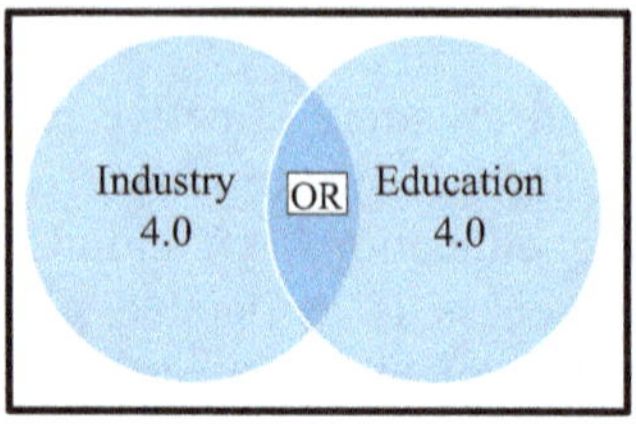

Figure 11.6 Boolean strategy: OR. Source: Self-made.

11.4.8 Ethics

The research process has been done by maintaining proper ethical codes in the proper way. The ideas and knowledge that are gathered from the research have not been misused. The provenance of collected data has been maintained. The researcher has accessed the data from authentic websites which are legal and government approved. Along with this, the journals and books that are used by the researcher have not been broken or deprived of further usage in terms of copyright issues. The language is properly maintained while conducting the research in order to avoid any inconveniences. Data sharing, storage, and compiling have been done by maintaining ethics.

11.5 Findings

11.5.1 Current engineering education in education 4.0 provides the requirements of industry 4.0

The modified industry 4.0 perished carries new cross-functional responsibilities with various skills and knowledge that can combine product knowledge and information technology. The universities and engineering departments play a vital role in the fulfilment of the basic requirements of technological purposes. Industry 4.0 becomes essential in terms of trending toward information exchange and manufacturing automation throughout the entire system of manufacturing [40]. It is the shift beyond automation to machines of cyber-physical purpose. The evaluation of educational objectives has been based on some precise classification regarding skills and knowledge areas offered by the current adaptation of engineering departments by implementing advanced technologies.

Figure 11.7 indicates the increasing value of education 4.0 in engineering education for improving the requirements of industry 4.0. Additionally, the value of education 4.0 increased by $750 million in 2020 [41]. On the other hand, the fourth evaluation of industry 4.0 has achieved a growth of 92% in 2020 based on the integration with technical advantages such as ***AI, machine learning***, and ***the IoT***. These have helped enough to improve creativity and performance of engineering growth, which indicates to deal with the critical challenges while developing industry 4.0. Additionally, ***cloud computing*** has also helped software companies to deal with the critical challenges in industry 4.0 while focusing on the improvement

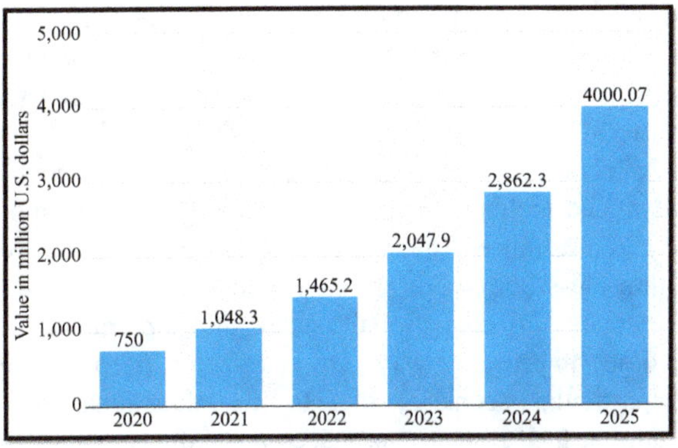

Figure 11.7 Value of education 4.0 in engineering education. Source: Statista [42].

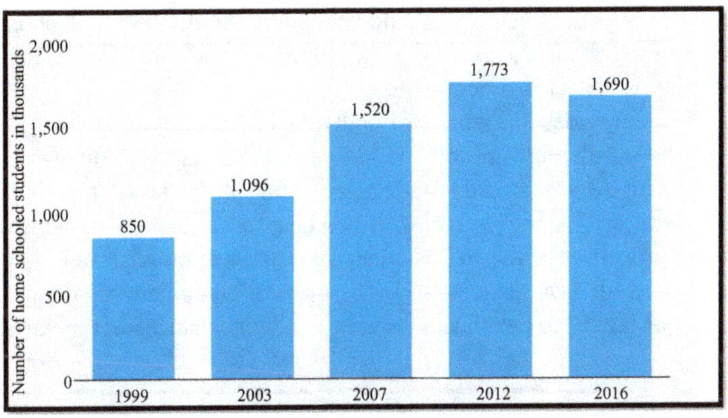

Figure 11.8 Growth in education 4.0 through digital tools. Source: Weforum [44].

of engineering education [43]. It also has been identified that "***public cloud service***" makes the growth of the cloud computing market and has amounted to $12 billion in 2020. This often has a market share of 4% within the "***global public cloud market***" and has improved industry 4.0 with integration with cloud computing.

Figure 11.8 provides the growth in education 4.0 with the help of digital tools during the era of the pandemic outbreak. This includes the increasing number of students of 1,773 based on the integration with digital tools. The overall performance also depends on the capabilities and understanding based on the use of digital tools within education 4.0 while improving engineering education [45]. However, cloud infrastructure includes an investment of £1.3 billion in 2019 for improving the knowledge skills of IT professionals within industry 4.0 [11]. Industry 4.0 refers to the generally used term regarding the consideration of the fourth industrial revolution which is recently underway and, in this regard, the effect of digital technologies like the IoT, robotics, additive manufacturing, AI, cloud computing, etc. become the hallmarks of the transformation. Education 4.0

deals with the purposeful approach and objectives of learning that can line up with this fourth industrial revolution by providing necessary requirements in terms of the future scope of education [46]. This scenario is basically about the transformation of the feasibility of industry 4.0 utilizing advanced technology as well as automation.

Figure 11.8 reflects the increasing number of applicants in education 4.0 based on the use of advanced technologies in universities. There are more than 63,690 applicants have taken admitted to universities due to the effective use of smart technologies within classrooms. For the universities in order to be regular in proceeding with the successful educational aspect, the implementation of advanced technologies becomes an effective way to modernize the purpose of education [47]. Regarding this particular scenario, this fourth educational revolution assists industry 4.0 in gaining the effective and necessary requirement of improvement in different areas as the industrial revolution mainly focuses on smart technologies. Industry revolution has been controlled by effective digital tools and therefore can introduce the future model of education by concentrating on smart, comprehensive, mobile, and virtual skill development and education. Along with this, education 4.0 can denote the modification, relevant to the fourth revolution of the industry along with responding to the global acquisition.

Figure 11.9 provides the share of individuals learning in online, which has increased by 46% for the age group of 15–24 years [48]. Starting from Smartphone to robotic equipment, AI has already started generating its presence that is felt in the industry of healthcare. Along with this, it has been progressively demonstrating the transformative properties of the IoT that can drive innovation regarding the improvement of associated medical devices [49]. The medical equipment regarding engineering education has related to healthcare devices. Gradual enhancement in the number of

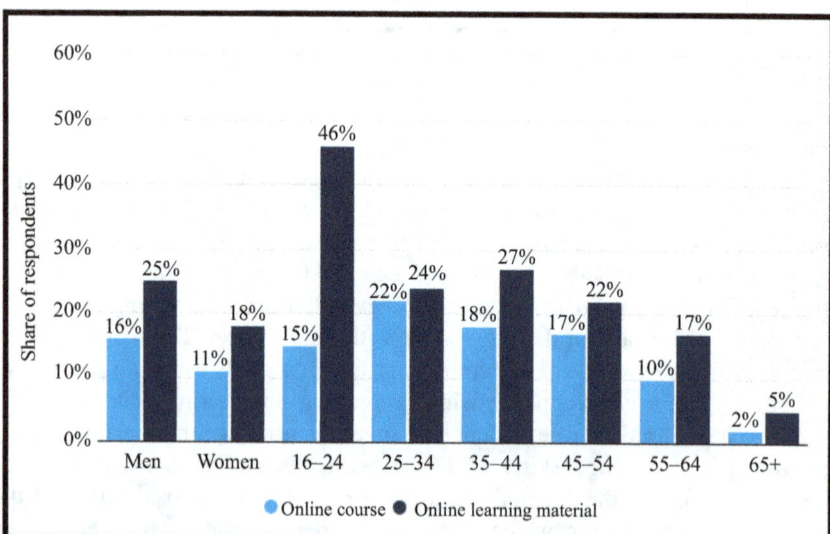

Figure 11.9 Share of individuals learning from online in UK. Source: Statista [48].

associated medical equipment with the advancement of technology helps in capturing as well as transmitting almost all types of medical-related information whenever and wherever needed to the respective area. Therefore, it has given birth to the "Internet-of-Medical-Things" (IoMT) in which IoT meets with healthcare. This technology helps in monitoring the behavior of patients and this further helps the medical educational purpose by helping the medical students in an effective way. Education 4.0 usually involves the utilization of technical equipment as supportive tools for the education sector and focuses on innovative and smart technology.

11.5.2 Education 4.0 in industry 4.0 enables personalized learning of students in engineering education

In this chapter, it is discussed how education 4.0 in industry 4.0 enabled personalized learning in engineering education. It is also discussed how it is influencing engineering education. It is allowing the students to adopt modern infrastructure and technologies to improve their modern education. It also helps in the development of the paradigms toward the innovation of modern technologies.

Education 4.0 is the modern version of learning and teaching which involves some innovative technologies. It involves collaborative learning along with information and communication technologies of learning. In this 4.0 education system, the evolution of the Internet along with information technologies has offered good learning outcomes. It involves some strategies, which are helping both education 4.0 and industry 4.0 is knowledge generation, new learning outcomes, and smart and sustainable infrastructure to improve the learning process in the industry [50].

Figure 11.10 illustrates the annual investment in digital operations aimed at improving Industry 4.0 through innovative practices. It can be said that these investments are crucial for operating Industry 4.0 businesses effectively in the digital realm. Sectors such as electronics, aerospace, defense and security, automotive, chemicals, engineering and construction, industrial manufacturing, transportation and logistics, metals, and others are necessary for the growth of the Industry 4.0 sector and to enhance digital operations.

New learning outcomes play a pivotal role in the development of Industry 4.0. They contribute to the advancement of learning techniques, resulting in improved learning outcomes. Furthermore, they facilitate the generation of innovative ideas and theories, which in turn contribute to better learning outcomes. The digital learning infrastructure is a smart and sustainable system that supports the learning process. It also promotes social and political development among students, positively influencing their overall personal growth, particularly those pursuing engineering education.

The IoT is helping the learning outcomes and significantly impacting learning. It helps in the digitalization of education to make learning active digitally. It also enhances the teaching-learning process. It also maintains a sustainable infrastructure within the education system. In the year 2020, due to the pandemic situation, most educational institutions have adopted the virtual mode of education that helps in the teaching-learning process.

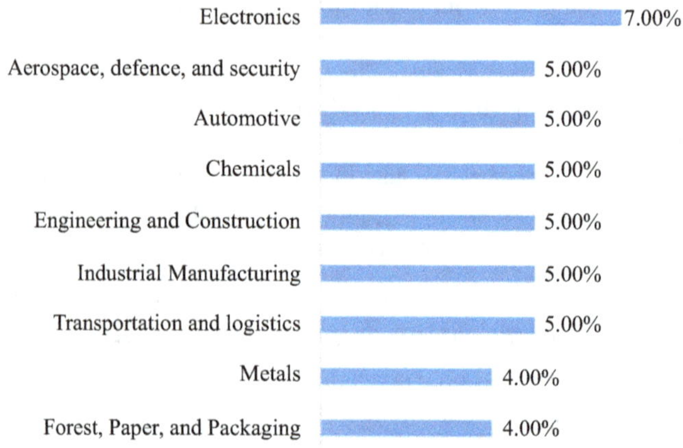

Figure 11.10 Investment of digital operations in industry 4.0. Source: Statista [51].

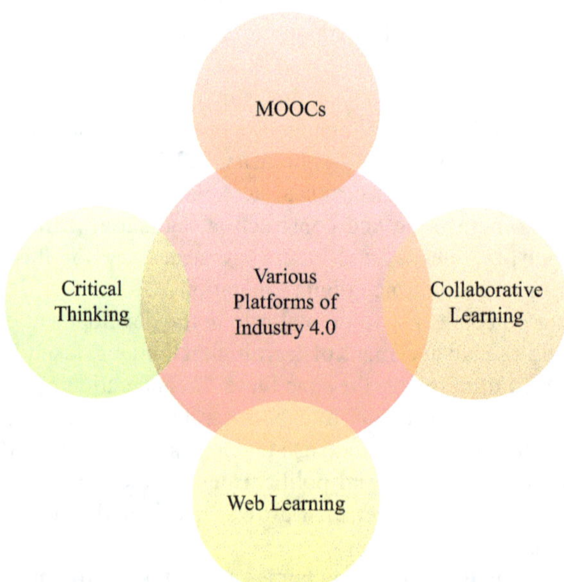

Figure 11.11 Various platforms of industry 4.0. Source: Self-created.

11.5.3 Medical equipment engineering provides a technical solution in education 4.0

Medical 4.0 develops strategies for the medical equipment to provide the technical solution in education 4.0. Medical 4.0 uses better strategies and modern technologies for the development of technical solutions in education 4.0. It uses modern technologies to connect with patients of hospitals by developing better technologies [52]. The medical 4.0 technologies are the most important part of the education which handles the individual in the hospital. Implications of digital technologies in different tools and equipment are the primary aspects of industry 4.0. It can be said that implementation of technologies, such as AI and IoT, has helped to make different technologies smarter. This aspect is crucial to gathering necessary data and act on them effectively. Prior to industry 4.0, most of the devices were analog and had to used manually; however, the current goal of industry 4.0 is to improve the usability of medical equipment, which is also applicable for educational purpose. Communication between the patients is the most important for the development of strong relationships between the patients and healthcare sectors. It also influences social media along with other online modes of communication.

There are 14% of the medical equipment that can be achieved through technical solutions, which has increased the overall efficiency as well [53]. Telemedicine or e-medicines are playing a major role in the healthcare sector which is helping in medical diagnosis. Sensors are also playing the most important role in the healthcare sector. It is also providing wireless sensors which are used for blood samples, and pharmaceuticals and also help in better treatment and prevention. They played the most important role in customer satisfaction which is the main aim for the development of the industry. The safety and quality of the patients depend upon the medical equipment used by the healthcare sector [54]. It is also maintaining the other infrastructure of the healthcare system which includes AI. AI has played the most important factors in the development of the industry. It also helps in improving the healthcare system. It also influences engineering education which decreases the risks and surgery in hospitals. It analyzes the data for the proper detection of the disease.

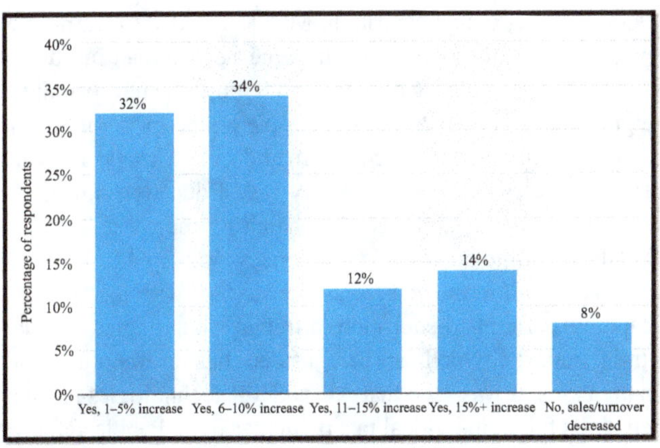

Figure 11.12 Growth of medical equipment through the technical solution. Source: Statista [55].

Data science also plays the most important part in the development of education 4.0. Various gadgets and models are used for examining crucial data. The IoT is used for data collection and also maintains the quality of the treatments. With the help of innovative technologies, the IoT can monitor treatments and improve the treatment's accuracy [7]. Besides, robotic technology also results in a low cost for implementing medical services in the healthcare sector. It also helps in the growth of industry 4.0 with the help of medical equipment.

11.5.4 Limitation and challenges for implementation

There are difficult challenges for the remaining medical equipment in engineering education. While developing technological productivity and security, it has faced price-related problems. It has also encountered high cost problems in product design and development in engineering education. According to the views of Wang *et al.* [57], challenges related to product quality and high recall rates are present in medical equipment engineering education. Consequently, the industry has encountered significant difficulties in further growth. Moreover, ensuring regulatory compliance poses a big challenge for the medical device industry. Product quality is another problem that must be addressed to run the medical industry successfully. According to Weforum [44], high cost is a major issue in running medical devices in emerging markets. Therefore, this study is limited to these challenges within the medical device industry. It is important to successfully run the medical device industry while mitigating all of these challenges.

11.6 Discussion

Today's educational sectors are very much significant for the development of digital learning. It also helps in the development of industry 4.0 which helps in the development of effective engineering education. The adoption of various innovative ideas and manufacturing systems helps in the development of the education system in industry 4.0. It mainly focuses on the IoT, online education, MOOCs, and web learning which help in collaboration within the education system. It is the new human resource management approach that helps in the flourishing of industry 4.0 [56]. The new paradigms of industry 4.0 focus on digital education which encourages the online mode of education.

Teachers are also getting privileges from the online mode of education which helps in flourishing the education in industry 4.0. Education 4.0 also helps in the development of learning institutions which also improves learning outcomes. Education 4.0 is the dynamic process that influences industry 4.0. There are changes in the digital world that result in the change in industry 4.0 with the help of technologies [57]. In medical engineering and education, different technologies of industry 4.0 have been used to train students, which can be considered as an important use of the technologies. In many cases, it was seen that AR and VR technologies has helped students to enhance their skills for an individual in a particular field. People get advantages from digital learning. Distance learning and communication also help in the development of industry 4.0 with the help of online learning tools. Knowledge is also playing the most

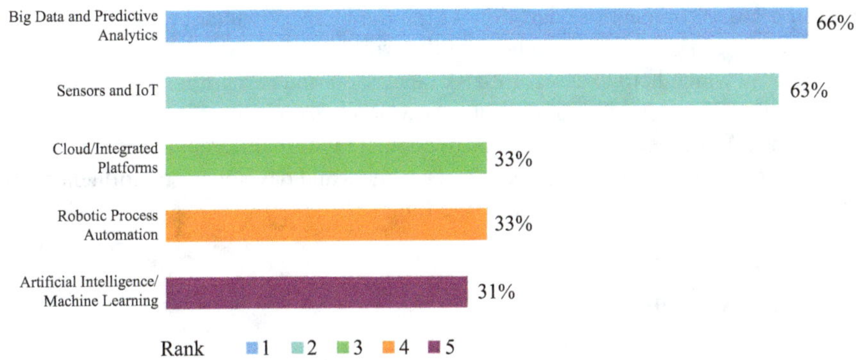

Figure 11.13 Investment in industry 4.0 based on digital transformation. Source: Statista [58].

important part in industry 4.0 which enhances the quality of knowledge. It also helps in the development of the knowledge level within industry 4.0 [44].

Figure 11.13 provides the overall investment in digital transformation for improving the efficiency of industry 4.0. This also includes that the rate of investment has increased by $2.5 million in 2022. The training and education centers have influenced industry 4.0. They adopted some innovative strategies and technologies for a better scope within industry 4.0. It also helps in the expertise in the particular field which helps to focus on the education within the industry 4.0. People are motivated by different innovative strategies which help in the development of industry 4.0. Industry 4.0 is based on digital technologies which focus on the online mode of communication [59].

Various educational methods are adopted for the development of industry 4.0 which also influences engineering students. Ethical consideration is also maintained while handling crucial information about people. It also helps in digital transformation with the help of innovative technologies; it also hampers the educational centers and training centers which help in the development of industrial growth. The Covid-19 situation changed the paradigm shift of the industry [60]. The world becomes competitive due to advanced technologies which help in the development of the industries. Surviving in this competitive world is not easy but adaptation within this industry helps to survive the competitive world. Information technologies are helping in the development of strategies to develop the strengths within the industry.

AI helps in the development of innovative ideas and technologies in this competitive world. The main objective is to reach the optimum production in industry 4.0 which helps in the development of industry 4.0. Digitalization helps the world to progress digitally with the help of modern technologies. The achievement of smart technologies is the main aim of the development of industry 4.0. The digital eras are based on online modes of communication. Though digital communication helps in the development of technologies, it also hampers the situation of progress.

The people also face problems due to the lack of technology which also hampers the connections between the people. In the future, the main aim is to enhance the power of the technologies with the help of special skills and knowledge [61]. It also helps in the development of education within the industry which helps in the development of industry 4.0. It is also helping the world to address the different levels of the economy which help to assess the risk factors. Various Smartphone apps are used to detect the ailing condition of the patients which helps to identify the conditions of the patients. A competitive world helps to compete within different industries, which helps in the progress of industry 4.0 [62]. Designers and developers are influenced by industry 4.0 which helps in change in the future.

11.7 Conclusion

The study has concluded the need for education 4.0 in the industrial revolution reimaging the medical equipment engineering education system. Industry revolution is majorly consisting of modernization in the flow of technologies and automation. The development of the advanced computer replacement into a cyber-physical system connects with the growth of advanced technology such as *the IoT, cloud computing, robotics, data sciences, machine learning, and virtual reality.* The impact of industrial 4.0 is not only in education but also in economics, business, national and global, and individual also. With the development of the industrial revolution, industrial 4.0 is the major part of the industry for growth.

The concept of education 4.30 in this study of the industrial revolution 4.0 has comparative methods that led in the sector of both industry and education. With the rise of the industrial revolution, the education system has selected a major step in terms of the concept of teaching and the process of industrialization. The changes in the education system highly impact digital technologies such as additive manufacturing, cloud computing, the IoT, and robotics. In this literature, the current system of medical equipment engineering education in the industry by considering various types of engineers such as *Robotics engineers, medical device design engineer, imaging engineers, and biomedical engineers* has been discussed with their vital roles in the medical field which is also connected to the industrial revolution.

This study also analyses the new model of engineering education and this model and is based on predictive maintenance and failure prevention. The researchers have identified the current situation of education 4.0 which has discussed how it is different from the current model of education. It has been clear that the future of education and the workplace will change. The method of this research has been discussed about the pattern and structure of the system, the post-positivism philosophy has been selected to complete this research in order to help the research strategy. The research is based on the secondary research method in which data are collected for secondary resources and the data collection method helps in gathering the prominent dates in an efficient manner which is necessary to complete this respective research. The major findings of this research are analyzing the current engineering education in education 4.0 which helps to provide the requirements of industry 4.0 and both education 4.0 and industry 4.0 enable personalized learning of students in the field of engineering education.

References

[1] Heredia-Rivera, U., Ferrer, I., and Vázquez, E. (2019). Ultrasonic moulding technology: recent advances and potential applications in the medical industry. *Polymers*, *11*(4), p. 667.

[2] Bongomin, O., Yemane, A., Kembabazi, B., *et al.* (2020). Industry 4.0 disruption and its neologisms in major industrial sectors: a state of the art. *Journal of Engineering*, *2020*, 1–45.

[3] Alammary, A., Alhazmi, S., Almasri, M., and Gillani, S. (2019). Blockchain-based applications in education: a systematic review. *Applied Sciences*, *9*(12), p. 2400.

[4] Ptes.edu.in (2021). Is Education 4.0 the Future Learning in the Digital Revolution. Available at: https://ptes.edu.in/is-education-4-0-the-future-learning-in-the-digital-revolution/ [accessed on 9 September 2022].

[5] Al-Qurabat, A.K.M. and Idrees, A.K. (2018). Energy-efficient adaptive distributed data collection method for periodic sensor networks. *International Journal of Internet Technology and Secured Transactions*, *8*(3), 297–335.

[6] Alloghani, M., Al-Jumeily, D., Hussain, A., Aljaaf, A.J., Mustafina, J., and Petrov, E. (2018). Healthcare services innovations based on the state of the art technology trend industry 4.0. In *11th International Conference on Developments in eSystems Engineering (DeSE)* (pp. 64–70). IEEE.

[7] Zhang, C. and Chen, Y. (2020). A review of research relevant to the emerging industry trends: industry 4.0, IoT, blockchain, and business analytics. *Journal of Industrial Integration and Management*, *5*(1), 165–180.

[8] Antony, J., McDermott, O. and Sony, M. (2021). Quality 4.0 conceptualisation and theoretical understanding: a global exploratory qualitative study. *The TQM Journal*.

[9] Bolander, W., Chaker, N.N., Pappas, A., and Bradbury, D.R. (2021). Operationalizing salesperson performance with secondary data: aligning practice, scholarship, and theory. *Journal of the Academy of Marketing Science*, *49*(3), 462–481.

[10] Brusakova, I., Mamina, R., and Kossukhina, M. (2020). Engineering education in the conditions of the digital economy. *In Proceedings of the III International Scientific and Practical Conference* (pp. 1–4).

[11] Salah, B., Abidi, M.H., Mian, S.H., Krid, M., Alkhalefah, H., and Abdo, A. (2019). Virtual reality-based engineering education to enhance manufacturing sustainability in industry 4.0. *Sustainability*, *11*(5), 1477.

[12] Busetto, L., Wick, W., and Gumbinger, C. (2020). How to use and assess qualitative research methods. *Neurological Research and Practice*, *2*(1), 1–10.

[13] Cevik Onar, S., Ustundag, A., Kadaifci, Ç., and Oztaysi, B. (2018). The changing role of engineering education in industry 4.0 era. In *Industry 4.0: Managing the Digital Transformation* (pp. 137–151). Springer, Cham.

[14] Chaka, C. (2020). Skills, competencies and literacies attributed to 4IR/ Industry 4.0: scoping review. *IFLA Journal*, *46*(4), 369–399.

[15] Chenoy, D., Ghosh, S.M., and Shukla, S.K. (2019). Skill development for accelerating the manufacturing sector: the role of 'new-age' skills for 'Make in India'. *International Journal of Training Research*, *17*(sup1), 112–130.

[16] Chong, S., Pan, G.T., Chin, J., Show, P.L., Yang, T.C.K., and Huang, C.M. (2018). Integration of 3D printing and Industry 4.0 into engineering teaching. *Sustainability*, *10*(11), 3960.

[17] Chute, C. and French, T., (2019). Introducing care 4.0: an integrated care paradigm built on industry 4.0 capabilities. *International Journal of Environmental Research and Public Health*, *16*(12), 2247.

[18] Correia, R.A., Ladle, R., Jarić, I., *et al.* (2021). Digital data sources and methods for conservation culturomics. *Conservation Biology*, *35*(2), 398–411.

[19] Das, S., Kleinke, D.K., and Pistrui, D. (2020). Reimagining engineering education: does industry 4.0 need education 4.0? In *ASEE Virtual Annual Conference Content Access*.

[20] De Propris, L. and Bailey, D. (2020). Disruptive industry 4.0. In *Industry 4.0 and Regional Transformations* (p. 1). Routledge, London.

[21] Di Sia, P. (2021). Industry 4.0 revolution: introduction. In *Handbook of Smart Materials, Technologies, and Devices: Applications of Industry 4.0* (pp. 1–20). Springer International Publishing, Cham.

[22] Dieck-Assad, G., Ávila-Ortega, A., and González Peña, O.I. (2021). Comparing competency assessment in electronics engineering education with and without industry training partner by challenge-based learning oriented to sustainable development goals. *Sustainability*, *13*(19), 10721.

[23] Frew, A., Weston, L.A., Reynolds, O.L., and Gurr, G.M. (2018). The role of silicon in plant biology: a paradigm shift in research approach. *Annals of Botany*, *121*(7), 1265–1273.

[24] Garraway, J. and Winberg, C. (2019). Reimagining futures of universities of technology. *Critical Studies in Teaching and Learning*, *7*(2), 38–60.

[25] Guile, D. and Mitchell, J., (2022). *Fusion Skills and Industry 5.0: Conceptions and Challenges*. Intech Open Books, London.

[26] Gupta, S. (2018). *Driving Digital Strategy: A Guide to Reimagining Your Business*. Harvard Business Press.

[27] Haleem, A. and Javaid, M. (2019). Additive manufacturing applications in industry 4.0: a review. *Journal of Industrial Integration and Management*, *4* (04), 1930001.

[28] Statista.com (2022). *Medical Technology – Worldwide Revenue*. https://www.statista.com/outlook/hmo/medical-technology/worldwide [Accessed 9 Sep 2022].

[29] Hernandez-de-Menendez, M., Escobar Díaz, C.A., and Morales-Menendez, R. (2020). Engineering education for smart 4.0 technology: a review. *International Journal on Interactive Design and Manufacturing (IJIDeM)*, *14*(3), 789–803.

[30] Hong, C. and Ma, W.W. (2020). Introduction: education 4.0: applied degree education and the future of work. *In Applied Degree Education and the Future of Work* (pp. 1–13). Springer, Singapore.

[31] Huang, C., Lu, J., Ho, D.W., Zhai, G., and Cao, J. (2020). Stabilization of probabilistic Boolean networks via pinning control strategy. *Information Sciences*, *510*, 205–217.

[32] Li, L. (2022). Reskilling and upskilling the future-ready workforce for industry 4.0 and beyond. *Information Systems Frontiers*, *13*, 1–16.

[33] Low, M.C., Lee, C.K., Sidhu, M.S., Lim, S.P., Hasan, Z., and Lim, S.C. (2021). Blended learning to enhanced engineering education using flipped classroom approach: an overview. *Electronic Journal of Computer Science and Information Technology*, *7*(1), 290–301.

[34] Miśkiewicz, R. and Wolniak, R. (2020). Practical application of the industry 4.0 concept in a steel company. *Sustainability*, *12*(14), 5776.

[35] Mogoş, R.I., Bodea, C.N., Dascălu, M.I., *et al.* (2018). Technology enhanced learning for industry 4.0 engineering education. *Revue Roumaine des Sciences Techniques. Série Électrotechnique et Énergétique*, *63*(4), 429–435.

[36] Molla, T. and Cuthbert, D. (2019). Calibrating the PhD for Industry 4.0: global concerns, national agendas and Australian institutional responses. *Policy Reviews in Higher Education*, *3*(2), 167–188.

[37] Muktiarni, M., Widiaty, I., Abdullah, A.G., Ana, A., and Yulia, C. (2019). Digitalisation trend in education during industry 4.0. *Journal of Physics: Conference Series, 1402*(7), 077070.

[38] Pang, T.Y., Pelaez Restrepo, J.D., Cheng, C.T., Yasin, A., Lim, H., and Miletic, M. (2021). Developing a digital twin and digital thread framework for an 'Industry 4.0' shipyard. *Applied Sciences*, *11*(3), 1097.

[39] Olivera, P., Danese, S., Jay, N., Natoli, G., and Peyrin-Biroulet, L. (2019). Big data in IBD: a look into the future. *Nature Reviews Gastroenterology and Hepatology*, *16*(5), 312–321.

[40] Pinto, C.M. and Mendonça, J. (2022). DriVE-MATH: reimagining education. *Open Education Studies*, *4*(1), 21–34.

[41] Podgórska, M. (2022). Challenges and perspectives in innovative projects focused on sustainable industry 4.0—a case study on polish project teams. *Sustainability*, *14*(9), 5334.

[42] Statista (2022). *Value of EdTech Industry Across*. https://www.statista.com/statistics/1278197/india-edtech-industry-value/ [Accessed on 5 Aug 2022].

[43] Rajendran, N. (2020). Overhauling research in Indian universities. In *Reimagining Indian Universities*, p. 331.

[44] Weforum (2020). *Digital Technologies are Increasingly Being Used to Deliver Lessons to Children at Home*. https://www.weforum.org/agenda/(2020)/04/coronavirus-homeschooling-technology-oecd/ [Accessed on 5 Aug 2022].

[45] Raparla, K., Modh, S., and Pandey, N. (2021). Looking beyond the pandemic: adoption of industry 4.0 in manufacturing industries. *Business Research and Innovation*, 432.

[46] Siedlecki, S.L. (2020). Understanding descriptive research designs and methods. *Clinical Nurse Specialist*, *34*(1), 8–12.

[47] Sima, V., Gheorghe, I.G., Subić, J., and Nancu, D. (2020). Influences of the industry 4.0 revolution on the human capital development and consumer behavior: a systematic review. *Sustainability*, *12*(10), 4035.

[48] Statista (2022). *Share of Individuals Using Online Learning Materials*. https://www.statista.com/statistics/882117/online-learning-in-the-uk-by-demographic/ [Accessed on 5 Aug 2022].

[49] Sitthipon, T., Kaewpuang, P., Jaipong, P., Sriboonruang, P., Siripipattanakul, S., and Auttawechasakoon, P. (2022). Artificial Intelligence (AI) adoption in

the medical education during the digital era: a review article. *Review of Advanced Multidisciplinary Sciences, Engineering and Innovation*, *1*(2), 1–7.

[50] Squitieri, L. and Chung, K.C. (2020). Deriving evidence from secondary data in hand surgery: strengths, limitations, and future directions. *Hand Clinics*, *36*(2), 231–243.

[51] Statista (2020). *Annual industry 4.0 investments in digital operations 2016-2020.* https://www.statista.com/statistics/548699/worldwide-industry4-survey-digital-operations-solutions-investments/ [Accessed on 5 Aug 2022].

[52] Žukauskas, P., Vveinhardt, J., and Andriukaitienė, R. (2018). Philosophy and paradigm of scientific research. *Management Culture and Corporate Social Responsibility*, *121*, 121–139.

[53] Statista (2022). *Spending on Digital Transformation Technologies*. https://www.statista.com/statistics/870924/worldwide-digital-transformation-market-size/ [Accessed on 5 Aug 2022].

[54] Yüceol, N. (2021). The steps to be taken in higher education for successful adaptation to industry 4.0. *Yükseköğretim Dergisi*, *11*(3), 563–577.

[55] Statista (2021). *Percentage of Medical Device Companies*. https://www.statista.com/statistics/938791/sales-increase-among-medical-device-companies/ [Accessed on: 05.08.2022].

[56] Venkatesh, D.A.N. (2019). Reimagining the future of healthcare industry through internet of medical things (IoMT), artificial intelligence (AI), machine learning (ML), big data, mobile apps and advanced sensors. In *Artificial Intelligence (AI), Machine Learning (ML), Big Data, Mobile Apps and Advanced Sensors,* October 28, 2019.

[57] Wang, R., Ji, W., Liu, M., *et al.* (2018). Review on mining data from multiple data sources. *Pattern Recognition Letters*, *109*, 120–128.

[58] EY Business Forum. (2020). Will the next transformation in manufacturing be led by digital? [Online]. Available at: https://www.ey.com/en_in/supply-chain/will-the-next-transformation-in-manufacturing-be-led-by-digital [accessed on: 15-08-2022].

[59] Van den Beemt, A., MacLeod, M., Van der Veen, J., Van de Ven, A., van Baalen, S., Klaassen, R., and Boon, M. (2020). Interdisciplinary engineering education: a review of vision, teaching, and support. *Journal of Engineering Education*, *109*(3), 508–555.

[60] Varga, P., Bácsi, S., Sharma, R., *et al.* (2022). Converging telco-grade solutions 5G and beyond to support production in industry 4.0. *Applied Sciences*, *12*(15), 7600.

[61] Takrouri, K., Causton, E., and Simpson, B. (2022). AR technologies in engineering education: applications, potential, and limitations. *Digital*, *2*(2), 171–190.

[62] Tripathi, S. and Gupta, M. (2021). Identification of challenges and their solution for smart supply chains in Industry 4.0 scenario: a neutrosophic DEMATEL approach. *International Journal of Logistics Systems and Management*, *40*(1), 70–94.

Chapter 12

Wireless communication technologies for medical equipment engineering

Wendy Wai Yeng Yeo[1] *and Chia Chao Kang*[2]

12.1 Introduction

Since the coronavirus disease (COVID-19) pandemic hits in year 2019, it has affected global health and economic crisis in almost all the countries in the world. This has prompted countries across the world to employ digital technologies to combat this global crisis using the wireless communication systems [1]. Wireless communication technology enables transmission of data or information without using wires, cables, or electrical conductors. This technology utilizes satellite, radio frequencies, infrared, Bluetooth, and others for wireless transmission of data which offers advantages including high transmission efficiency, long transmission distance, low wear rate as well as high reliability and flexibility [2,3].

During the COVID-19 pandemic, wireless communication technology plays a crucial role to support public-health response to COVID-19 worldwide. Herein, the medical equipment engineering integrates engineering discipline into healthcare systems from diagnosis, treatments, monitoring, rehabilitation, and patient care. The wireless technology helps to connect patients, healthcare professionals, sensors, computers, and medical devices via Wireless Body Area Network (WBAN), Wireless Personal Area Network (WPAN), Radio Frequency Identification (RFID), general packet radio service/Universal Mobile Telecommunication System (GPRS/UMTS), wireless local area network (LAN) (802.11), and sensor networks [4].

Wireless communication has always been backbone of smart healthcare system even before the pandemic as to provide various health services to the patients and healthcare providers within hospitals and remotely [3]. The wireless use is expected to expand in the healthcare systems with the collaboration of the Internet of Things (IoT) coupled with low-power wide-area network (LPWAN). The wireless healthcare market shows compound annual growth rate (CAGR) of 21.2% over the forecast period 2021–2026 as shown in Figure 12.1.

[1]School of Pharmacy, Monash University Malaysia, Jalan Lagoon Selatan, Malaysia
[2]Department of Electrical and Electronics Engineering, Xiamen University Malaysia, Malaysia

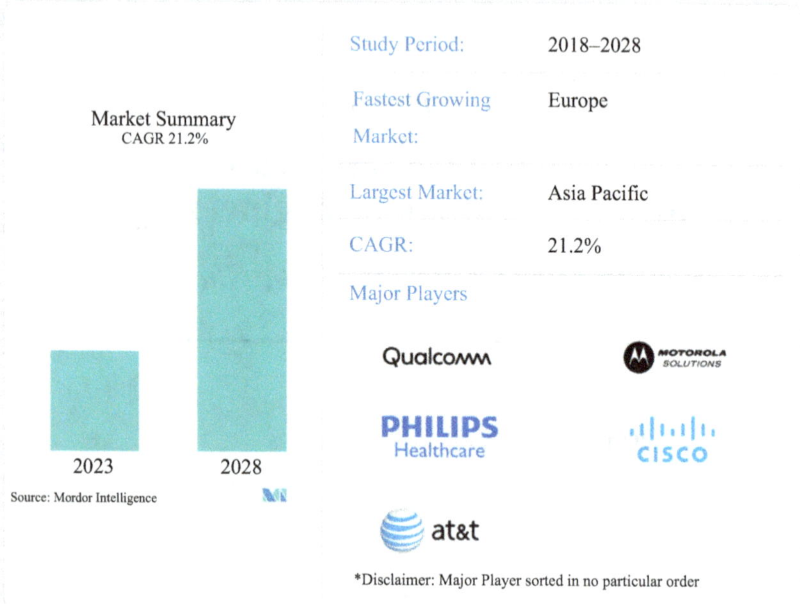

Figure 12.1 Overview of wireless healthcare industry. Source: [5].

12.2 Development of wireless communication technology in medical equipment engineering

The healthcare system that has been going through a technology evolution has evolved from point-to-point communication systems to smart sensor technology. This development was made possible by the evolution of wireless communication technologies which has become a powerful enabler for medical equipment engineering. The evolution of wireless communication technology has evolved in several stages.

Early on in the advent of wireless communication, it was mainly used to transmit patient data from a medical equipment to the healthcare professional. In early 1920, a "wired wireless" electronic stethoscope was developed by the U.S. Army Signal Corps which was utilized for ship-to-shore transmission of cardiac sounds [6] as shown in Figure 12.2. The information travels from source to the receiver through point-to-point communication system which were not connect to the Internet.

At the intermediate stage, the healthcare system has been going through a technology evolution. The modern medical equipment uses wireless communication technology which offers significant convenience, accessibly, and accuracy to transfer information. It supports real-time data access and collection as well as facilitates patient monitoring [7]. The wireless communications are essential to

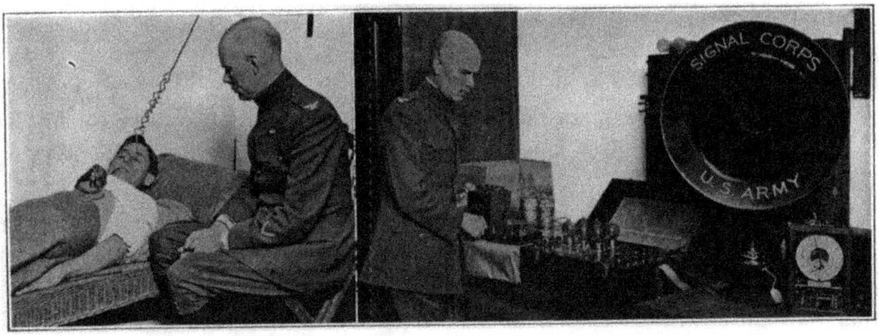

Figure 12.2 The transmitter (left) and amplifier (right) used in sending out by wireless the heart record of a patient on board a ship where there is no doctor. Source: [6].

connect medical equipment to hospital networks besides establishing a seamless integration and interconnection with all the stakeholders inside and outside the premises [4].

During the advanced stage, the wireless sensor network (WSN) has a significant impact on healthcare especially during the COVID-19 pandemic. The wireless medical sensors network that is deployed to monitor patient's conditions such as vital parameters (body temperature, oxygen saturation, heartbeat, blood pressure, and respiratory rate) has reduced threat of communicable diseases [8]. Together with the advance of semiconductor technology, tiny sensors are embedded with integrated chips which enables the transmission of information wirelessly to receiving device and then to a central database [9].

In the beginning of this decade, adoption of Internet of Things (IoT) and 5G technology together with wireless communication technology has become possible to connect not only limited to medical equipment but also to wearables, connected implants, smart tags and smart cards which enable remote monitoring, diagnosis, and treatment [10,11]. The current stage of wireless communications enables digital health and better healthcare system in real-time for the development of personalized medicine [12]. Information disseminates via wireless communication technology in a digitally enabled and integrated public-health system have played an essential role in a comprehensive response especially during an infectious-disease outbreak, a lesson which we have learned during COVID-19 pandemic [13].

Generally, wireless communication technologies for medical equipment can be divided into machine-to-human and machine-to-machine (M2M) communications which will be discussed in this chapter.

12.3 Machine-to-human communication technologies

Interestingly, one of the current increasing trendy fashion accessories is the wearable wireless devices that are used across different areas including sports, child monitoring as well as healthcare. These wearable devices are designed to collect data of user's vital signs and act as fitness tracker for daily activities by syncing to various smartphone applications [14]. The robust, dynamic, and proficient WBAN is commonly utilized to support such sensor platform with requires extremely low power requirements which is suitable for day-to-day wearables [15] as shown in Figure 12.3.

Meanwhile, doctors and nurses could also keep track of patients' real-time vital signs distant over the WBAN through this remote patient monitoring system. This recent advancement in wearable devices has made substantial contributions to reduce the burdens of hospitals and patients, who need frequent hospital visits for monitoring their diseases [16]. Furthermore, this technology is useful to send data to help doctors to make appropriate decision at that real time which is vital for chronic diseases patients such as diabetes people to meet their administer therapy programs such as diabetes patients [16]. Sometimes although some wearable applications may not be commonly use in real time, the data obtained from it may provide early medical alerts for the risk diagnosis of the patients' conditions [15].

On top of that, these sensing devices can be attached to patients' bodies for the collection of significant health information such as electrocardiogram (ECG), blood pressure, and others. Typically, ECG system is a non-invasive method to

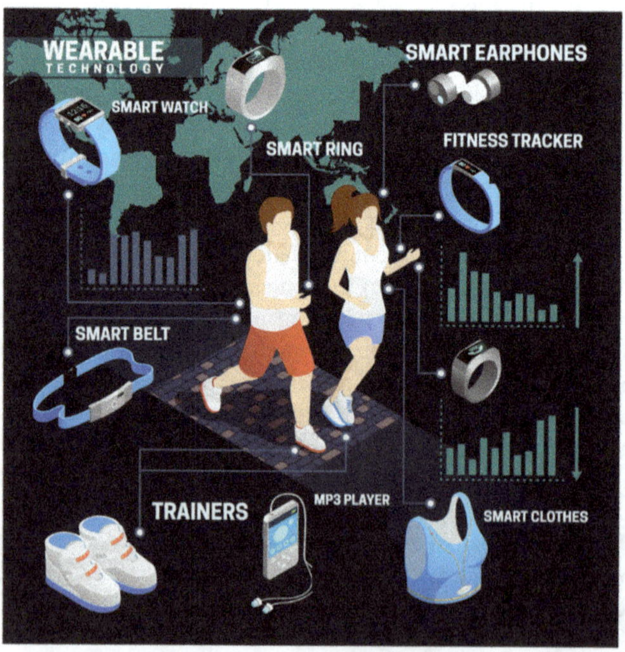

Figure 12.3 The wearable technology is greatly impacted by the growth of wireless communication technology. Wearable devices, such as smartwatches and fitness trackers are using the wireless connectivity to obtain health data (image by Macrovector on Freepik).

check heart's rhythm and electrical activity by placing electrodes on human body surface, which are linked to the ECG monitoring device via cables [17]. The advancement of wireless technologies has allowed the implementation of wireless ECG monitoring via Bluetooth and Zigbee transmission protocols based on Wireless Sensor Network (WSN) applications [17]. Findings have shown that smartphone wireless ECGs provide accurate, non-invasive, and real-time monitoring the abnormal rhythm on routine ECG in pediatric patients [18] as shown in Figure 12.4.

The current Fourth Industrial Revolution (4IR) is expected to change how we communicate using the artificial intelligence (AI)-driven wireless technologies. For example, the artificial intelligence (AI)-powered text messaging systems are widely used by healthcare organizations to confirm patient appointment times and refill prescriptions. As shown in Figure 12.5, integration of chatbots applications for telehealth, mental health, and others is becoming more common to ease the burden on medical professionals for (1) medication management, (2) organization of patient pathways, (3) helping with first aid, and (4) solving simpler medical issues [20,21]. Hereby, the AI is fueling the future wireless network transmission using machine learning to transform various aspects of patient care and also administrative processes within the healthcare provider as well as pharmaceutical organizations.

An emerging field of augmented reality (AR) and virtual reality (VR) have set off a new technology paradigm of 5G networks for medical equipment engineering (Figure 12.6). The VR is created via the combination of realistic sounds, images, and other sensations using tools including VR headsets/protective caps, gloves, and

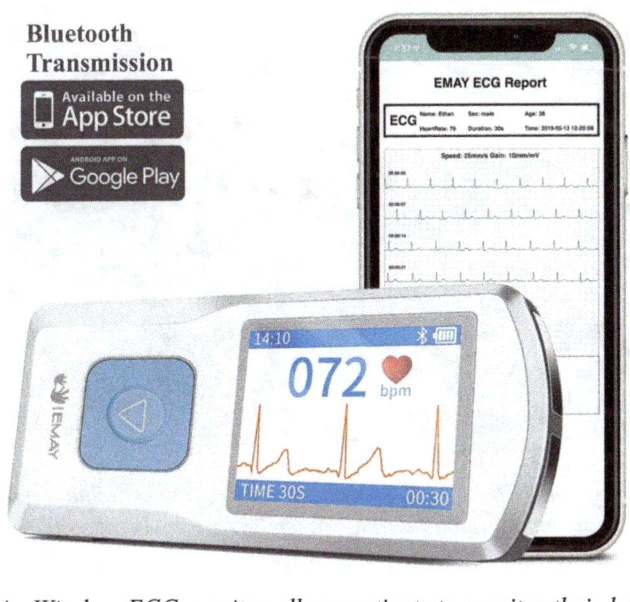

Figure 12.4 Wireless ECG monitor allows patients to monitor their heart health remotely and share the data with healthcare providers. Source: [19].

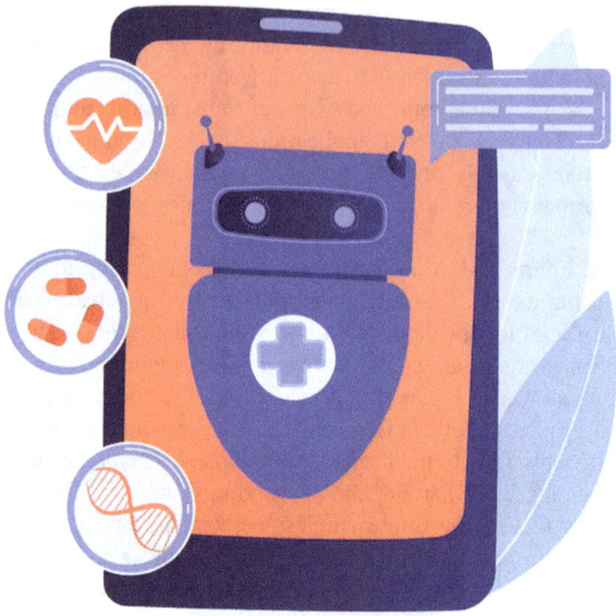

Figure 12.5 Chatbot provides information to assist with scheduling appointments and prescription refills (image by Vectorjuice on Freepik)

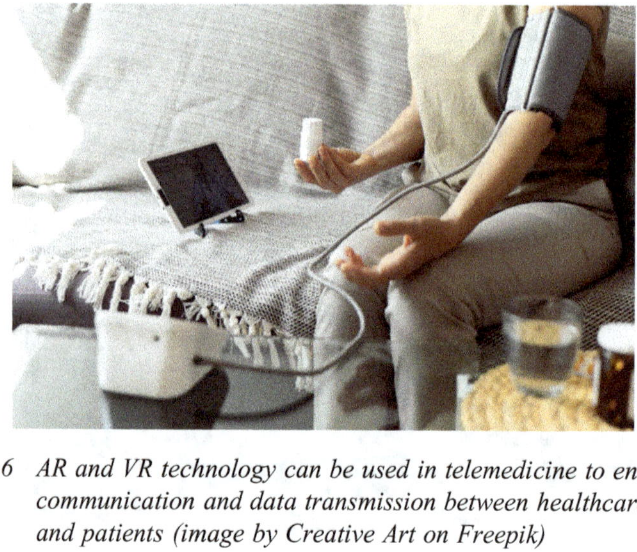

Figure 12.6 AR and VR technology can be used in telemedicine to enhance communication and data transmission between healthcare providers and patients (image by Creative Art on Freepik)

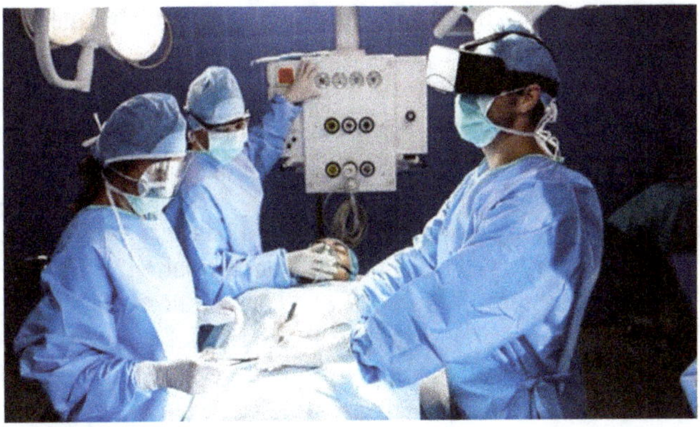

Figure 12.7 Surgical applications of augmented reality and virtual reality. Source: [28].

sensors of body locators [22]. The wireless VR-based application that simulates surgical procedures is widely utilized by surgeons for a safe and realistic method to practice and improve their surgical skills [23] as shown in Figure 12.7. Likewise, AR which integrates digital information with the user's environment in real time is becoming more accessible for medical education, surgical simulation, and planning [24,25]. With the help of wireless communication technology, AR and VR can be used in telemedicine to transmit data and communication between patients and healthcare providers as an option for remote consultations and treatments, in which their demands were escalated amid COVID-19 [26,27].

12.4 Machine-to-machine communication technologies

The machine-to-machine (M2M) communications have profound effect on the medical device field which bring a whole new dimension to patient care, patient monitoring, and also making an efficient medical supply chain. The M2M communications permit autonomous networking among devices or sensors to capture an event (e.g., the heart rate of a person), which is relayed through a network to an application (software), and finally translating the captured event into usable information, without human intervention. With regard to this, the AI technologies and big data analytics have also bridged between wireless networks with the medical devices. Alongside, there is an intelligent software application which is utilized to support the big data analytics and provide the end user with a set of smart services and a practical interface including efficient parameter estimation and interactive decision making [29].

With the rising number of chronic diseases and global population is ageing, the deployment of IoT enables autonomous networking among devices without human intervention. The IoT platform enables healthcare professionals to integrate medical devices such as pumps, monitors, cart systems, and other instrumentations with hospital facilities for seamless, and continuous patient monitoring [4,10]. These

M2M devices are usually wearable on body such as smart bandage for monitoring and treatment of chronic wounds [30] or medical actuators such as insulin pump [31] that are implantable or in human body which are capable of establishing wireless communication links [29]. A recent study reported that wearable biosensor patch with skin-conformal attachment and multiple biosensor integration is designed to monitor different vital signs including body temperature, blood pressure, and electrocardiography using IoT-connected healthcare platform [32].

One of the core drivers of healthcare transformation is Radio Frequency Identification (RFID) system (Figure 12.8). The wireless sensor networks and RFID are often seen as the prerequisites for the IoT [33,34]. The RFID refers to an auto identification technology whereby information of a uniquely RFID tagged object are captured by a reader which uses radio waves at several different frequencies to transfer data [33]. In order to facilitate access to quality information in real-time, RFID is adopted in clinical practice. For instance, a wearable RFID tag which is embedded with body temperature monitoring sensor, automatic identification and localization was designed for real-time emergency notification [35]. Other applications include RFID tag antenna-based wireless sensing which is attached to a transfusion bag/bottle for automated monitoring of the fluid level in the transfusion bag/bottle [36] and a wireless monitoring of RFID-sensorized facemask of newborns breath temperature during mild hypothermia treatment without interfering their treatments or specific diagnostic tests [37].

Wireless technology equips the healthcare personnel to perform their works more efficiently with the easy access to various information resources, electronic health records (EHRs), as well as viewing and reporting patient data [16]. With the current of huge clinical data generated through wearable medical devices, wireless EHRs are crucial to track down patient's previous medical records and provide up-to-date and accurate patient information through remote access instantly [38,39]. The RFID is also broadly implemented to keep medical devices that are all labeled with RFID tags under surveillance as

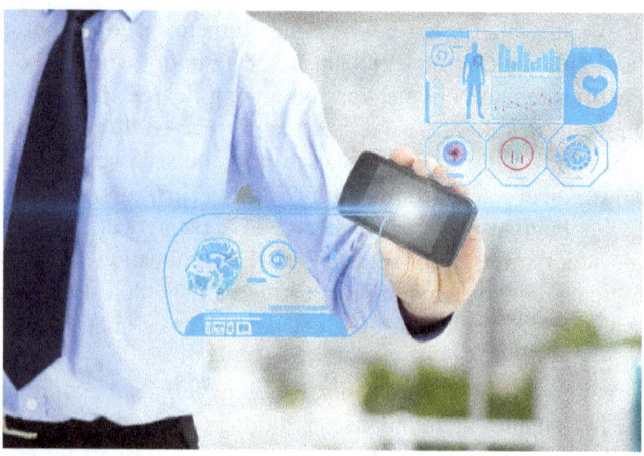

Figure 12.8 RFID technology is widely used in healthcare which help to improve patient safety, reduce medical errors, and increase the efficiency of healthcare operations (image by Creative Art on Freepik)

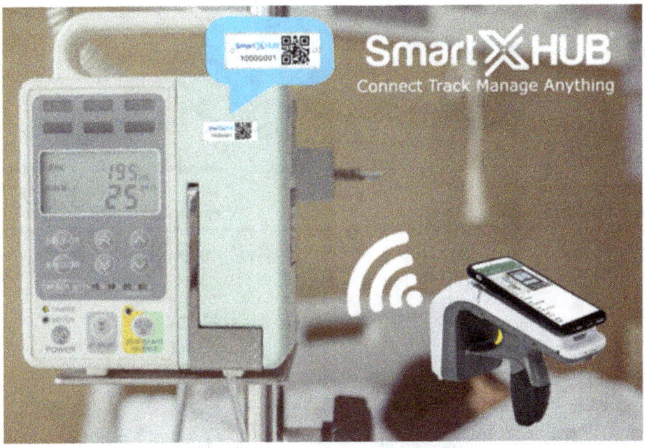

Figure 12.9 The use of RFID technology to track and manage medical devices such as surgical instruments, equipment, and implants. Source: [42].

part of an effective medical device management system as shown in Figure 12.9. Besides that, RFID has been used for monitoring of traceability and consumption of high value surgical supplies [40] and also deployment of a pharmaceutical formulary validation [41]. This M2M networks offer seamless device interconnection via smartphone application, website service, database server, and mobile gateway without the need of human interaction [32]. Figure 12.10 shows the applications and advantages of wireless communication technologies for medical equipment engineering in healthcare system.

12.5 Challenges of using wireless technologies in medical equipment engineering

Moving forward, wireless communications improve our current healthcare systems that ensure safe and efficient healthcare services within the hospitals and remote areas. However, there are challenges deploying wireless in medical devices like the technique issues such as sensor nodes, wireless transmission, energy efficiency, and safety [43].

Due to improper maintenance, manufacturing defects or malfunctions of digital components such as relays, contactors, and blown fuses may occur. Interference from radio frequency (RF) sources such as local area networks (LANs), metallic detectors, and Bluetooth gadgets may interfere with the function of these medical equipment and restrict the use of Wi-Fi networks [3]. Besides that, electromagnetic interference can additionally have an effect on the operation of implantable gadgets and stationary digital devices [3].

The space of the healthcare facilities equipped with modern technologies and numerous communications technologies such as IoT, sensors, and wireless medical equipment or devices needs to be considered as well. This is because the physical structure of these buildings may limit the penetration of signals through walls, resulting in limited coverage areas and poor connectivity [3]. In addition, with the growing of wireless networks at the healthcare facilities contributes to spectrum

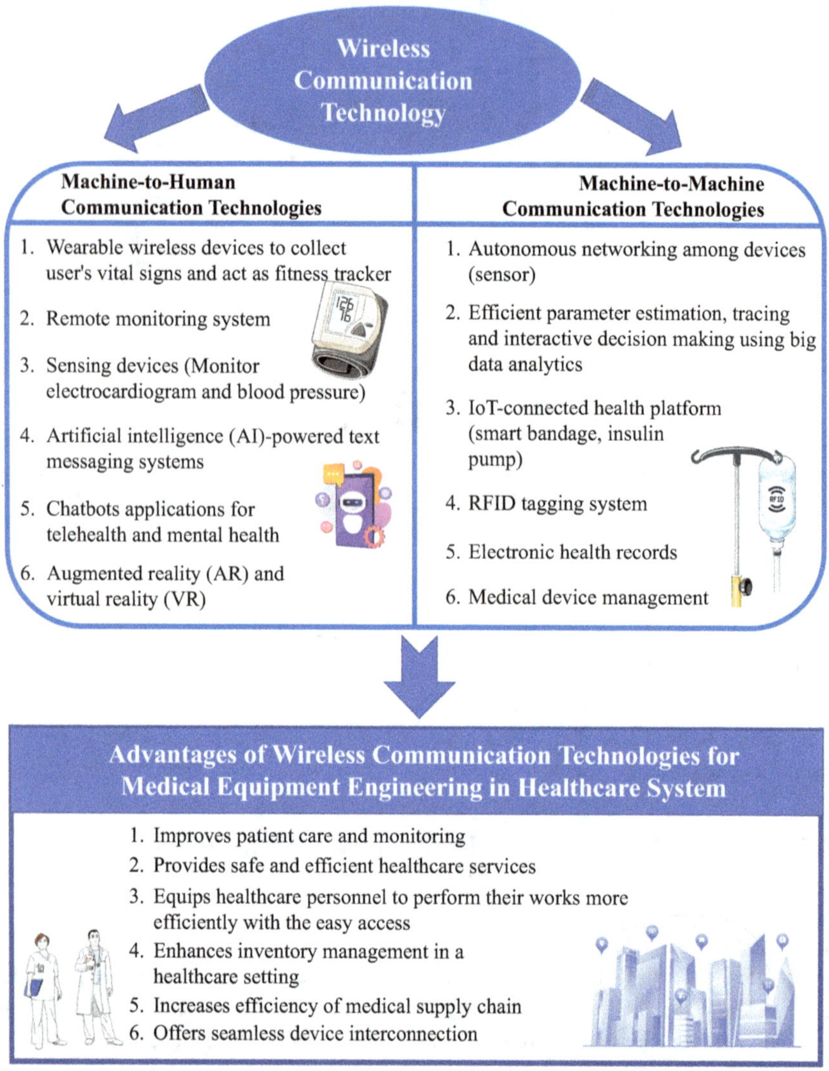

Figure 12.10 Applications of wireless communication technologies for medical equipment engineering and their advantages in healthcare system. Figure was modified using Servier Medical Art templates, which are licensed under a Creative Commons Attribution 3.0 Unported License (https://creativecommons.org/licenses/by/3.0/).

congestion and energy efficiency, typically for radio-based communications systems [4]. The inadequacy of wireless networks to support capacity and connectivity requirements of the real-time health records monitoring due to high usage could lead to delay and irreversible serious consequences in case of emergencies [3].

Next, data integrity is another main concern in this fast-growing healthcare system in pace with the proliferation of wireless technology advancements. There is a possibility for the wireless communication systems to lose data or errors occurred during data transmission [44]. Therefore, it is crucial to enhance the network security to protect patient's privacy for ethics and legal reasons as well as to protect from unauthorized access, disclosure, modification or destruction [45]. In addition, there are chances for the unauthorized users to interrupt with data transmission, perform malicious activities, eavesdrop acts, and also remotely extract sensitive health information from medical devices [46].

12.6 Conclusion

A fast, stable, and reliable network security of the wireless networking infrastructure is important for communications, medical data transmission, patient monitoring, and inventory management in a healthcare setting. Therefore, improving fault-tolerance and maximizing energy-efficiency of the system lifetime, protection of data as well as strong network security are the key elements to be considered with the increasing number of patients. Meanwhile, medical devices and equipment should be able to provide accurate and secure data protection with precision and speed. Lastly, cost-effectiveness and sustainability approaches need to be thought of in order to prolong the network lifetime to bring forward wireless technologies in the healthcare industry to the next level.

References

[1] N. Saeed, A. Bader, T. Y. Al-Naffouri, and M.-S. Alouini, "When wireless communication responds to COVID-19: combating the pandemic and saving the economy," *Front. Commun. Networks*, vol. 1, no. November, pp. 1–15, 2020, doi: 10.3389/frcmn.2020.566853.

[2] J. Li, "Research progress of wireless power transmission technology and the related problems," *AIP Conf. Proc.*, vol. 1820, no. 2017, pp. 1–5, 2017, doi:10.1063/1.4977407.

[3] M. B. Janjua, A. E. Duranay, and H. Arslan, "Role of wireless communication in healthcare system to cater disaster situations under 6G vision," *Front. Commun. Networks*, vol. 1, no. December, pp. 1–10, 2020, doi: 10.3389/frcmn.2020.610879.

[4] I. Ahmed, H. Karvonen, T. Kumpuniemi, and M. Katz, "Wireless communications for the hospital of the future: requirements, challenges and solutions," *Int. J. Wirel. Inf. Networks*, vol. 27, no. 1, pp. 4–17, 2020, doi: 10.1007/s10776-019-00468-1.

[5] "Wireless healthcare market – growth, trends, Covid-19 impact, and forecasts (2023–2028)." Industry Reports. Accessed: Jan. 30, 2023. https://www.mordorintelligence.com/industry-reports/global-wireless-healthcare-market-industry?gclid=Cj0KCQiAz9ieBhCIARIsACB0oGJQQx4VU4E9dWtH2wc1JYTqISwD1By27LpqMobWmeTHz-0mnfivAIsaAkAqEALw_wcB.

[6] S. R. Winters, "Diagnosis by wireless," *Sci. Am.*, vol. 124, no. 24, pp. 465–465, 1921, doi: 10.1038/scientificamerican06111921-465a.

[7] E. Kartsakli, A. S. Lalos, A. Antonopoulos, *et al.*, *Machine-to-Machine (M2M) Communications for e-Health Applications*, no. July 2012. New York, NY: Elsevier Ltd., 2015, doi:10.1016/B978-1-78242-102-3.00020-4.

[8] R. Saher and M. Anjum, "Role of technology in COVID-19 pandemic," in *Researches and Applications of Artificial Intelligence to Mitigate Pandemics*. New York, NY: Elsevier, 2021, pp. 109–138, doi: 10.1016/B978-0-323-90959-4.00005-5.

[9] S. Ali, R. P. Singh, M. Javaid, *et al.*, "A review of the role of smart wireless medical sensor network in Covid-19," *J. Ind. Integr. Manag.*, vol. 5, no. 4, pp. 413–425, 2020, doi: 10.1142/S2424862220300069.

[10] H. Taleb, A. Nasser, G. Andrieux, N. Charara, and E. Motta Cruz, "Wireless technologies, medical applications and future challenges in WBAN: a survey," *Wirel. Networks*, vol. 27, no. 8, pp. 5271–5295, 2021, doi: 10.1007/s11276-021-02780-2.

[11] S. M. Asiful Huda, M. Y. Arafat, and S. Moh, "Wireless power transfer in wirelessly powered sensor networks: a review of recent progress," *Sensors*, vol. 22, no. 8, 2022, doi: 10.3390/s22082952.

[12] D. Ho, S. R. Quake, E. R. B. McCabe, *et al.*, "Enabling technologies for personalized and precision medicine," *Trends Biotehnol.*, vol. 38, no. 5, pp. 497–518, 2021, doi: 10.1016/j.tibtech.2019.12.021.Enabling.

[13] J. Budd, B. S. Miller, E. M. Manning, *et al.*, "Digital technologies in the public-health response to COVID-19," *Nat. Med.*, vol. 26, no. 8, pp. 1183–1192, 2020, doi: 10.1038/s41591-020-1011-4.

[14] M. E. Haveman, M. C. van Rossum, R. M. E. Vaseur, *et al.*, "Continuous monitoring of vital signs with wearable sensors during daily life activities: validation study," *JMIR Form. Res.*, vol. 6, no. 1, pp. 1–16, 2022, doi: 10.2196/30863.

[15] C. A. Tavera, J. H. Ortiz, O. I. Khalaf, D. F. Saavedra, and T. H. H. Aldhyani, "Wearable wireless body area networks for medical applications," *Comput. Math. Methods Med.*, vol. 2021, Article ID 5574376, 2021, doi: 10.1155/2021/5574376.

[16] N. El-Rashidy, S. El-Sappagh, S. M. Riazul Islam, H. M. El-Bakry, and S. Abdelrazek, "Mobile health in remote patient monitoring for chronic diseases: principles, trends, and challenges," *Diagnostics*, vol. 11, no. 4, pp. 1–33, 2021, doi: 10.3390/diagnostics11040607.

[17] N. Dey, A. S. Ashour, F. Shi, S. J. Fong, and R. S. Sherratt, "Developing residential wireless sensor networks for ECG healthcare monitoring," *IEEE Trans. Consum. Electron.*, vol. 63, no. 4, pp. 442–449, 2017, doi: 10.1109/TCE.2017.015063.

[18] M. R. F. Gropler, A. S. Dalal, G. F. Van Hare, and J. N. A. Silva, "Can smartphone wireless ECGs be used to accurately assess ECG intervals in pediatrics? A comparison of mobile health monitoring to standard 12-lead ECG," *PLoS One*, vol. 13, no. 9, pp. 1–9, 2018, doi: 10.1371/journal.pone.0204403.

[19] "Wireless EKG monitor". Emaycare.com. Accessed: Jan. 30, 2023. https://www.emaycare.com/products/wireless-ekg-monitor-blue

[20] T. Davenport and R. Kalakota, "The potential for artificial intelligence in healthcare," *SSRN Electron. J.*, vol. 6, no. 2, pp. 94–98, 2020, doi: 10.2139/ssrn.3525037.

[21] F. Frangoudes, M. Hadjiaros, E. C. Schiza, M. Matsangidou, O. Tsivitanidou, and K. Neokleous, "An overview of the use of chatbots in medical and healthcare education," in *Lecture Notes on Computer Science (including Subser. Lect. Notes Artif. Intell. Lect. Notes Bioinformatics)*, vol. 12785 LNCS, no. July, pp. 170–184, 2021, doi: 10.1007/978-3-030-77943-6_11.

[22] A. Shetty, G. S. Kulkarni, R. B. Sn, and P. M. Paarakh, "A review on: metaverse in health care and pharma," *J. Community Pharm. Pract.*, no. 01, pp. 1–11, 2023.

[23] G. T. Yamamoto and D. Altun, "Virtual reality technology in healthcare," *Pearson J. Soc. Sci. Humanit.*, vol. 6, no. 13, pp. 92–104, 2021, doi: http://dx.doi.org/10.46872/pj.282.

[24] S. Wang, M. Parsons, J. Stone-McLean, *et al.*, "Augmented reality as a telemedicine platform for remote procedural training," *Sensors*, vol. 17, no. 10, pp. 1–21, 2017, doi: 10.3390/s17102294.

[25] T. Morimoto, H. Hirata, M. Ueno, *et al.*, "Digital transformation will change medical education and rehabilitation in spine surgery," *Medicina*, vol. 58, no. 4, 2022, doi: 10.3390/medicina58040508.

[26] M. Kenoui, "Telemedicine meets augmented reality: healthcare services delivery and distance training," in *ISIA 2020 – Proceedings, 4th Int. Symp. Informatics its Appl.*, pp. 20–24, 2020, doi: 10.1109/ISIA51297.2020.9416532.

[27] A. Gasmi and R. Benlamri, *Augmented Reality, Virtual Reality and New Age Technologies Demand Escalates Amid COVID-19*. New York, NY: Elsevier Inc., 2022. doi: 10.1016/B978-0-323-90054-6.00005-2.

[28] "Augmented reality and virtual reality in medical devices". *Medical Devices*. Accessed: Jan. 24, 2023. https://www.fda.gov/medical-devices/digital-health-center-excellence/augmented-reality-and-virtual-reality-medical-devices

[29] E. Kartsakli, A. S. Lalos, A. Antonopoulos, *et al.*, "A survey on M2M systems for mhealth: a wireless communications perspective," *Sensors (Switzerland)*, vol. 14, no. 10, pp. 18009–18052, 2014, doi: 10.3390/s141018009.

[30] P. Mostafalu, A. Tamayol, R. Rahim, *et al.*, "Smart bandage for monitoring and treatment of chronic wounds," *Small*, vol. 14, no. 33, pp. 1–9, 2018, doi: 10.1002/smll.201703509.

[31] X. Hei, X. Du, S. Lin, I. Lee, and O. Sokolsky, "Patient infusion pattern based access control schemes for wireless insulin pump system," *IEEE Trans. Parallel Distrib. Syst.*, vol. 26, no. 11, pp. 3108–3121, 2015, doi: 10.1109/TPDS.2014.2370045.

[32] D. T. Phan, C. H. Nguyen, T. D. P. Nguyen, *et al.*, "A flexible, wearable, and wireless biosensor patch with internet of medical things applications," *Biosensors*, vol. 12, no. 3, p. 139, 2022, doi: 10.3390/bios12030139.

[33] H. Landaluce, L. Arjona, A. Perallos, F. Falcone, I. Angulo, and F. Muralter, "A review of IoT sensing applications and challenges using RFID and wireless sensor networks," *Sensors (Switzerland)*, vol. 20, no. 9, pp. 1–18, 2020, doi: 10.3390/s20092495.

[34] X. Jia, Q. Feng, T. Fan, and Q. Lei, "RFID technology and its applications in Internet of Things (IoT)," in *2012 2nd International Conference on Consumer Electronics, Communications and Networks, CECNet 2012 – Proceedings*, pp. 1282–1285, 2012, doi: 10.1109/CECNet.2012.6201508.

[35] Y. C. Chen, H. M. Sun, and R. S. Chen, "Design and implementation of wearable RFID tag for real-time ubiquitous medical care," in *BioWireleSS 2014 – Proceedings of the 2014 IEEE Topical Conference on Biomedical Wireless Technologies, Networks, and Sensing Systems*, pp. 25–27, 2014, doi: 10.1109/BioWireleSS.2014.6827735.

[36] Z. Jiang, Z. Fu, and F. Yang, "RFID tag antenna based wireless sensing method for medical transfusion applications," in *2012 IEEE International Conference on RFID-Technologies and Applications. RFID-TA 2012*, pp. 126–130, 2012, doi: 10.1109/RFID-TA.2012.6404496.

[37] N. Panunzio, V. Olivieri, F. Montecchia, P. Papoff, and G. Marrocco, "RFID-sensorized facemask for wireless monitoring of newborn breath temperature during mild hypothermia treatment," in *2022 7th International Conference on Smart and Sustainable Technologies, SpliTech 2022*, pp. 1–5, 2022, doi: 10.23919/splitech55088.2022.9854380.

[38] S. M. Shah and R. A. Khan, "Secondary use of electronic health record: opportunities and challenges," *IEEE Access*, vol. 8, pp. 136947–136965, 2020, doi: 10.1109/ACCESS.2020.3011099.

[39] G. Assenza, C. Fioravanti, S. Guarino, and V. Petrassi, "New perspectives on wearable devices and electronic health record systems," in *2020 IEEE International Workshop on Metrology for Industry 4.0 & IoT- Proc.*, pp. 740–745, 2020, doi: 10.1109/MetroInd4.0IoT48571.2020.9138170.

[40] M. del Carmen León-Araujo, E. Gómez-Inhiesto, and M. T. Acaiturri-Ayesta, "Implementation and evaluation of a RFID smart cabinet to improve traceability and the efficient consumption of high cost medical supplies in a large hospital," *J. Med. Syst.*, vol. 43, no. 6, p. 178, 2019, doi: 10.1007/s10916-019-1269-6.

[41] P. H. Frisch, "RFID in today's intelligent hospital enhancing patient care optimizing hospital operations," in *2019 IEEE International Conference on RFID Technology and Applications. RFID-TA 2019*, pp. 458–463, 2019, doi: 10.1109/RFID-TA.2019.8892070.

[42] "Rapidly identify and access essential healthcare equipment." Smartxhub.com. Accessed: Jan. 30, 2023. https://smartxhub.com/healthcare-asset-tracking-using-rfid/

[43] L. Zhong, S. He, J. Lin, *et al.*, "Technological requirements and challenges in wireless body area networks for health monitoring: a comprehensive survey," *Sensors*, vol. 22, no. 9, 2022, doi: 10.3390/s22093539.

[44] X. Shi, J. Cao, T. Lu, and V. Chang, "A survey on RFID security and privacy in smart medical: threats and protections," in *IoTBDS 2019 – Proceedings of the International Conference on Internet of Things, Big Data and Security*, no. IoTBDS, pp. 278–285, 2019, doi: 10.5220/0007713402780285.

[45] S. B. Sadkhan and N. A. Abbas, "Privacy and security of wireless communication networks," *Mob. Networks Cloud Comput. Converg. Progress. Serv. Appl.*, no. January, pp. 58–78, 2013, doi: 10.4018/978-1-4666-4781-7.ch004.

[46] L. Kibona and H. Ganame, "Wireless network security: challenges, threats and solutions. a critical review," *Int. J. Acad. Multidiscip. Res.*, vol. 2, no. 4, pp. 19–27, 2018, www.ijeais.org/ijamr

Chapter 13

Human–robot interaction in medical equipment manufacturing

R. Kamalakannan[1], Dadapeer Doddamani[2], P. Sivakumar[3], S. Nagarajan[4] and J. Vairamuthu[5]

The market for medical devices includes implants, tools, and equipment used for treatment, observation, and diagnosis. Implantable cardiac and diabetes monitoring are among them, as well as reconstructive equipment like hip and knee replacements.

Typically, the use of robots has moved fast from industrial to social reasons. Because of this, robots can now communicate with humans in a natural way. With the on-demand adjustable manufacture of complicated geometries, additive manufacturing (AM) techniques have been significantly reshaping the medical sectors, particularly medical equipment manufacturing, tissue engineering and implantable medical devices. Robots not only make AM easier but they also take care of 3D printers, which are also robots, automate post-processing for AM, and let architects come up with creative, adaptive ways to build the environment around us. To closely monitor the process before, during, and after the construction, active head control and dynamic deposition measurement are utilised.

13.1 Robotic AM for medical equipment

The AM revolution is affecting more than just how we construct things. As a result, the way designers think is changing. They must set aside the constraints imposed by traditional manufacturing techniques and consider the design options.

Possibilities that are anticipated to propel the global market for AM to $20 billion by 2025. All of these are digital manufacturing techniques that include

[1]Department of Mechanical Engineering, M. Kumarasamy College of Engineering, India
[2]Mechanical & Industrial Engineering Section, Higher College of Technology, Sultanate of Oman
[3]Mechanical and Industrial Engineering, University of Technology and Applied Sciences, Sultanate of Oman
[4]Department of Mechanical Engineering, College of Engineering and Technology, Mettu University, Ethiopia
[5]Department of Mechanical Engineering, Sethu Institute of Technology, India

building up layers of material, whether it be liquid, powder, sheet, or another kind of material, using CAD data to produce a 3D product, even tissue from humans. AM is used to build a variety of constructions, including bridges, innovative aviation components, and dental appliances. It might also be creative. One method builds each tiny layer repeatedly using a steady, repeating action. The repeatability and control of the other technologies are well known. It seems as though they were meant to be together. The future of manufacturing and disruptive technologies is a match made in heaven. In addition to facilitating AM robots are also tending 3D printers, which are also robotic, automating post-processing for AM, and enabling architects to imagine novel, adaptable methods to construct the world around us increasing our potential.

13.1.1 Six-axis articulated robot

The procedure uses a six-axis articulated robot to create metal pieces on an existing substrate layer by layer using a combination of hot wire deposition and a laser. Exotic metals are quickly and precisely deposited to create prototypes and small quantities of highly complicated, expensive items. Therefore, a metallurgical link is created between the wire and substrate. The distinction is that a hot wire technique is used in this procedure. The process employs the appropriate amount of laser energy to melt the substrate beneath the wire, which is already molten, to create a solid link is shown in Figure 13.1. When you are not aiming to melt the wire and the substrate, you can use less laser power [1]. With the hot wire, you may increase deposition while applying less heat to the part. A substrate is always the first step in the process. It is a cylinder in the demonstration involving the propeller. It could be a big steel plate or block with other parts.

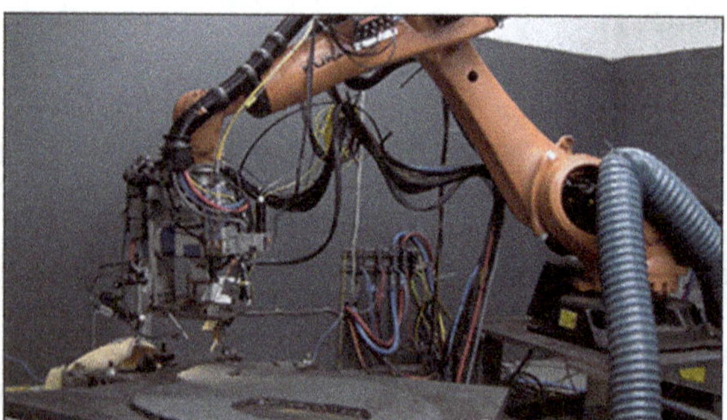

Additive manufacturing process uses a robot equipped with a laser head and hot wire deposition to build a metal part layer by layer. (Courtesy of Midwest Engineered Systems Inc.)

Figure 13.1 Robot equipped with a laser head

13.1.1.1 Wire and laser plus robot

The essential parts of this process are a high-precision industrial robot, a laser system, an integrated MIG wire and laser head, and the MWES controls system. To closely monitor the process before, during, and after the construction, active head control and dynamic deposition measurement are utilised [2].

CAD/CAM software is used to import the CAD data and prepare it for the AM process. The robot path is then generated offline once the part has been "sliced" into layers. Process data can be manually edited or added automatically. The post-processor automatically translates the generated path and process information before sending it to the robot controller. The programme is then carried out by the robot, which layers the part together. The KUKA KR 90 HA (high accuracy) six-axis long-reach robot used by the ADDere system offers path flexibility and a sizable operating envelope. With a multi-axis part positioner, it is combined. Working ranges of 2 m × 8 m × 40 m, according to Woida, are feasible as shown in Figure 13.2.

Depending on the rate of deposition, tolerances between ± 0.5 mm and ± 1.5 mm are achievable. Typically, post-processing involves some machining. Soft metal needs to be annealed as well because the AM process turns the material into a harder form.

13.1.1.2 Freeform fabrication, less waste

The advantages of the system include quick design modifications without additional tooling costs, rapid development of new metal parts, and low initial manufacturing costs [3]. Woida lists the ability to integrate many part subassemblies into a single unit as one of the main advantages. The use of different metals on different areas of the item to produce tailored features particular to an application is made possible by MWES'

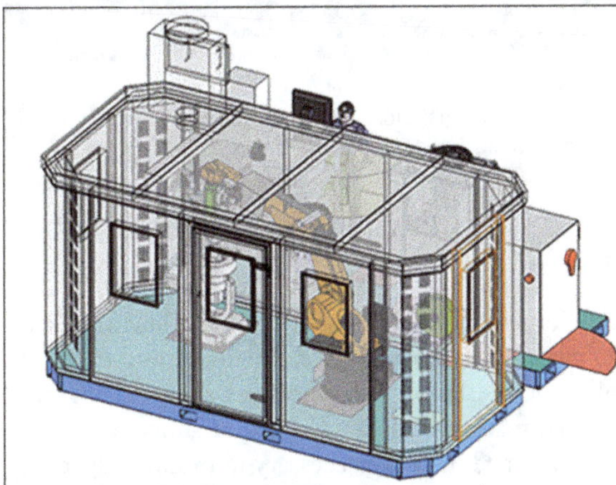

Proprietary additive manufacturing system comprises a six-axis articulated robot, integrated laser and hot wire deposition, and sophisticated controls system in a laser safety enclosure. (*Courtesy of Midwest Engineered Systems Inc.*)

Figure 13.2 Six-axis articulated robot

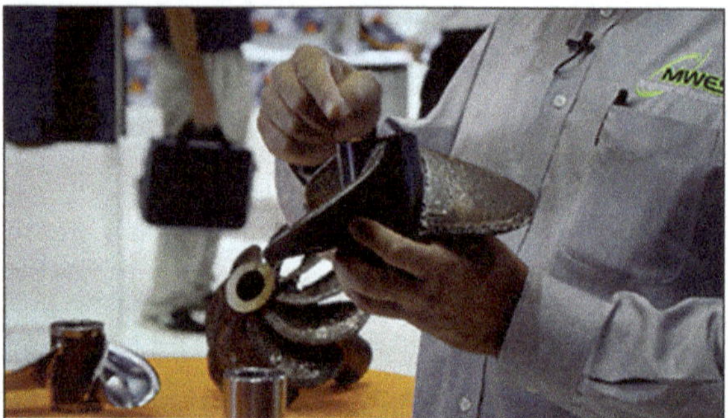

Propeller blades built with a robotic laser additive manufacturing process shown near net shape before finishing. (*Courtesy of Midwest Engineered Systems Inc.*)

Figure 13.3 Robotic laser AM

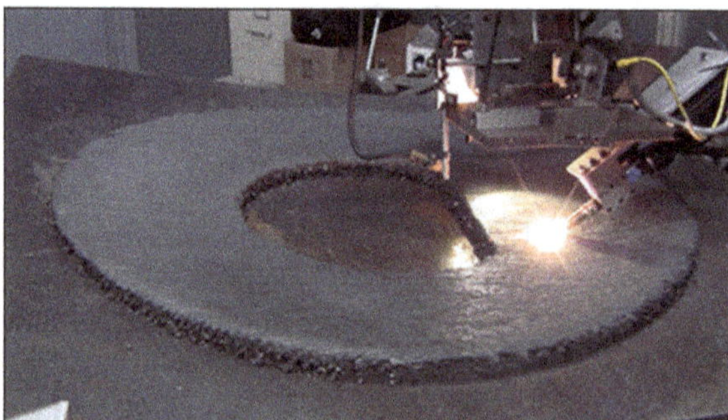

Robotic laser additive manufacturing testbed builds an 1,800-pound bulkhead one layer at a time. (*Courtesy of Midwest Engineered Systems Inc.*)

Figure 13.4 Robotic laser AM for testbed

ADDere technology for solid freeform manufacturing. This is especially cost-effective when you want to clad a less expensive metal with a more exotic metal for specific attributes like high wear resistance. The process as shown in Figure 13.3 can also be used for repairs by first machining a part to a robust structure and then rebuilding the item back to its original state. It is not necessary to machine the entire component.

13.1.1.3 High-value parts, exotic metals

The AM technology can be used to make equipment for the military, oil and gas, construction, mining, agricultural, drive train, and suspension industries. Tungsten alloy, stainless steel, titanium, Inconel and aluminium are the ideal materials used for this application as indicated in Figure 13.4.

13.1.1.4 Metal casting

The metal casting industry is likewise entering a brand-new digital era thanks to AM and robotic automation [4]. Once more, technological advancements are allowing design engineers to see a future filled with new options. The history of additive must first start at the MIT which is called as Massachusetts Institute of Technology, the birthplace of 3D printing. The process of dispensing sporadic layers of powdered materials and liquid binder in a predetermined pattern to create a 3D object is known as three-dimensional printing. Today, the terms 3D printing and AM are frequently used interchangeably, and the term now refers to a wide range of procedures as shown in Figure 13.5.

13.1.1.5 Medical equipment's 3D printing with robots

Using a standard four-axis ABB IRB460 robot, the pending patent approach creates sand moulds and cores for metal castings [5]. Sand is distributed throughout the robot by a powdered material feeder and a printer head that pours a liquid binder into the mixed sand. By occasionally spreading sand and dispensing binder, the robotic 3D printer builds the mould layer by layer. Sand can make the print head rather heavy when it is full of it. According to the procedure, four-axis robots are preferred to six-axis robots since they can support more weight. The only way that these printing parts actually work is when they are held horizontally. The print head moves on a plane and rises up quite gradually. Four-axis is appropriate because they must frequently travel on an aeroplane, at the very least with their wrists. It is accurate and capable of supporting a lot of weight as shown in Figure 13.6.

13.1.2 AM Technology using robot

Figure 13.7 shows a schematic illustration of the use of AM technologies for tissue engineering and regenerative medicine.

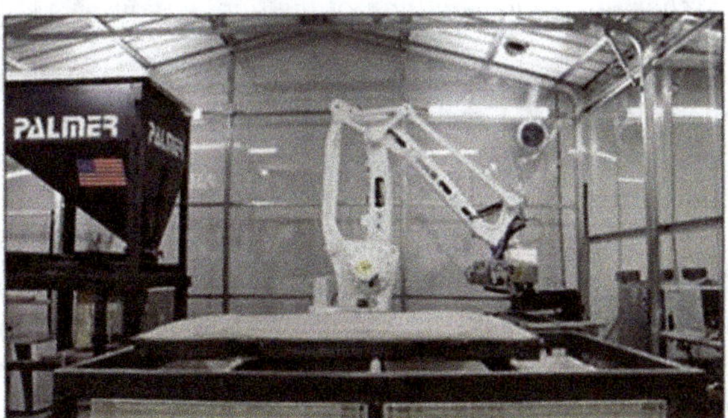

Robotic additive manufacturing system uses a proprietary 3D printing process to produce sand molds and cores for the metal casting industry. (*Courtesy of Viridis3D*)

Figure 13.5 Robotic AM for metal casting

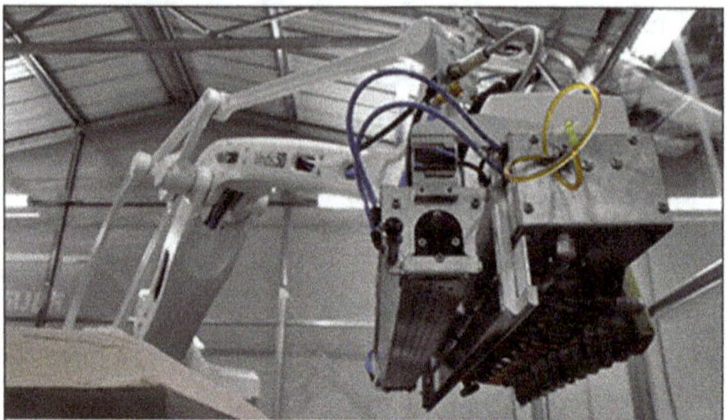

Close-up of robot-mounted 3D print head that dispenses sand and binder up to 2-1/2 inches per hour to create molds for sand casting. (*Courtesy of Viridis3D*)

Figure 13.6 Robotic laser AM for medical equipment

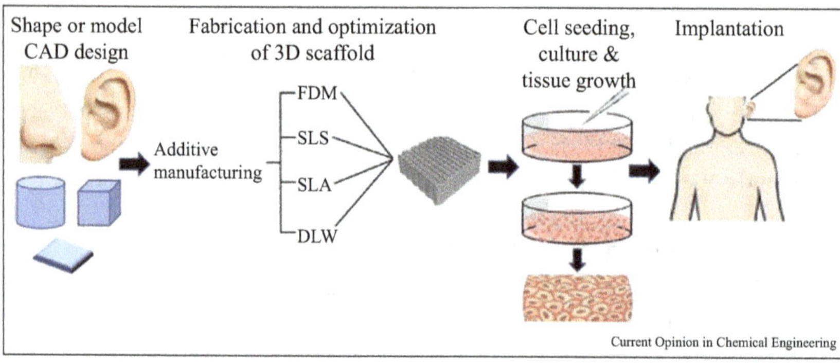

Figure 13.7 Schematic representation of the application of AM technologies

Future applications of AM technology include individualized treatment that can lower the need for medication, as well as tissue engineering and regenerative medicine. Reducing the patients' daily polypill load to one and improving patient adherence. The production of complicated heterogeneous tissues like the heart, liver, kidney, and bone, which can significantly ease the problem of organ transplant, has advanced greatly thanks to AM technology [6]. Additionally, the utilisation of 3D-printed organ models in the drug discovery and cosmetics business can put a stop to animal suffering as shown in Figure 13.7.

13.2 Human–robot interface in medical equipment

There are numerous definitions for "human–robot interaction." By way of illustration, Human–Robot Interaction (HRI) is described by Scheutz [6] as a field of study concerned with understanding, developing, and evaluating robotic systems for use by or in conjunction with people as represented in Figure 13.8. This definition of interaction states that it is the act of collaborating with others to achieve a shared goal. HRI is especially interested in how well robots can perform tasks that currently require people [7]. There are numerous ways in which a person and a robot can communicate. In this context, a team is any combination of people or robots working together to achieve a single goal [8]. However, the robot team may consist of both distinctive and comparable types of robots. Table 13.1 shows the different forms of interaction in robot human interaction. The structure of human–robot interactions is shown in Figure 13.8.

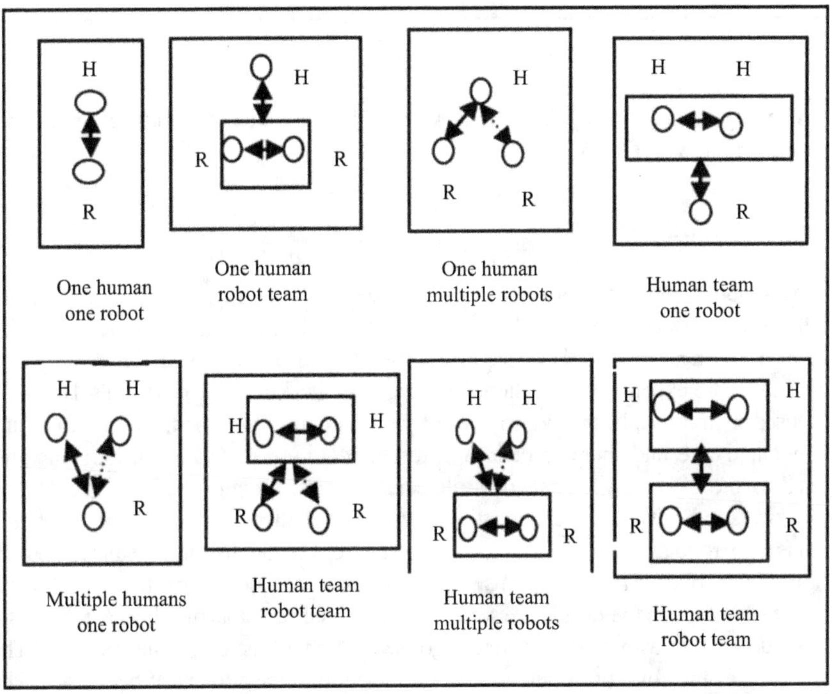

Figure 13.8 Forms of interaction in human–robot interaction

Table 13.1 An analysis of some social robots in medical equipment manufacturing

Medical robot	Interaction type	Level of autonomy	Role
Davinci Surgicals System	Proximate & remote	Non-autonomous	Human is supervisor here and operator, humans, and robots are team
Robotic Wheel Chair	Proximate	Non-autonomous	Humans and robots are team

(Continues)

Table 13.1 (*Continued*)

Medical robot	Interaction type	Level of autonomy	Role
Pearl	Proximate & remote	Non-autonomous	Human is supervisor here robots and human are team
Paro	Proximate	Non-autonomous	Robots and human are team
Guide	Proximate	Non-autonomous	Robots and human are team
Autom	Proximate	Non-autonomous	Robots and human are team

The hope that someday RFID tags would take the place of the current bar codes across all business sectors [9].

13.3 Conclusion

"Human–robot interaction" is a recent and active field that examines how people and social robots interact in specific contexts. Human–robot interaction is quickly gaining traction in the healthcare industry as a result of the expanding vulnerable populations, rising healthcare expenses, and a shortage of qualified healthcare professionals. HRI have been used in the healthcare industry to provide human company, medical treatments, rehabilitative care, and entertainment. As a result, HRI improves patient health outcomes as well as the efficiency of patient healthcare services. Despite the many benefits of social robots in healthcare, there are still a number of challenges in interactions between humans and robots. These include privacy, culture, dishonesty, trust, safety, and the design of the robot. These problems primarily result in a decline in the use of social robotic technology in the healthcare sector. The essential concepts of robots are discussed in this study, along with how they are categorised in light of the duties they perform. This study assesses the concept of human–robot interaction in the context of healthcare. This study also looks at usability and ethical concerns affecting human–robot interaction in healthcare. The ethical problems were viewed in the context of the Beauchamp and Childress's ethics principles. This study suggests that when humans and robots engage in healthcare, it is important to consider the human component, patient privacy, permission, robot safety, healthcare professional safety, and patient safety.

References

[1] T.W. Fong, I. Nourbakhsh, and I.K. Dautenhahn, A survey of socially interactive robots: concepts, design, and applications, *Robotics and Autonomous Systems*, vol. 42, pp. 142–166, 2002.

[2] J. Złotowski, D. Proudfoot, K. Yogeeswaran, and C. Bartneck, Anthropomorphism: opportunities and challenges in human–robot interaction, *International Journal of Social Robots*, vol. 7, pp. 347–360, 2015.

[3] J. Vincent, S. Taipale, B. Sapio, G. Lugano, and L. Fortunati, *Social Robots from a Human Perspective,* New York, NY: Springer, 2015.

[4] R.A. Cohen, Health insurance coverage: early release of estimates from the national health interview survey, *National Health Interview Survey Program*, http://www.cdc.gov/nchs/data/nhis/earlyrelease/insur201605.pdf, 2015.

[5] O.G. Iroju and J.O. Olaleke, Ethical issues in interoperability of electronic healthcare systems, In *Communications on Applied Electronics*, New York, NY: MECS Press, pp. 12–18, 2015.

[6] M. Scheutz, The inherent dangers of unidirectional emotional bonds between humans and social robots, In *Human-Robot Interaction Laboratory Cognitive Science Program*, Bloomington, IN: Indiana University Bloomington, 2015

[7] K.G. Engelhardt and R.A. Edwards, Human robot integration for service robotics, In M. Rahimi and W. Karwowki (eds.) (Eds.), *Human–Robot Interaction*, London: Taylor & Francis Ltd., 1992, pp. 315–346.

[8] M.O. Qureshi and R.S. Syed, The impact of robotics on employment and motivation of employees in the service sector, with special reference to health care, *Safety and Health at Work*, vol. 5, pp. 198–202, 2014.

[9] I. Olaronke, O. Oluwaseun, and I. Rhoda, State of the art: a study of human-robot interaction in healthcare. *International Journal Information Engineering and Electronic Business*, vol. 3, pp. 43–55, 2017. Published Online May 2017 in MECS Press (http://www.mecs-press.org/), doi:10.5815/ijieeb.2017.03.06.

Chapter 14

Trends in medical equipment engineering for additive manufacturing in the Industry 4.0 era

Ramesh Raju[1], Sivakumar Paramasivam[2], Tan Koon Tat[3], N. Manikandan[4], D. Giridhar[5] and P. Thejasree[6]

Medical field is creating a pathway for the holistic life as well as meeting the demands for well-being of the society. The sustainability of medical field becomes possible with the development of new and advanced medical devices and components. The technology upgradation is true with proper knowledge and awareness within medical equipment engineering. The medical field is witnessing tremendous growth in the year after year, it always becomes possible with inheritance of latest technologies every time. The present era is for Industry 4.0, it leads the world into perfect digitalization. Every single component of the system inside the digitization process is used to be interconnected and enabled the space for virtual representation.

The process makes many things very simple and even more flexible. The software-controlled system can help us to overcome any common errors made in the traditional manual system. Here the automation process enjoys the advancements in the information technology and communication process to transform the normal devices into the smart device. This Industry 4.0 setting up the smart technologies to make the paradigm shift towards advancements in the medical equipment engineering. The process of additive manufacturing which is also refereed as rapid prototyping or 3D printing comes under the part of Industry 4.0, it helps to achieve higher the level of precision and flexible to produce more intricated shapes of medical devices. The present chapter is intended to discuss more about the additive manufacturing concepts and their impact in the recent developments in the medical equipment engineering.

[1]Department of Mechanical Engineering, Sree Vidyanikethan Engineering College, India
[2]Department of Mechanical and Industrial Engineering, University of Technology & Applied Sciences, Oman
[3]Wawasan Open University, Malaysia
[4]Department of Mechanical Engineering, Mohan Babu University, India
[5]Product Management, Alarvy Technologies Private Limited, India
[6]Department of Mechanical Engineering, Mohan Babu University, India

14.1 Introduction

The medical sector becomes inevitable part of human life, the post COVID era proved the importance of healthcare sector to product human body. It demands the special attention towards maintaining optimal conditioning of healthcare systems, which is built over several years by respective societies [1–3]. The study of healthcare systems also falls under the medical equipment engineering, where several other things namely information technology, communication and computing technologies integrated with each other build a sustainable medical system [4,5]. It consistently demands the adoption of day-to-day technological advancements around the world [6]. In this connection, the recent technological advancements such as digitalization, the fourth industrial revolution, Industry 4.0 get incorporated majorly in the medical equipment engineering.

Industry 4.0, the fourth industrial revolution created a revolution in the industrial sectors and improvised the production operations and its efficiency. The process majorly focused on industrial automation through integration between heterogeneous as well as information data in terms of knowledge transition [8,9]. This Industry 4.0 is a kind of cyber physical model which integrated many technologies like Internet of Things, Cyber security, Cloud computing, digital twinning, additive manufacturing and so on. Figure 14.1 shows the architecture of the Industry 4.0 technology. To overall it makes the possibility of machine-to-machine interface without human interaction, it makes the normal process into smart process

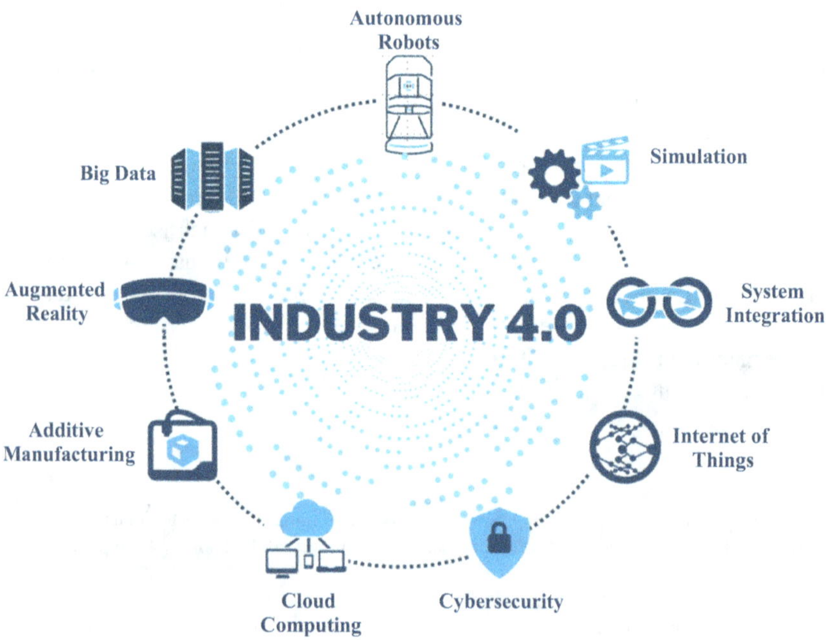

Figure 14.1 The architecture of Industry 4.0 technology [7]

[10–12]. The digitalization process helped in detailed research on materials technologies, which helped to bring out mew materials as well as methods through the additive manufacturing approach.

The additive manufacturing pointedly ensures the perfection in the design as well as manufacturing processes, Figure 14.2 shows the various processes under additive manufacturing technology. The study of additive manufacturing is very essential in order to improvise medical parts manufactured and any other practical implementations [14,15]. Additive manufacturing technique uses the layered manufacturing concepts controlled by the computer aided drawing and design programs. The process mainly ensures the fabrication of the complex structures in addition with lesser material wastage. The parts that can be produced in a short period through these techniques also ensures very cost effective. It also gives more freedom to the designer; hence, the technique was represented as manufacturing for design [16–19]. The same reasons, it attracted applications in various sectors starting from automotive to aerospace. In recent times, the biomedical field is also getting more benefit out of these techniques. The customized products can be easily manufactured through this technology; hence, it gives more attraction in biomedical sectors. It contributed to the fabrication of medical and surgical devices based on customer-specific designs and other customized implants through 3D printing process. Not only in the devices but also in the tissue engineering, human body internal organs including blood vessels are possible to create using 3D printing technology [20–23]. The 3D printing as part of additive manufacturing technology greatly overcomes the limitations and rules over the conventional human body organ donation process.

The human body organ transplantation becomes very easy through 3D printing technology, as the necessity to hire proper organ donors is eradicated. The human body organs like heart, kidneys and so on can easily be 3D printed with customized

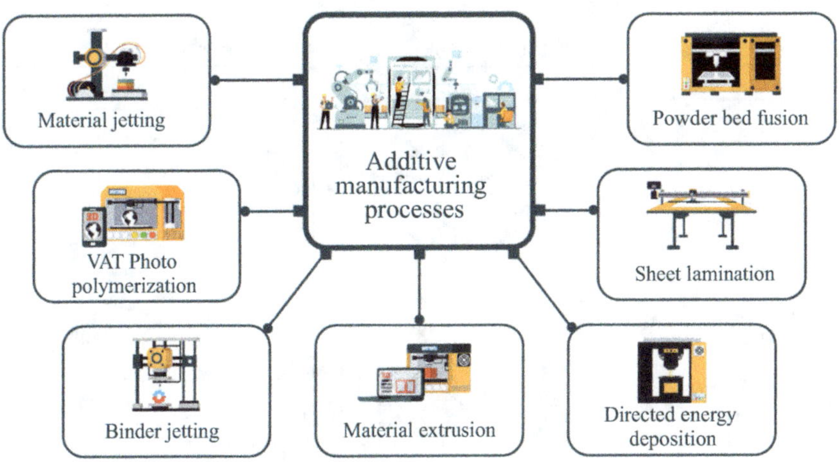

Figure 14.2 Additive manufacturing processes [13]

designs [24]. The printed parts with the support of advanced techniques like artificial intelligence and machine learning process can function like original body organs. This bio printing process is a boon to victims suffering with skin issues, as the skin tissues can easily be 3D printed up to a full thickness of the skin. With the arrival of additive manufacturing, tissue engineering witnesses a lot of advantages in the grafting then repair process. Likewise, 3D printed surgical devices and implants are getting highlighted which makes even complex orthopedic surgeries into very easy. The operation time was reduced at great extent as well as the post-operation difficulties in the conventional process were considerably reduced with this approach [25–27]. Overall, the additive manufacturing reduced many complications over conventional biomedical issues, however, the 3D printed parts also required some more attention over the biodegradability and adaptability. As the tissue engineering and 3D printing technology together can help the growth of tissue culture, the post-process like transportation of body fluids and migration of cells are still the challenging one which should obey the genetic rules of the recipient [24,28,29].

Bio-printing is most widely used along with stereolithography and inkjet bio-printing in the biomedical field, however, laser-assisted printing is also more frequently used now a days. The 3D printing technology came to limelight from Stereolithography process, the first in its kind, Figure 14.3 shows the various bio-medical components printed through 3D printing technology. This technology used thermoset polymers as work materials and produces the desired shaped components through solidification process. The ceramic bio-medical devices are mostly fabricated by this technique and similar fashion the selective laser sintering and selective

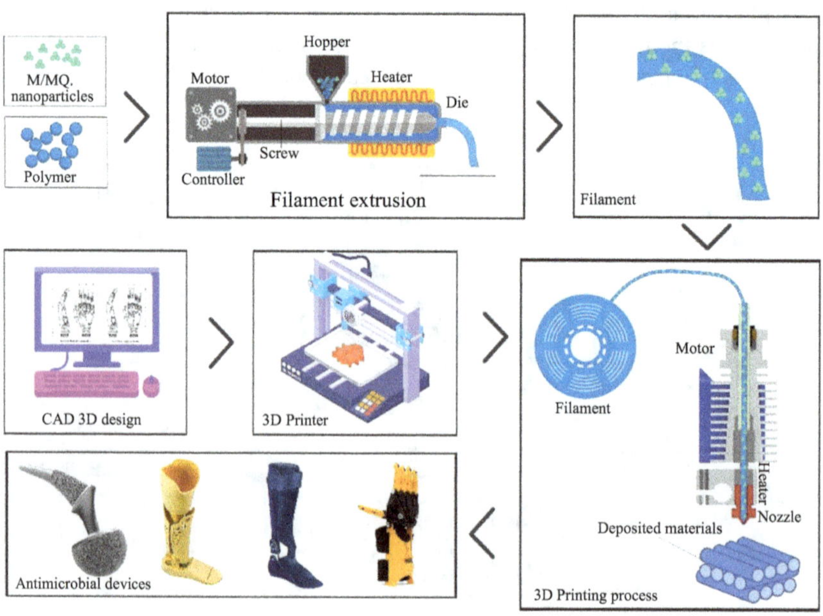

Figure 14.3 3D printing of bio-medical components [30]

laser melting processes are used to fabricate the bio-medical implants [30–32]. The selective laser ablation process was most popularly suggested for the fabrication of dental implants. There are many materials – metals to polymers and ceramics can be used in the additive manufacturing technology for the medical implants. The study of medical equipment engineering further speaks about the advantages of additive manufacturing process over other techniques [33,34]. The major advantages like 3D bio-printed devices exhibit superior thermal and mechanical properties than other conventional fabricated components [33–35]. The present work is mainly focused on to elaborate the influence of Industry 4.0 and the applications of additive manufacturing in the biomedical field.

14.2 The Industry 4.0 model

The fourth industrial revolution was the outcome of joint initiatives from several associations across Germany. The reference architecture model for the same is also created to give basic understanding about the existing standards and technological implementations [36,37]. The reference model contains several layers from asset layer to business layer, Figure 14.4 shows various layers in the Industry 4.0 architecture. Each layer is dedicated to perform several tasks. The first layer is Asset Layer, which emphasizes the corporal components connected within the system.

All these components were connected with cyber system for effective communication with outside systems and this layer is represented as Integration layer. Next comes the communication layer, which takes the job of data dispatch and delivery from internal systems to external systems and vice versa. The communication layer is the predominant layer works along with integration layer for attaining uniformity in data transfer. Information layer is taking care of converting the available data into useful information and carry forward to the next level via the functional layer. The data integrity of the system mainly depends on this layer, and it takes care of system integrity with virtual access. The last layer, business layer, empowers the connection between various

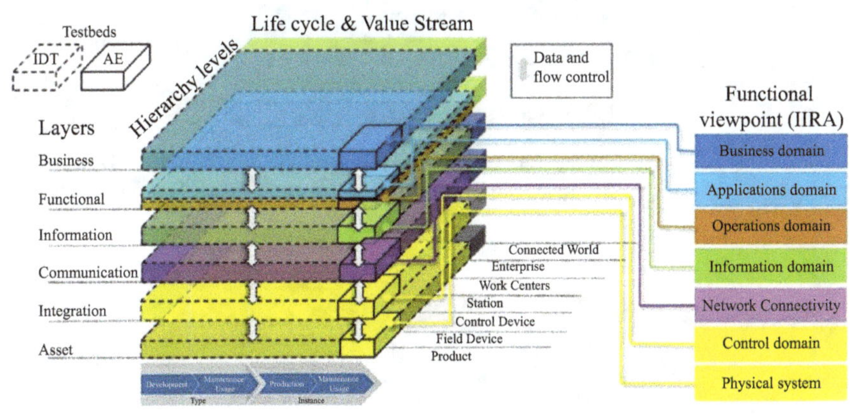

Figure 14.4 Industry 4.0 (RAMI 4.0) architecture for the IDT and AE testbeds [38]

business models [39–42]. The integration of all layers helps to meet the objective of Industry 4.0, the impending machines and respective manufacturing setups. The Industry 4.0 structure importunately consists of a few building blocks such as industrial IoT, Cloud computing, augmented reality, cyber security, and additive manufacturing [43,44].

14.2.1 Industrial Internet of Things

The primary sector of Industry 4.0 evolves through the Internet protocol connections, which makes each and every part of the systems stay interconnected within the developed model. The buzzword Internet rules the entire world by connecting anything together. The objects or the human everyone is well connected and can communicate anything very instant [45,46]. The revolution in the Internet world made possible to transport any data into anywhere through this network. The technology converts any information into the digital forms with the help of cyber-physical as well as virtual technologies. Hence, the entire system, for example the manufacturing units along with machineries, can be brought into the virtual world and controlled very easily [47,48]. This industrial IoT benefits the systems to attain a state where the works can be decentralized and assorted. The architecture of IoT consists of four layers and they are Sensing, Network, Service and Interface layers [49,50].

Figure 14.5 shows the various layers of IoT architecture, the first layer sensing layer integrated with many technical gadgets like sensors and actuators to identify the object status. Here objects could be anything and the identified or predicted

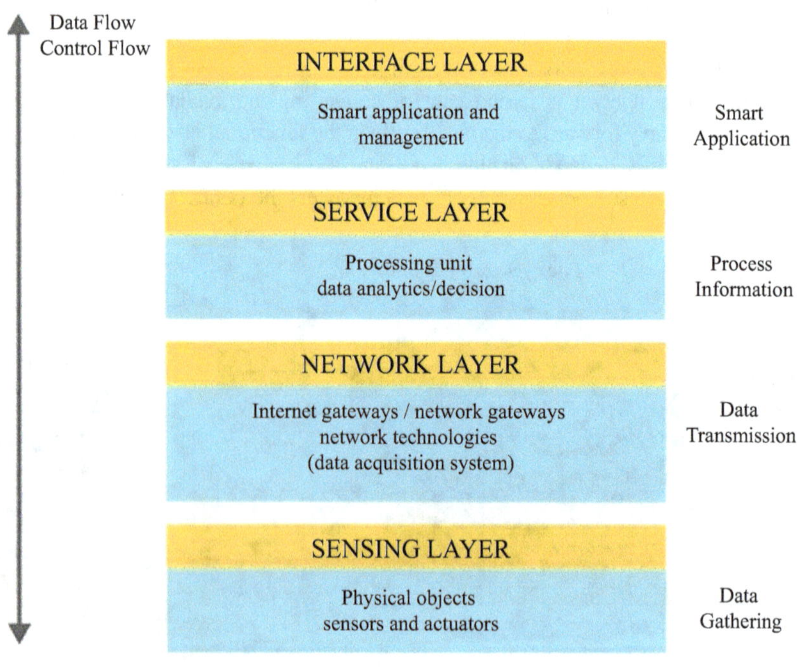

Figure 14.5 Architecture of the IoT with different layer levels

information will be sent to the next layer for further processing. The network layer takes care of the effective transformation of data between sensing and service layers. The optimal network connections are made in this layer to transfer the data without any loss. The service layer acts like a storage database where it stores all the received information and can retrieve the stored information based on requirements. This layer is intended to support the entire architecture and system with respect to the data handling and usage by adopting the middleware technology. The last layer is the interface layer, which takes care of the integration of end-to-end system, through internal connections it allows the end user to access the required information from the system [51–55]. The industrial IoT has proved as one of the valuable assets to recent technology specially to improve the performance efficiency of the system.

14.2.2 Cloud computing

Cloud computing is a technological gift to the present-day era for the majority of the companies. Cloud computing is a resource sharing with speedy and flexible service technique. The cloud computing service became a mandatory self-service with its broad Internet access. The cloud computing offers resource mobilization facilities with a mountable computing facilitator to interconnect any instruments which are connected in the network through internet service all over the world. The cloud offers different services based on the end user's requirement [56]. In general, services can be either a public domain where everyone can have the access to the data or a private domain which limits to a particular group with more benefits. At some instances, the combination of both public and private can be offered in the name of hybrid domain and some cases like community domains [57,58].

The cloud services are further defined as infrastructure, platform and software services. Figure 14.6 represents the different layers under cloud architecture. The

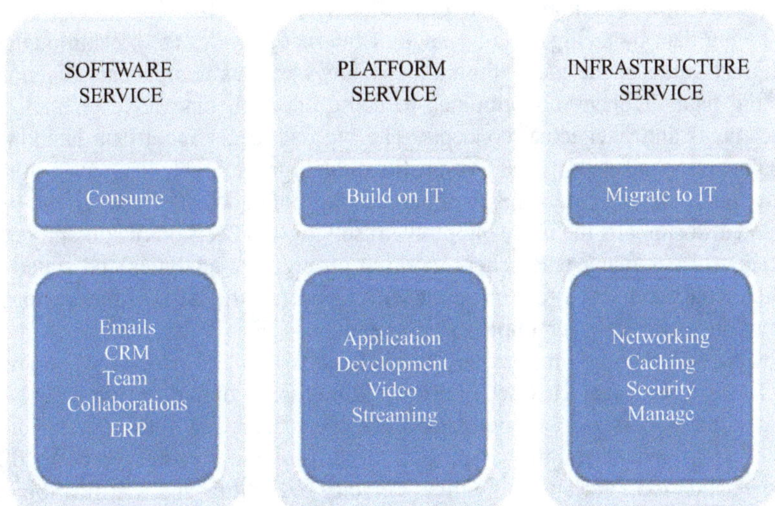

Figure 14.6 Architecture of the cloud computing with different service levels

infrastructure service represents the virtual space which is provided to the end user. The virtual space acts like a server and user can deploy and retrieve their data. The end users develop and run any applications in the next service which is referred as platform service. The development and deployment of programming will take place at platform service [58,59]. The place helps to achieve speedy processes with more storage capacity also it is totally free and users no need to bother about the maintenance. The place where programming languages are getting executed is referred as software service. The virtual connection enables the end users to execute their software applications by operating their systems from different location. It greatly helps to eliminate the additional spaces required for launching the software applications in the local devices. The user can easily afford the ownership for any software applications through this process. By combining all these infrastructure, platform and software services a cloud manufacturing perception was created [60].

The cloud manufacturing acts like demand-based solution provider in every stage of manufacturing which enables it to service based methodology. It changes the perception of conventional manufacturing from production based to service based approach. The technology enables the sustainable engineering process by means of balancing the providers and the users. The data can be safer and more secured while adopting hybrid domain in this approach [60,61]. The general data can be accessed in the public cloud domain while the important data can be secured by allotting them to the private cloud domain.

14.2.3 Big data

Big data characterizes the handling of bulk amount of data generated through various operations. The data can be any form like organized, partially organized and chaotic which customarily needs more attention. Handling such a type of data attracts more time and money in a conventional approach [62–64].

The big data by taking the advantage of Internet provides the breakthrough and offers great value to the users, Figure 14.7 shows various components functioning under big data. It opens opportunities to come out with innovative technological advancements and intellectual concepts. The big data deals about data handling as well as analysis and with the help of artificial intelligence it acts like smart solution provider [64]. The big data helps to attain a fool proof and cost-effective state to the users and also supports the user with problem solving and decision-making processes.

Recent times many researchers working on big data analytics and stated that still there is a good scope to work on it with respect to the state-of-the-art form of information processing for improved perceptions. The big data can be primarily categorized based on volume, variety and velocity within the structured framework [65]. These three categories act like three dimensions of the big data analytics. Similarly, to process most complicated data, there are a few more dimensions in terms of accuracy and stability coming to the picture and they are represented like Vision, Validation, Variability, Value, Veracity, Volatility and Verification. The big data process can be restrained and assessed by all its dimensions, and one needs cutting-edge analytics to discover more.

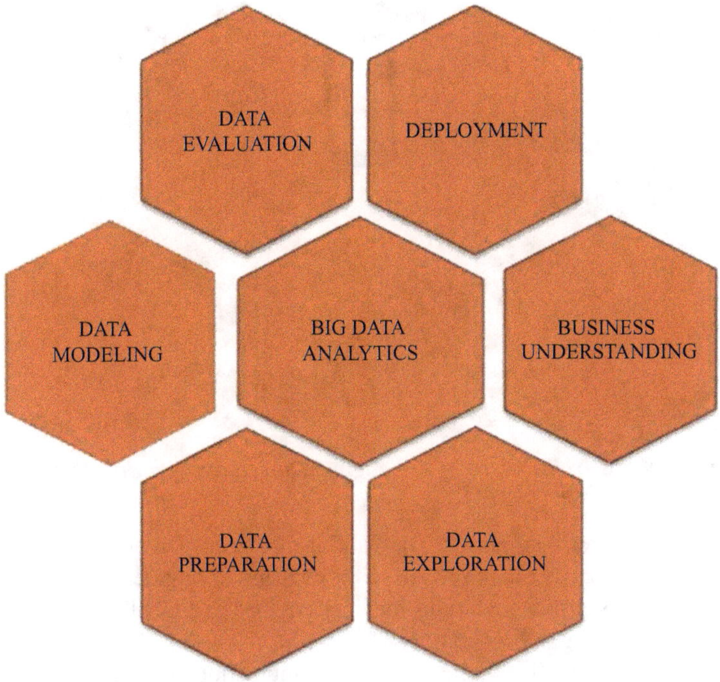

Figure 14.7 Architecture of the Big data with different components

The big data along with cloud computing offers the great advantages, the data can be processed and mined very well. This advanced big data can facilitate best solutions to the end user for any kind of complicated tailback situations. The paradigm shift towards smart technology was made possible by the IoT-assisted big data. It reveals that big data can assist the users to make coherent, well-versed and approachable decision-making. The medical equipment engineering affordability in the worldwide market is improved by these big data characteristics. The data flow from bottom most level plays a significant role in the engineering process, hence, the data should be more accurate and analyzed in a very distinctive way [65–67]. Further it is very well noted that the big data is a main part of digital engineering.

14.2.4 Augmented reality

The augmented reality assists with human to enhance their performance by guiding with data as well as desired information to accomplish any specific job. The human to machine interface becomes easy with this innovative technology. Nowadays the application of this technology is started increasing from manufacturing sectors to medical sectors and so on [68,69]. The augmented reality provides solution to many of the day-to-day problems by means of providing lot of additional artificial information. The augmented reality inbuilds the ability to simulate and reproduce any task with the help of artificial information and digital data. The insight of the

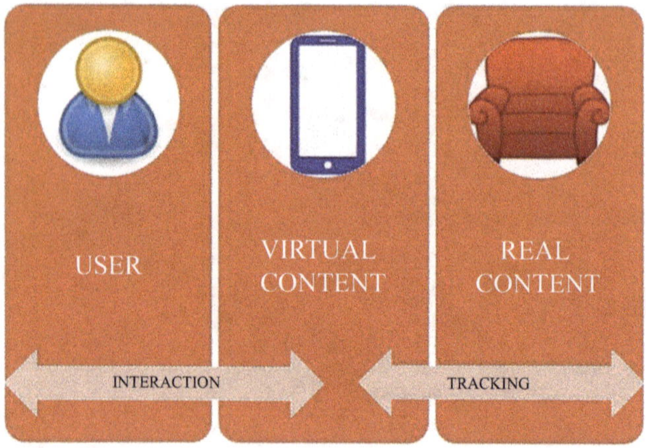

Figure 14.8 Architecture of the augmented reality with different levels

users behaves smarter than normal way, and it makes easy to accomplish any task with a more efficient manner [69,70]. The concept of augmented reality started increasing in every sector including medical engineering to fill the technological gaps between planning and operations [71].

The augmented reality works with the combination of digital processing as well as artificial intelligent, Figure 14.8 shows the flow and interactions inside the process. The user gets into the feel of the environment in terms of its reality in addition to the artificial intelligence-based guidance. The guidance can be associated as 2- or 3-dimensional objects with respect to the surroundings. This augmented reality provides on-time solutions to the users which can suppress most of technical glitches in the real time environment [70–72]. The hardware and software components used in the augmented reality might be chosen in accordance with the environmental conditions, which differ for every application, e.g., the augmented reality in medical environment depends on remote assistances connections, differing from the real-time military applications [69–71,73,74].

14.2.5 Cybersecurity

The Internet era is bringing every device to under single roof and the count is always increasing in order. As the devices are getting linked with global network, the chances of vulnerabilities attack to the user data are also getting increased. The possibilities to compromise on user information lead to uncertainty in the real-time applications and faithfulness on the technology. In this connection, the industries set up an advanced level of security system to protect the user information, as the security is defined for the virtual world it was named cyber security [75,76]. The cybersecurity runs on IoT and offers complete protection over data theft and any untoward occurrences. The IoT-based cybersecurity can respond and defends to any type of cyber-attacks and confirms safer communication between the facilitators. The Industry 4.0 environment would be very safer and always protected under this cybersecurity. This industry-based cybersecurity has superior controls over data acquisition and processing systems as well as programming logic control units. However, the growing number of IoT devices may become easy target for vulnerabilities attacks, the cybersecurity in such cases supposed to be strengthened with more controlling features [77,78].

The data security and information protection play a significant role in any industrial sectors, Figure 14.9 represents the different features. The authentication process is very important and so the veracity and information dada must be established. The cybersecurity should possess security to the system architecture as well as design, it greatly reduces the complications over system integration. The industrial sectors with weak cybersecurity may be easily targeted and prone to be attacked. These attacks lead to changes in the entire system architecture and designs which may lead to complete change in the system operations [78,79]. Also, it may further lead to a chance of losing the total control over system, such that user have to face severe consequences like money loss, delay in the process and finally result in customer loss due to no trust.

The cyber-attack from internal sources generally occurs, as there are more possibilities to communicate with outside through unprotected channels. Sometimes the wireless connection and weak firewall system may open a fair chance, as it may access the external sources or outside data port. To avoid any such cases the cybersecurity has to be automated [77–80]. The automation can be offered through cloud

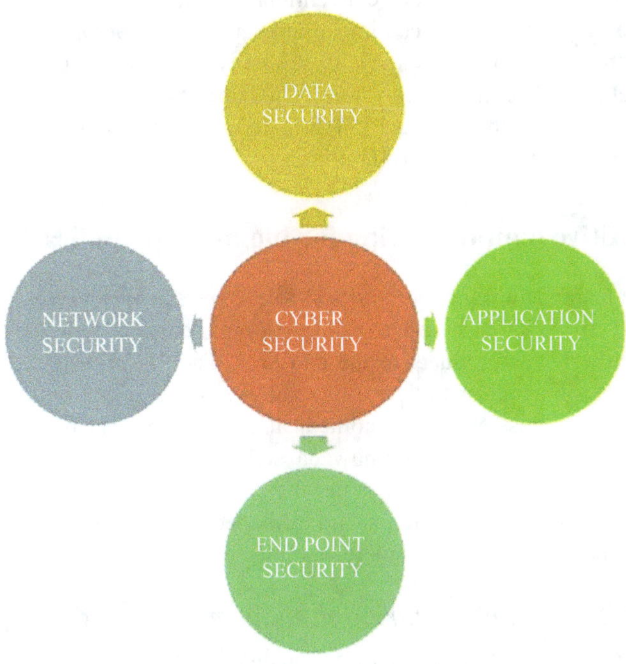

Figure 14.9 Architecture of the cybersecurity with different security features

architecture, software-defined network, and network function virtualization. It improves the cyber network in a greater extent with respect to the visibility, capability and functionality aspects.

14.2.6 Additive manufacturing

The Industry 4.0 deals all pre-processes through virtual manner by using digital technology, next comes as real-time fabrication. Here, the industry again needs a smart technology to exhibit whatever the things previously planned. The smart technology has to continue the same momentum created by previous virtual processes [81]. The additive manufacturing is one such technology which fulfils the demand created here. Additive manufacturing is a technology in demand all over the world, as the users are having complete freedom over the fabrication of their desired components. It enhanced the flexibility over new designs, new materials and new products which created a healthy livelihood for the end user. The technology also offered low or almost no wastage of raw materials, the fabrication will take place as an additive process, layer by layer development [82,83]. The word 3D printing in additive manufacturing became very popular by the way the products were built over. The complicated shape product can be easily fabricated in this process in passionate manner. The process is speedy compared with conventional fabrication process; hence, it is also referred as rapid prototyping, digital manufacturing processes.

The additive manufacturing process starts with design stage where the user having complete freedom to come out with any design shape or model. The freedom is not available in any other conventional fabrication process [82–84]. The design further processed and sliced into a number of layers before delivering to the printing control unit. It made possible to print any materials up to any scale, e.g., bioprinting at a level of micro/nano scale. The fabrication will take place at higher resolution level on multi-materials [84–86]. In a day-to-day life, the technology further improvised to the level of 4D printing.

14.3 Additive manufacturing for biomedical applications

The additive manufacturing plays a critical role in the scientific development in the medical field. It works with largest dataset towards enhanced engineering design and delivers the better products to the end user. The 3D printing becomes most inevitable part of smart manufacturing and the same fashion, the technology brought several progressions in the biomedical applications. The printing of various biomaterials became very common nowadays. The human tissues and body organs can be easily designed and printed as per the customized design. Also, the human body implants like vascular stents and orthopedic implants were successfully modeled and fabricated through this technology.

14.3.1 Additive manufacturing in tissue engineering

The human bone is having regenerative quality by nature, still the quality may change with respect to any injuries on the bone. The injured bone may lag with regenerative process leading to permanent damages like bone cancer. In such cases, most often traditional methods are used to recover from the damage and sometimes it will suggest for bone replacement. Tables 14.1–14.6 give the clarity about various materials processed under different 3D printing techniques and their outcomes.

The metals and polymers were used to prepare a support structure while performing bone replacement. And a lot of conventional methods were used to prepare such a support structure in the previous days, however, the control over metallurgical properties of the materials is very difficult. Controlling the metallurgical properties like pore size is more important while preparing for bone replacement. The 3D printing technology proved that control over such properties is no more difficult in the present days. The support structures and tissues are getting developed and replaced with defected bones inside the human body, the adoptability of such materials shows a great progress and one can witness the growth of new tissues over there [84,85].

The 3D printed materials always show very good metallurgical and mechanical properties also show biocompatible with human body. As these are the essential properties for the healing and cell growth, fabrication of such support structures cannot be compromised on its quality part. The metallurgical property of the fabricated structure plays a significant role in cell transportation and orientation. The medical records indicates that the lower the pore sizes like 100–700 μm gives better nutrient flow through the

Table 14.1 Various materials processed through fused deposition modeling-based 3D printing technique and their properties

Materials	Property and performance
Bioactive glasses	The printed bioactive glass composite scaffolds components produced a favourable result under laboratory test conditions [87].
Polymer-bioactive Glass Composite Filaments	The FDM proved as an effective method to fabricate PLA-BG composite scaffolds which was best suited for bone tissue engineering [88].
Poly (butylene adipate-co-terephthalate) (PBAT)/niobium containing bioactive glasses (BAGNb) scaffolds	The properties and shape of the 3D printed scaffolds were most satisfying and further recommended as best alternative to fabricate bioactive materials for bone regeneration [89].
Bioceramic scaffolds	The 3D fabricated component exhibited superior compressive strength and filigree structure with moderate porosity [90].
Phosphate glass	The FDM offered superior quality and the better layer resolutions [91].
Biphasic calcium phosphate	The BCP/ZrO2 scaffold blended with slurry foams was fabricated successfully through FDM technology. The sintering process was further implemented to remove the blending materials from the fabricated structure. The fabricated structure exhibited with the desired pore characteristics, porosity and dimension [92].

Table 14.2 Various materials processed through steriolithography-based 3D printing technique and their properties

Materials	Performance
Mesoporous bioactive glasses (MBGs)	The SLA process significantly achieved improvement in the processing of bioactive materials and made easy to preserve the textural and functional properties of MBGs. The fabricated scaffolds exhibited superior mechanical properties [93].
Nanocomposite hydrogel	The nanocomposite hydrogel scaffold was fabricated. The fabricated structures witnessed excellent biocompatibility and bioactive properties. The tissue-specific growth factors show a coactive effect with respect to the increased cell adhesion and directed stem cell differentiation [94].
GelMA/PCL and dECM/ PCL resins	The bio resin material dECM/PCL-MA hydrogels were fabricated by 3D printing processes. The fabricated components exhibited excellent qualities which made it suitable to replace the conventional ECM (dECM-MA) hydrogels [95].
Calcium-phosphate	The SLA fabricated CaP-based scaffolds show better quality and compatibility, however, still there was a scope left for improvising the accuracy and biomimetic scaffolds materials [96]

Table 14.3 Various materials processed through digital light processing-based 3D printing technique and their properties

Materials	Property and performance
Cell-seeding hydrogel	The mechanical property, elastic modulus increased 60% through the 3D fabrication [97].
Poly l-lactic acid synthesis	The DLP based 3D printing shows optimal quality to fabricate synthesized polymer-based bio materials for scaffolds with intricate structures [98].
Silica-doped HAp ceramic	The fabricated ceramic scaffold exhibited superior mechanical strength as well as vitro bioactive [99].
β-Tricalcium phosphate	The DLP 3D printing process shows significant performance for bone regeneration [100].
GelMA/HAp porous composite	The fabricated GelMA/HAp porous composite scaffolds revealed superior mechanical properties and osteogenic activity [101].

Table 14.4 Various materials processed through powder sintering-based 3D printing technique and their properties

Materials	Property and performance
Poly (3-hydroxybutyrate) scaffolds	The fabricated structures show ability to sustain cell growth to support tissue formation [102].
Polymeric scaffolds	The 3D-printed structures exhibited excellent qualities and made them more suitable for next generation polymeric scaffolds [103].
Bio ceramic scaffolds	The 3D fabrication technology suits well for the fabrication of bone scaffolds used in vitro models [104].

Table 14.5 Various materials processed through electron beam melting-based 3D printing technique and their properties

Materials	Property and performance
Metal scaffolds	EBM was recognized as a capable technology for fabricating complex non-stochastic metallic scaffolds [105].
Titanium scaffolds	The fabricated artificial organs shown very good biocompatibility with the connective tissues. The process was also recommended for dental implants [106].
Ti6Al4V scaffolds	The mechanical property of the fabricated components was improved also the pore size and the porosity of the scaffold matched with bone tissues [107].
Ti-6Al-4V	The fabricated scaffold structure possessed improved fatigue life [108].
Anisotropic Ti-6Al-4V gyroid scaffolds	The fabricated metallic structure exhibited with mixed mode of ductile and brittle behavior under test conditions [109].
Ti2448 scaffolds	The fabricated implant structure shows significantly improved biological functionalities [110].

Table 14.6 Various materials processed through binder jetting-based 3D printing technique and their properties

Materials	Property and performance
Tricalcium phosphate scaffolds	The fabricated MgO/ZnO-TCP scaffold shows improved mechanical and biological properties, which is most preferred for orthopedic and dental applications [114].
Tricalcium phosphate-bioactive glass	The fabricated TCP-BG scaffolds exhibited with superior mechanical and dissolution properties [115].
Biphasic calcium phosphate, Polycaprolactone Scaffold	The fabricated PCL/BCP composite scaffold exhibited superior mechanical properties like high compressive strength, moduli, and toughness [116].
Biodegradable Fe-Mn-Ca/Mg alloys	The fabricated Fe-Mn and Fe-Mn-1Ca alloys shows its feasibility as hypothetically feasible bone structures [117].
Ceramic bone scaffolds	The fabricated bone scaffolds shows a biocompatibility, very good mechanical strength and dimensional accuracy [118].
Ceramic bone scaffolds	The fabricated ceramic bone scaffolds exhibited good compressive strength as well as decent percentage of porosity level [119].

support structures [84,86]. Fabrication of such a sensitive structure is always possible with 3D printing technology, also, the fabricated structures possess a similar quality to the existing neighboring tissues in the same human body. In a similar way, the mechanical properties like roughness and wettability of the structure play a vital role in

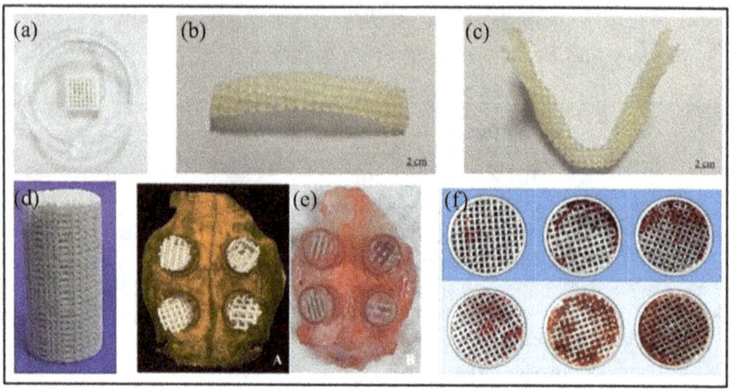

Figure 14.10 Scaffold images of different materials produced by different 3D printing techniques: (a) 3D-printed bone scaffold by FDM [111]; (b) and (c) pure UV-cured resin using SLA [112]; (d) 3D printed scaffold via SLS [102]; (e) 3D-printed HA/TCP scaffolds using DLP [113]; (f) graphene-reinforced biodegradable resin composites for stereolithographic 3D printing of bone structure scaffolds [107]

the bio activeness inside the human body. Fabrication of such a structure will be done by different 3D printing processes based on the materials to be possessed, Figure 14.10 represents various scaffolds fabricated using different 3D printing technologies.

14.3.2 Additive manufacturing in medical devices and implants

The additive manufacturing made a remarkable achievement in the scaffold fabrication, in the same manner, the technology proved as a best alternative for the fabrication of human implants and other medical devices. The implants act as replacement inside the human body, in such cases, the implants must be custom designed with more accuracy and quality. Like scaffold, the implants also should possess very good mechanical and metallurgical properties along with. The medical implants surface should be bio acceptable and biocompatible with human body tissues and cells, as the implant performance is highly depending on the cell adhesion. For all these reasons, biodegradable materials are mostly preferred for the fabrication of such implants [120–122]. The additive manufacturing has shown a promising approach towards fabrication of such implants without compromising the material properties and accuracy. Different kinds of implants are already fabricated through additive manufacturing route, e.g., knee joints, dental implants, and femur and fibula implants. Many researchers reported the significant achievements made in the development of human implants through 3D printing approach [122,123]. The printed implants have shown good fatigue strength and very good corrosion resistance properties. The different structural formation in the combinations of cubic and octahedral also been reported by many researchers. All those fabricated structures possessed superior mechanical strength, reasonable pore size, and porosity [122–125].

The materials used in the implants must be compatible with human body tissues, hence, metal powders are used for the fabrication of such implants. The 3D fused powder deposition technique is most suitable for the fabrication of powder-based materials. The polymer-based materials such as polyether ether ketone (PEEK) are also recommended for medical implants. The PEEK exhibited superior mechanical and metallurgical qualities and made them best suitable for spinal as well as orthopedic implants [130–132]. The PEEK-based implants were experimented by many researchers and reported that the PEEK-based implants show great biocompatibility which are very effective for the cell adhesion and helped to attain fast recovery in the treatment process [133]. There are metallic implants made by titanium alloys like Ti6Al4V can be 3D printed through EBM techniques. The implants made by titanium-based alloys possess an acceptable level of compatibility with human body. Similarly, many nano composites also used for the fabrication of biomedical implants [134–136]. Figure 14.11

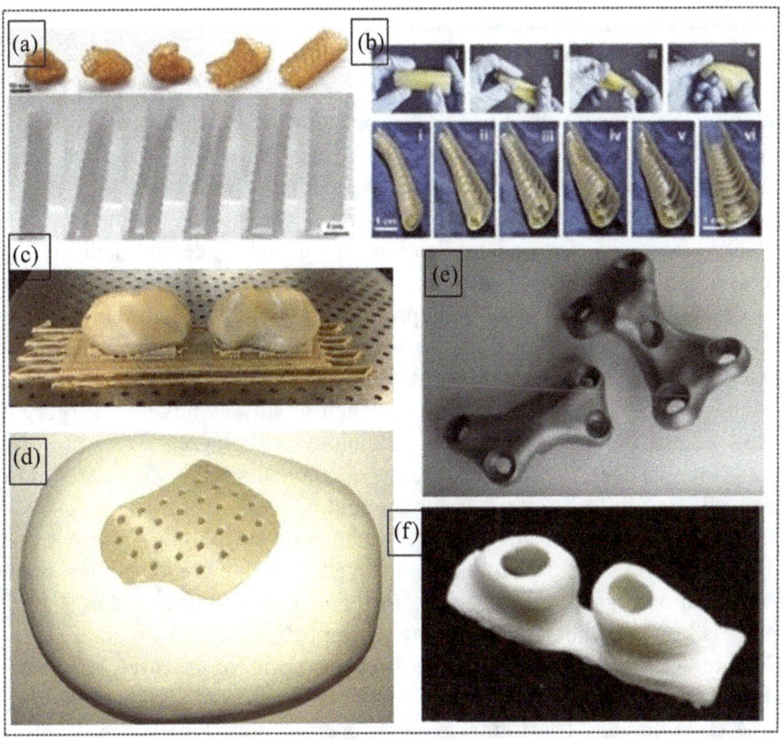

Figure 14.11 Medical implants produced by various 3D printing processes: (a) shape-memory stent prototypes from PCL photopolymers. (b) Shape-memory tracheal stent from poly(propylene glycol)-PCL block photopolymers [126]. (c) Prosthetic implant for scaphoid bone replacement. (d) PEEK cranioplasty PSI [127]. (e) EBM printed titanium bone implants made from Ti–6Al–4V [128]. (f) FDM fabricated PLA-based personalized nasal support [129].

illustrates the various medical implants fabricated from different biomaterials using different 3D printing technologies.

The additive manufacturing technique is also used in the fabrication of medical devices which are mostly polymer-based materials. The 3D printing technology is more pioneer in the fabrication of polymer materials, it makes the technique more suitable for the fabrication of medical devices in recent times. The material epoxy resins are used to produce hearing aids in biomedical devices which can be fabricated through SLA technology, as the fabrication is very cost effective also offers increased product life [137]. The other devices like medical stethoscopes, eye glasses and lenses can be fabricated in an effective manner using this technology. The recent pandemic situation made the FDM and SLS technology to move forwards towards fabrication of many medical emergency kits like face shields, antibacterial face masks and so on. The swabs used for testing were fabricated by this technology and the fabricated kit shows good accuracy and superior mechanical qualities [138–141].

14.4 Conclusion

The additive manufacturing is one of the research areas which are growing very rapidly in a recent time. The technology is most suited for the fabrication of medical engineering devices in accordance with the custom-made design and development. The technique attracted many researchers in the biomedical field as because the necessity for the fabrication of custom-made biomedical support structures, implants and devices is more. The fabrication of prostheses and implants was successfully made by various 3D printing technologies. The fabricated structures were exhibited excellent qualities with respect to the mechanical and metallurgical properties. The biocompatibility of such structures with human body tissues and cells is also quite impressive which greatly avoids post-surgery complications in the human body. The technology offers great freedom towards designing such devices and implants, as the components can be fabricated into any custom-made design to fit into any human bodies.

The human organ fabrication through additive manufacturing processes opens a great channel for organ transplantation in the medical field. The biomedical materials can be printed on organic and inorganic materials makes very easy for bioprinting. The process used for the fabrications of biocompatible human organs reduces the complications of waiting for organ donors in the majority of the cases. However, still there is lot of scope for working on the 3D printing parameters such as printing speed and time consumption. The future research opens a door for many researchers to work on progressive aspect of 3D fabrications of biomedical devices.

References

[1] Bai C, Dallasega P, Orzes G, and Sarkis J. Industry 4.0 technologies assessment: a sustainability perspective. *International Journal of Production Economics*. 2020;229:107776.

[2] Tang YM, Chau KY, Fatima A, and Waqas M. Industry 4.0 technology and circular economy practices: business management strategies for environmental sustainability. *Environmental Science and Pollution Research*. 2022;29(33):49752–69.

[3] Nascimento DL, Alencastro V, Quelhas OL, *et al.* Exploring Industry 4.0 technologies to enable circular economy practices in a manufacturing context: a business model proposal. *Journal of Manufacturing Technology Management*. 2019;30(3):607–27.

[4] Ibarra D, Ganzarain J, and Igartua JI. Business model innovation through Industry 4.0: a review. *Procedia Manufacturing*. 2018;22:4–10.

[5] Nagy J, Oláh J, Erdei E, Máté D, and Popp J. The role and impact of Industry 4.0 and the internet of things on the business strategy of the value chain—the case of Hungary. *Sustainability*. 2018;10(10):3491.

[6] Marcucci G, Antomarioni S, Ciarapica FE, and Bevilacqua M. The impact of operations and IT-related Industry 4.0 key technologies on organizational resilience. *Production Planning & Control*. 2022;33(15):1417–31.

[7] Web Reference: https://www.calsoft.com/what-is-industry-4-0/

[8] Buer SV, Strandhagen JO, and Chan FT. The link between Industry 4.0 and lean manufacturing: mapping current research and establishing a research agenda. *International Journal of Production Research*. 2018;56(8):2924–40.

[9] Ozkan-Ozen YD and Kazancoglu Y. Analysing workforce development challenges in the Industry 4.0. *International Journal of Manpower*. 2022;43 (2):310–33.

[10] Frederico GF, Garza-Reyes JA, Kumar A, and Kumar V. Performance measurement for supply chains in the Industry 4.0 era: a balanced scorecard approach. *International Journal of Productivity and Performance Management*. 2021;70(4):789–807.

[11] Frederico GF, Garza-Reyes JA, Kumar A, and Kumar V. Performance measurement for supply chains in the Industry 4.0 era: a balanced scorecard approach. *International Journal of Productivity and Performance Management*. 2021;70(4):789–807.

[12] Javaid M, Haleem A, Singh RP, Suman R, and Gonzalez ES. Understanding the adoption of Industry 4.0 technologies in improving environmental sustainability. *Sustainable Operations and Computers*. 2022;3:203–217.

[13] Web Reference: https://www.symmetryelectronics.com/blog/defining-additive-manufacturing/

[14] Singh P, Singari RM, and Mishra RS. A review of study on modeling and simulation of additive manufacturing processes. *Materials Today: Proceedings*. 2022;56:3594–603.

[15] Mahadevan S, Nath P, and Hu Z. Uncertainty quantification for additive manufacturing process improvement: recent advances. *ASCE-ASME Journal of Risk and Uncertainty in Engineering Systems, Part B: Mechanical Engineering*. 2022;8(1):010801.

[16] de Pastre MA, Quinsat Y, and Lartigue C. Effects of additive manufacturing processes on part defects and properties: a classification review.

International Journal on Interactive Design and Manufacturing (IJIDeM). 2022;16(4):1471–96.

[17] Korkmaz ME, Waqar S, Garcia-Collado A, Gupta MK, and Krolczyk GM. A technical overview of metallic parts in hybrid additive manufacturing industry. *Journal of Materials Research and Technology*. 2022;18:384–395.

[18] Brenken B, Barocio E, Favaloro A, Kunc V, and Pipes RB. Development and validation of extrusion deposition additive manufacturing process simulations. *Additive Manufacturing*. 2019;25:218–26.

[19] Salmi M. Additive manufacturing processes in medical applications. *Materials*. 2021;14(1):191.

[20] Germaini MM, Belhabib S, Guessasma S, Deterre R, Corre P, and Weiss P. Additive manufacturing of biomaterials for bone tissue engineering – a critical review of the state of the art and new concepts. *Progress in Materials Science*. 2022;130:100963.

[21] Yousef H, Harris BT, Elathamna EN, Morton D, and Lin WS. Effect of additive manufacturing process and storage condition on the dimensional accuracy and stability of 3D-printed dental casts. *The Journal of Prosthetic Dentistry*. 2022;128(5):1041–6.

[22] Yu JR, Navarro J, Coburn JC, *et al.* Current and future perspectives on skin tissue engineering: key features of biomedical research, translational assessment, and clinical application. *Advanced Healthcare Materials*. 2019;8(5):1801471.

[23] Veeman D, Sai MS, Sureshkumar P, *et al.* Additive manufacturing of biopolymers for tissue engineering and regenerative medicine: an overview, potential applications, advancements, and trends. *International Journal of Polymer Science*. 2021;2021:1–20.

[24] Radenkovic D, Solouk A, and Seifalian A. Personalized development of human organs using 3D printing technology. *Medical Hypotheses*. 2016;87:30–3.

[25] Ventola CL. Medical applications for 3D printing: current and projected uses. *Pharmacy and Therapeutics*. 2014;39(10):704.

[26] Hussain MK, Mirza R, Bagarish A, *et al.* A study about 3D printing technology and its effects on organ transplant. *Health Sciences*. 2021;10(7):149–62.

[27] Bozkurt Y and Karayel E. 3D printing technology; methods, biomedical applications, future opportunities and trends. *Journal of Materials Research and Technology*. 2021;14:1430–50.

[28] Yan Q, Dong H, Su J, *et al.* A review of 3D printing technology for medical applications. *Engineering*. 2018;4(5):729–42.

[29] Hann SY, Cui H, Esworthy T, *et al.* Recent advances in 3D printing: vascular network for tissue and organ regeneration. *Translational Research*. 2019;211:46–63.

[30] Abdullah T, Qurban RO, Bolarinwa SO, Mirza AA, Pasovic M, and Memic A. 3D printing of metal/metal oxide incorporated thermoplastic nanocomposites with antimicrobial properties. *Frontiers in Bioengineering and Biotechnology* 2020;8:568186. doi: 10.3389/fbioe.2020.568186.

[31] Charbe N, McCarron PA, and Tambuwala MM. Three-dimensional bio-printing: a new frontier in oncology research. *World Journal of Clinical Oncology*. 2017;8(1):21.

[32] Du X. 3D bio-printing review. In *IOP Conference Series: Materials Science and Engineering*, 2018, vol. 301, no. 1, p. 012023. Bristol: IOP Publishing.

[33] Kantaros A. Bio-inspired materials: exhibited characteristics and integration degree in bio-printing operations. *American Journal of Engineering and Applied Sciences*. 2022;15(4):255–63.

[34] Beheshtizadeh N, Lotfibakhshaiesh N, Pazhouhnia Z, Hoseinpour M, and Nafari M. A review of 3D bio-printing for bone and skin tissue engineering: a commercial approach. *Journal of Materials Science*. 2020;55(9):3729–49.

[35] Habib A and Khoda B. Development of clay based novel hybrid bio-ink for 3D bio-printing process. *Journal of Manufacturing Processes*. 2019;38:76–87.

[36] Sony M and Naik S. Key ingredients for evaluating Industry 4.0 readiness for organizations: a literature review. *Benchmarking: An International Journal*. 2020;27(7):2213–32.

[37] Ghobakhloo M. Industry 4.0, digitization, and opportunities for sustainability. *Journal of Cleaner Production*. 2020;252:119869.

[38] Pai DM. Interoperability between IIC architecture & industry 4.0 reference architecture for industrial assets. *Technical Report*, 1, pp. 1–12, 2016.

[39] Bag S, Gupta S, and Kumar S. Industry 4.0 adoption and 10R advance manufacturing capabilities for sustainable development. *International Journal of Production Economics*. 2021;231:107844.

[40] Masood T and Sonntag P. Industry 4.0: adoption challenges and benefits for SMEs. *Computers in Industry*. 2020;121:103261.

[41] Xu X, Lu Y, Vogel-Heuser B, and Wang L. Industry 4.0 and Industry 5.0—inception, conception and perception. *Journal of Manufacturing Systems*. 2021;61:530–5.

[42] Müller JM, Buliga O, and Voigt KI. The role of absorptive capacity and innovation strategy in the design of industry 4.0 business models – a comparison between SMEs and large enterprises. *European Management Journal*. 2021;39(3):333–43.

[43] Schumacher A, Nemeth T, and Sihn W. Roadmapping towards industrial digitalization based on an Industry 4.0 maturity model for manufacturing enterprises. *Procedia Cirp*. 2019;79:409–14.

[44] Oztemel E and Gursev S. Literature review of Industry 4.0 and related technologies. *Journal of Intelligent Manufacturing*. 2020;31:127–82.

[45] Malik PK, Sharma R, Singh R, *et al.* Industrial Internet of Things and its applications in industry 4.0: state of the art. *Computer Communications*. 2021;166:125–39.

[46] Serror M, Hack S, Henze M, Schuba M, and Wehrle K. Challenges and opportunities in securing the industrial internet of things. *IEEE Transactions on Industrial Informatics*. 2020;17(5):2985–96.

[47] Tange K, De Donno M, Fafoutis X, and Dragoni N. A systematic survey of industrial Internet of Things security: requirements and fog computing

opportunities. *IEEE Communications Surveys & Tutorials*. 2020;22 (4):2489–520.

[48] Pivoto DG, de Almeida LF, da Rosa Righi R, Rodrigues JJ, Lugli AB, and Alberti AM. Cyber-physical systems architectures for industrial internet of things applications in Industry 4.0: a literature review. *Journal of Manufacturing Systems*. 2021;58:176–92.

[49] Khalil RA, Saeed N, Masood M, Fard YM, Alouini MS, and Al-Naffouri TY. Deep learning in the industrial internet of things: potentials, challenges, and emerging applications. *IEEE Internet of Things Journal*. 2021;8 (14):11016–40.

[50] Tabaa M, Monteiro F, Bensag H, and Dandache A. Green Industrial Internet of Things from a smart industry perspectives. *Energy Reports*. 2020;6:430–46.

[51] Gong Y, Zhang L, Liu R, Yu K, and Srivastava G. Nonlinear MIMO for industrial Internet of Things in cyber-physical systems. *IEEE Transactions on Industrial Informatics*. 2020;17(8):5533–41.

[52] Boyes H, Hallaq B, Cunningham J, and Watson T. The industrial internet of things (IIoT): an analysis framework. *Computers in Industry*. 2018;101:1–2.

[53] Sadeghi AR, Wachsmann C, and Waidner M. Security and privacy challenges in industrial internet of things. In *Proceedings of the 52nd Annual Design Automation Conference* 2015 Jun 7, pp. 1–6.

[54] Wan J, Tang S, Shu Z, Li D, Wang S, Imran M, and Vasilakos AV. Software-defined industrial internet of things in the context of industry 4.0. *IEEE Sensors Journal*. 2016;16(20):7373–80.

[55] Jeschke S, Brecher C, Meisen T, Özdemir D, and Eschert T. *Industrial Internet of Things and Cyber Manufacturing Systems*. New York, NY: Springer International Publishing, 2017.

[56] Höfer CN and Karagiannis G. Cloud computing services: taxonomy and comparison. *Journal of Internet Services and Applications*. 2011;2(2):81–94.

[57] Dastbaz M. Industry 4.0 (i4. 0): the hype, the reality, and the challenges ahead. In *Industry 4.0 and Engineering for a Sustainable Future*. Cham: Springer, 2019, pp. 1–11.

[58] Majstorovic VD and Stojadinovic SM. Cloud computing: virtualization, simulation and cybersecurity–cloud manufacturing issue. In *Enabling Technologies for the Successful Deployment of Industry 4.0*. London: CRC Press, 2020 Apr 16, pp. 85–104.

[59] Varela ML, Putnik GD, Manupati VK, Rajyalakshmi G, Trojanowska J, and Machado J. Integrated process planning and scheduling in networked manufacturing systems for I4. 0: a review and framework proposal. *Wireless Networks*. 2021;27:1587–99.

[60] Pedone G and Mezgár I. Model similarity evidence and interoperability affinity in cloud-ready Industry 4.0 technologies. *Computers in Industry*. 2018;100:278–86.

[61] Nain G, Pattanaik KK, and Sharma GK. Towards edge computing in intelligent manufacturing: past, present and future. *Journal of Manufacturing Systems*. 2022;62:588–611.

[62] Xu LD and Duan L. Big data for cyber physical systems in industry 4.0: a survey. *Enterprise Information Systems*. 2019;13(2):148–69.

[63] Lee J, Kao HA, and Yang S. Service innovation and smart analytics for industry 4.0 and big data environment. *Procedia Cirp*. 2014;16:3–8.

[64] Qi Q and Tao F. Digital twin and big data towards smart manufacturing and industry 4.0: 360 degree comparison. *IEEE Access*. 2018;6:3585–93.

[65] Li D, Tang H, Wang S, and Liu C. A big data enabled load-balancing control for smart manufacturing of Industry 4.0. *Cluster Computing*. 2017;20: 1855–64.

[66] Yin S and Kaynak O. Big data for modern industry: challenges and trends [point of view]. *Proceedings of the IEEE*. 2015;103(2):143–6.

[67] Mourtzis D, Vlachou E, and Milas NJ. Industrial big data as a result of IoT adoption in manufacturing. *Procedia Cirp*. 2016;55:290–5.

[68] De Pace F, Manuri F, and Sanna A. Augmented reality in industry 4.0. *American Journal of Computer Science and Information Technology*. 2018;6 (1):17.

[69] Gattullo M, Scurati GW, Fiorentino M, Uva AE, Ferrise F, and Bordegoni M. Towards augmented reality manuals for industry 4.0: a methodology. *Robotics and Computer-Integrated Manufacturing*. 2019;56:276–86.

[70] Masoni R, Ferrise F, Bordegoni M, *et al.* Supporting remote maintenance in industry 4.0 through augmented reality. *Procedia Manufacturing*. 2017;11:1296–302.

[71] Pierdicca R, Frontoni E, Pollini R, Trani M, and Verdini L. The use of augmented reality glasses for the application in industry 4.0. In *Augmented Reality, Virtual Reality, and Computer Graphics: 4th International Conference, AVR 2017*, Ugento, Italy, June 12–15, 2017, *Proceedings*, Part I 4 2017. New York, NY: Springer International Publishing, pp. 389–401.

[72] Angrisani L, Arpaia P, Esposito A, and Moccaldi N. A wearable brain–computer interface instrument for augmented reality-based inspection in industry 4.0. *IEEE Transactions on Instrumentation and Measurement*. 2019;69(4):1530–9.

[73] Damiani L, Demartini M, Guizzi G, Revetria R, and Tonelli F. Augmented and virtual reality applications in industrial systems: a qualitative review towards the industry 4.0 era. *IFAC-PapersOnLine*. 2018;51(11):624–30.

[74] de Souza Cardoso LF, Mariano FC, and Zorzal ER. A survey of industrial augmented reality. *Computers & Industrial Engineering*. 2020;139:106159.

[75] Lezzi M, Lazoi M, and Corallo A. Cybersecurity for Industry 4.0 in the current literature: a reference framework. *Computers in Industry*. 2018;103:97–110.

[76] Corallo A, Lazoi M, and Lezzi M. Cybersecurity in the context of industry 4.0: a structured classification of critical assets and business impacts. *Computers in Industry*. 2020;114:103165.

[77] Ustundag A, Cevikcan E, Ervural BC, and Ervural B. Overview of cyber security in the industry 4.0 era. In *Industry 4.0: Managing the Digital Transformation*. 2018: 267–84.

[78] Süzen AA. A risk-assessment of cyber attacks and defense strategies in industry 4.0 ecosystem. *International Journal of Computer Network & Information Security*. 2020;12(1):1–12.

[79] Benias N and Markopoulos AP. A review on the readiness level and cyber-security challenges in industry 4.0. In *2017 South Eastern European Design Automation, Computer Engineering, Computer Networks and Social Media Conference (SEEDA-CECNSM)*. IEEE, 2017 Sep 23, pp. 1–5.

[80] Tsuchiya A, Fraile F, Koshijima I, Ortiz A, and Poler R. Software defined networking firewall for industry 4.0 manufacturing systems. *Journal of Industrial Engineering and Management (JIEM)*. 2018;11(2):318–33.

[81] Dilberoglu UM, Gharehpapagh B, Yaman U, and Dolen M. The role of additive manufacturing in the era of industry 4.0. *Procedia Manufacturing*. 2017;11:545–54.

[82] Haleem A and Javaid M. Additive manufacturing applications in industry 4.0: a review. *Journal of Industrial Integration and Management*. 2019;4 (04):1930001.

[83] Hernandez Korner ME, Lambán MP, Albajez JA, Santolaria J, Ng Corrales LD, and Royo J. Systematic literature review: integration of additive manufacturing and industry 4.0. *Metals*. 2020;10(8):1061.

[84] Sepasgozar SM, Shi A, Yang L, Shirowzhan S, and Edwards DJ. Additive manufacturing applications for industry 4.0: a systematic critical review. *Buildings*. 2020;10(12):231.

[85] Parmar H, Khan T, Tucci F, Umer R, and Carlone P. Advanced robotics and additive manufacturing of composites: towards a new era in Industry 4.0. *Materials and Manufacturing Processes*. 2022;37(5):483–517.

[86] Elhoone H, Zhang T, Anwar M, and Desai S. Cyber-based design for additive manufacturing using artificial neural networks for Industry 4.0. *International Journal of Production Research*. 2020;58(9):2841–61.

[87] Dukle A, Murugan D, Nathanael AJ, Rangasamy L, and Oh TH. Can 3D-printed bioactive glasses be the future of bone tissue engineering? *Polymers*. 2022;14(8):1627.

[88] Distler T, Fournier N, Grünewald A, *et al.* Polymer-bioactive glass composite filaments for 3D scaffold manufacturing by fused deposition modeling: fabrication and characterization. *Frontiers in Bioengineering and Biotechnology*. 2020;8:552

[89] Ulbrich LM, Balbinot GD, Brotto GL, *et al.* 3D printing of poly (butylene adipate-co-terephthalate)(PBAT)/niobium containing bioactive glasses (BAGNb) scaffolds: characterization of composites, in vitro bioactivity, and in vivo bone repair. *Journal of Tissue Engineering and Regenerative Medicine*. 2022;16(3):267–78.

[90] Esslinger S and Gadow R. Additive manufacturing of bioceramic scaffolds by combination of FDM and slip casting. *Journal of the European Ceramic Society*. 2020;40(11):3707–13.

[91] Zaki RM, Strutynski C, Kaser S, *et al.* Direct 3D-printing of phosphate glass by fused deposition modeling. *Materials & Design*. 2020;194:108957.

[92] Sa MW, Nguyen BN, Moriarty RA, Kamalitdinov T, Fisher JP, and Kim JY. Fabrication and evaluation of 3D printed BCP scaffolds reinforced with ZrO2 for bone tissue applications. *Biotechnology and Bioengineering*. 2018;115(4):989–99.

[93] Baino F and Fiume E. 3D printing of hierarchical scaffolds based on mesoporous bioactive glasses (MBGs)—fundamentals and applications. *Materials*. 2020;13(7):1688.

[94] Castro NJ, O'Brien J, and Zhang LG. Integrating biologically inspired nanomaterials and table-top stereolithography for 3D printed biomimetic osteochondral scaffolds. *Nanoscale*. 2015;7(33):14010–22.

[95] Elomaa L, Keshi E, Sauer IM, and Weinhart M. Development of GelMA/PCL and dECM/PCL resins for 3D printing of acellular in vitro tissue scaffolds by stereolithography. *Materials Science and Engineering: C*. 2020;112:110958.

[96] Le Guéhennec L, Van Hede D, Plougonven E, *et al.* In vitro and in vivo biocompatibility of calcium-phosphate scaffolds three-dimensional printed by stereolithography for bone regeneration. *Journal of Biomedical Materials Research Part A*. 2020;108(3):412–25.

[97] Xue D, Zhang J, Wang Y, and Mei D. Digital light processing-based 3D printing of cell-seeding hydrogel scaffolds with regionally varied stiffness. *ACS Biomaterials Science & Engineering*. 2019;5(9):4825–33.

[98] Saed AB, Behravesh AH, Hasannia S, Ardebili SA, Akhoundi B, and Pourghayoumi M. Functionalized poly l-lactic acid synthesis and optimization of process parameters for 3D printing of porous scaffolds via digital light processing (DLP) method. *Journal of Manufacturing Processes*. 2020;56:550–61.

[99] Zhang C, Yuan Y, Zeng Y, and Chen J. DLP 3D printed silica-doped HAp ceramic scaffolds inspired by the trabecular bone structure. *Ceramics International*. 2022;48(19):27765–73.

[100] Liu S, Mo L, Bi G, *et al.* DLP 3D printing porous β-tricalcium phosphate scaffold by the use of acrylate/ceramic composite slurry. *Ceramics International*. 2021;47(15):21108–16.

[101] Song P, Li M, Zhang B, *et al.* DLP fabricating of precision GelMA/HAp porous composite scaffold for bone tissue engineering application. *Composites Part B: Engineering*. 2022;244:110163.

[102] Saska S, Pires LC, Cominotte MA, *et al.* Three-dimensional printing and in vitro evaluation of poly (3-hydroxybutyrate) scaffolds functionalized with osteogenic growth peptide for tissue engineering. *Materials Science and Engineering: C*. 2018;89:265–73.

[103] Kondiah PP, Choonara YE, Kondiah PJ, *et al.* Recent progress in 3D-printed polymeric scaffolds for bone tissue engineering. In *Advanced 3D-Printed Systems and Nanosystems for Drug Delivery and Tissue Engineering*. Woodhead Publishing, 2020, pp. 59–81.

[104] Lin K, Sheikh R, Romanazzo S, and Roohani I. 3D printing of bioceramic scaffolds—barriers to the clinical translation: from promise to reality, and future perspectives. *Materials*. 2019;12(17):2660.

[105] Ataee A, Li Y, Song G, and Wen C. Metal scaffolds processed by electron beam melting for biomedical applications. In *Metallic Foam Bone*. Woodhead Publishing, 2017, pp. 83–110.
[106] Lee UL, Yun S, Cao HL, *et al.* Bioprinting on 3D printed titanium scaffolds for periodontal ligament regeneration. *Cells*. 2021;10(6):1337.
[107] Qiao S, Sheng Q, Li Z, *et al.* 3D-printed Ti6Al4V scaffolds coated with freeze-dried platelet-rich plasma as bioactive interface for enhancing osseointegration in osteoporosis. *Materials & Design*. 2020;194:108825.
[108] Liu F, Gan D, Zhang K, *et al.* A selective strategy for determining suitable structure and fatigue behavior study of minimal surface scaffolds fabricated by EBM. *International Journal of Fatigue*. 2023;167:107380.
[109] Ataee A, Li Y, Fraser D, Song G, and Wen C. Anisotropic Ti-6Al-4V gyroid scaffolds manufactured by electron beam melting (EBM) for bone implant applications. *Materials & Design*. 2018;137:345–54.
[110] Xu Q, Bai Y, Misra RD, *et al.* Improving biological functions of three-dimensional printed Ti2448 scaffolds by decoration with polydopamine and extracellular matrices. *ACS Applied Bio Materials*. 2022;5(8):3982–90.
[111] Kim CG, Han KS, Lee S, Kim MC, Kim SY, and Nah J. Fabrication of biocompatible polycaprolactone–hydroxyapatite composite filaments for the FDM 3D printing of bone scaffolds. *Applied Sciences*. 2021;11(14):6351.
[112] Feng Z, Li Y, Hao L, *et al.* Graphene-reinforced biodegradable resin composites for stereolithographic 3D printing of bone structure scaffolds. *Journal of Nanomaterials*. 2019;2019:1–3.
[113] Lim HK, Hong SJ, Byeon SJ, *et al.* 3D-printed ceramic bone scaffolds with variable pore architectures. *International Journal of Molecular Sciences*. 2020;21(18):6942.
[114] Ke D and Bose S. Effects of pore distribution and chemistry on physical, mechanical, and biological properties of tricalcium phosphate scaffolds by binder-jet 3D printing. *Additive Manufacturing*. 2018;22:111–7.
[115] Bose S, Bhattacharjee A, Banerjee D, Boccaccini AR, and Bandyopadhyay A. Influence of random and designed porosities on 3D printed tricalcium phosphate-bioactive glass scaffolds. *Additive Manufacturing*. 2021;40:101895.
[116] Ahn JH, Kim J, Han G, *et al.* 3D-printed biodegradable composite scaffolds with significantly enhanced mechanical properties via the combination of binder jetting and capillary rise infiltration process. *Additive Manufacturing*. 2021;41:101988.
[117] Hong D, Chou DT, Velikokhatnyi OI, *et al.* Binder-jetting 3D printing and alloy development of new biodegradable Fe-Mn-Ca/Mg alloys. *Acta Biomaterialia*. 2016;45:375–86.
[118] Sahu KK and Modi YK. Multi response optimization for compressive strength, porosity and dimensional accuracy of binder jetting 3D printed ceramic bone scaffolds. *Ceramics International*. 2022;48(18):26772–83.
[119] Lee G, Carrillo M, McKittrick J, Martin DG, and Olevsky EA. Fabrication of ceramic bone scaffolds by solvent jetting 3D printing and sintering: towards load-bearing applications. *Additive Manufacturing*. 2020;33:101107.

[120] Petrovic V, Haro JV, Blasco JR, and Portolés L. Additive manufacturing solutions for improved medical implants. *Biomedicine.* 2012;2012:147–80.
[121] Al-Tamimi AA, Almeida H, and Bartolo P. Structural optimisation for medical implants through additive manufacturing. *Progress in Additive Manufacturing.* 2020;5:95–110.
[122] Velu R, Calais T, Jayakumar A, and Raspall F. A comprehensive review on bio-nanomaterials for medical implants and feasibility studies on fabrication of such implants by additive manufacturing technique. *Materials.* 2019;13(1):92.
[123] Salmi M. Additive manufacturing processes in medical applications. *Materials.* 2021;14(1):191.
[124] Javaid M and Haleem A. Additive manufacturing applications in medical cases: a literature based review. *Alexandria Journal of Medicine.* 2018;54 (4):411–22.
[125] Salmi M, Tuomi J, Paloheimo KS, *et al.* Patient-specific reconstruction with 3D modeling and DMLS additive manufacturing. *Rapid Prototyping Journal.* 2012;18(3):209–14.
[126] Bao Y, Paunović N, and Leroux JC. Challenges and opportunities in 3D printing of biodegradable medical devices by emerging photopolymerization techniques. *Advanced Functional Materials.* 2022;32(15):2109864
[127] Honigmann P, Sharma N, Okolo B, Popp U, Msallem B, and Thieringer FM. Patient-specific surgical implants made of 3D printed PEEK: material, technology, and scope of surgical application. *BioMed Research International.* 2018;2018.
[128] Popov VV, Muller-Kamskii G, Kovalevsky A, *et al.* Design and 3D-printing of titanium bone implants: brief review of approach and clinical cases. *Biomedical Engineering Letters.* 2018;8:337–44.
[129] Domsta V and Seidlitz A. 3D-Printing of drug-eluting implants: an overview of the current developments described in the literature. *Molecules.* 2021;26(13):4066
[130] Vaezi M and Yang S. Extrusion-based additive manufacturing of PEEK for biomedical applications. *Virtual and Physical Prototyping.* 2015;10(3):123–35.
[131] Wang Y, Müller WD, Rumjahn A, and Schwitalla A. Parameters influencing the outcome of additive manufacturing of tiny medical devices based on PEEK. *Materials.* 2020;13(2):466.
[132] Haleem A and Javaid M. Polyether ether ketone (PEEK) and its manufacturing of customised 3D printed dentistry parts using additive manufacturing. *Clinical Epidemiology and Global Health.* 2019;7(4):654–60.
[133] Tilton M, Lewis GS, and Manogharan GP. Additive manufacturing of orthopedic implants. *Orthopedic Biomaterials: Progress in Biology, Manufacturing, and Industry Perspectives.* 2018:21–55.
[134] Lyons R, Newell A, Ghadimi P, and Papakostas N. Environmental impacts of conventional and additive manufacturing for the production of Ti-6Al-4V knee implant: a life cycle approach. *The International Journal of Advanced Manufacturing Technology.* 2021;112:787–801.

[135] Safdar A, He HZ, Wei LY, Snis A, and de Paz LE. Effect of process parameters settings and thickness on surface roughness of EBM produced Ti-6Al-4V. *Rapid Prototyping Journal*. 2012;18:401–408.

[136] Hrabe N, Gnäupel-Herold T, and Quinn T. Fatigue properties of a titanium alloy (Ti–6Al–4V) fabricated via electron beam melting (EBM): effects of internal defects and residual stress. *International Journal of Fatigue*. 2017;94:202–10.

[137] Radfar P, Bazaz SR, Mirakhorli F, and Warkiani ME. The role of 3D printing in the fight against COVID-19 outbreak. *Journal of 3D Printing in Medicine*. 2021;5(1):51–60.

[138] Rybicki FJ. 3D printing in medicine: coronavirus disease 2019 testing with 3D printed nasopharyngeal swabs. *Clinical Infectious Diseases*. 2021;73 (9):e3033–5.

[139] Oland G, Garner O, and de St Maurice A. Prospective clinical validation of 3D printed nasopharyngeal swabs for diagnosis of COVID-19. *Diagnostic Microbiology and Infectious Disease*. 2021;99(3):115257.

[140] Salmi M, Akmal JS, Pei E, Wolff J, Jaribion A, and Khajavi SH. 3D printing in COVID-19: productivity estimation of the most promising open source solutions in emergency situations. *Applied Sciences*. 2020;10 (11):4004.

[141] Callahan CJ, Lee R, Zulauf KE, *et al.* Open development and clinical validation of multiple 3D-printed nasopharyngeal collection swabs: rapid resolution of a critical COVID-19 testing bottleneck. *Journal of Clinical Microbiology*. 2020;58(8):e00876–20.

Chapter 15

Application of e-platforms in physiotherapy education

Surya Vishnuram[1], Vinodhkumar Ramalingam[1] and Prathap Suganthirababu[1]

E-platforms, such as online learning management systems and virtual reality simulations, can be used in physiotherapy education to enhance the learning experience for students. Online learning management systems can be used to deliver course content, provide interactive activities, and facilitate communication between students and instructors. Virtual reality simulations can be used to provide students with hands-on experience in a safe and controlled environment, allowing them to practice clinical skills and procedures before working with real patients. Additionally, e-platforms can also be used for remote physiotherapy consultation, telehealth and telerehabilitation. This can be particularly useful in situations where patients are unable to visit a physiotherapy clinic in person due to mobility or other issues [1–3].

Any service and communication tool that is available on or uses the Internet, such as social networks, web-based resources, and discussion forums, is referred to as an online technology. Internet technologies now play a crucial role in the lives of professors and students in higher education, impacting learning methodologies. Students in the health professions appear to regularly utilize the Internet, participating in a variety of online activities, mostly on social media platforms [4]. Many students studying for careers in the health professions now rely mostly on the Internet due to the quick development of web-based information platforms, and social media in particular [5].

Evidence-based, solid pedagogical strategies that are innovative, engaging, affordable, accessible, and sustainable are needed to train the upcoming health workforce. E-learning offers one method, or enabler, for universities to successfully upgrade capacity in this area. E-learning is described as "an approach to teaching and learning, representing all or part of the applied educational model, based on the use of electronic media and devices as tools for improving access to training, communication, and interaction, and that facilitates the adoption of new ways of understanding and developing learning" [6].

[1]Saveetha College of Physiotherapy, SIMATS, India

15.1 Role of e-platforms in physiotherapy education

E-platforms, or electronic platforms, have become an increasingly important tool in the field of physiotherapy education. These platforms refer to a variety of digital tools and technologies that can be used to facilitate learning and collaboration among students and educators. This includes everything from online learning management systems and virtual reality simulations to video conferencing and telerehabilitation.

The application of e-platforms in physiotherapy education is driven by several factors. One of the main reasons is the increasing demand for flexibility and accessibility in learning. With the rise of online, blended and distance learning, e-platforms as shown in Figure 15.1, allow students to access course materials and participate in class discussions from anywhere and at any time. This can be especially beneficial for students who have busy schedules or who live in remote areas [7].

Another reason for the use of e-platforms in physiotherapy education is the growing focus on hands-on, practical learning experiences. E-platforms can provide students with access to virtual reality simulations and other interactive tools that can help them to better understand and apply the concepts they are learning [8,9]. This can help to enhance their learning experience and improve their understanding of the subject matter.

15.2 Physiotherapy online education and COVID-19

During the COVID-19 pandemic, e-platforms have played a critical role in physiotherapy education by allowing students and instructors to continue learning and teaching remotely [10].

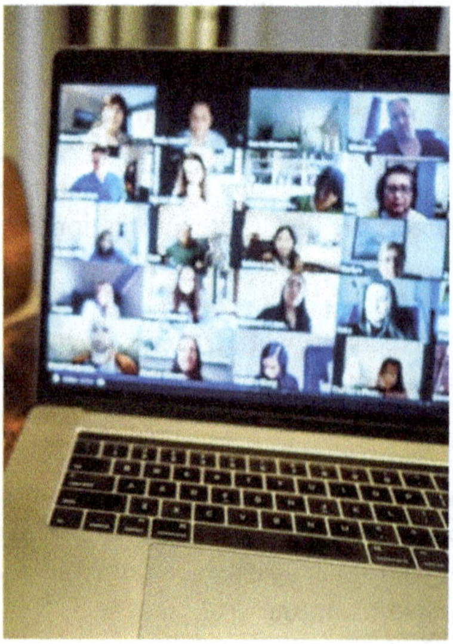

Figure 15.1 Online class in e-platform

Online learning management systems have been used to deliver course content and facilitate communication between students and instructors. This has allowed students to continue their education even when traditional in-person classes were not possible. Virtual reality simulations have also been used to provide students with hands-on experience in a safe and controlled environment. This has been particularly useful for students who were unable to complete their clinical hours due to restrictions on in-person learning [8,9].

Additionally, e-platforms have also been used for remote physiotherapy consultation and telerehabilitation during the COVID-19 pandemic. This has allowed patients to receive physiotherapy treatment remotely, which is especially beneficial for patients who are at high risk of contact with and exposure to COVID-19 or are unable to visit a physiotherapy clinic in person [11].

Overall, the use of e-platforms in physiotherapy education during the COVID-19 pandemic has helped to minimize disruptions to learning and ensure that students and patients continue to receive their care they need.

15.3 Types of online education in physiotherapy

There are several types of online education, including the following.

15.3.1 Synchronous learning

This type of online education takes place in real-time, with students and instructors participating in live virtual classes. Synchronous learning refers to a learning mode in which students and instructors participate in learning activities at the same time and in the same virtual space. In other words, synchronous learning happens in real-time, where students and instructors interact and engage with each other simultaneously. This mode of learning is typically facilitated through the use of technology, such as video conferencing, webinars, or chat tools.

Synchronous learning is becoming increasingly popular due to the rapid advancement of technology and its ability to create virtual classrooms that simulate face-to-face interactions. It provides a sense of community and collaboration, making it ideal for group projects, discussions, and debates. Moreover, synchronous learning helps to create a more structured and disciplined learning environment that can be helpful for students who may struggle with self-regulated learning [12].

15.3.2 Asynchronous learning

This type of online education allows students to complete coursework on their own schedule, without the need for real-time participation.

Asynchronous learning refers to a mode of learning where students can access learning materials and participate in learning activities at their own pace and on their own schedule. In other words, it is a self-paced learning mode where students can work through the course materials independently without having to follow a fixed schedule. This mode of learning is facilitated through various digital tools such as learning management systems, online discussion forums, video lectures, podcasts, and other pre-recorded materials [13].

Asynchronous learning is becoming increasingly popular in today's fast-paced world because it provides the flexibility and convenience that many learners need to balance their work, family, and personal responsibilities. This mode of learning is also ideal for learners who have different learning styles or who require extra time to process and understand the course material.

The simple concept of synchronous and asynchronous learning can be understood easily by looking at Figure 15.2.

15.3.3 Self-paced learning

This type of online education allows students to move through course material at their own pace, with no set schedule or deadlines.

Self-paced learning refers to a mode of learning where students have the freedom to work through course materials at their own pace and on their own schedule. In other words, students can take as much time as they need to understand the material, review concepts, and complete assignments. Self-paced learning is typically facilitated through online platforms, such as learning management systems or educational websites [14].

Self-paced learning is becoming increasingly popular in today's fast-paced world because it provides the flexibility and convenience that many learners need to balance their work, family, and personal responsibilities. This mode of learning is also ideal for learners who have different learning styles or who require extra time to process and understand the course material.

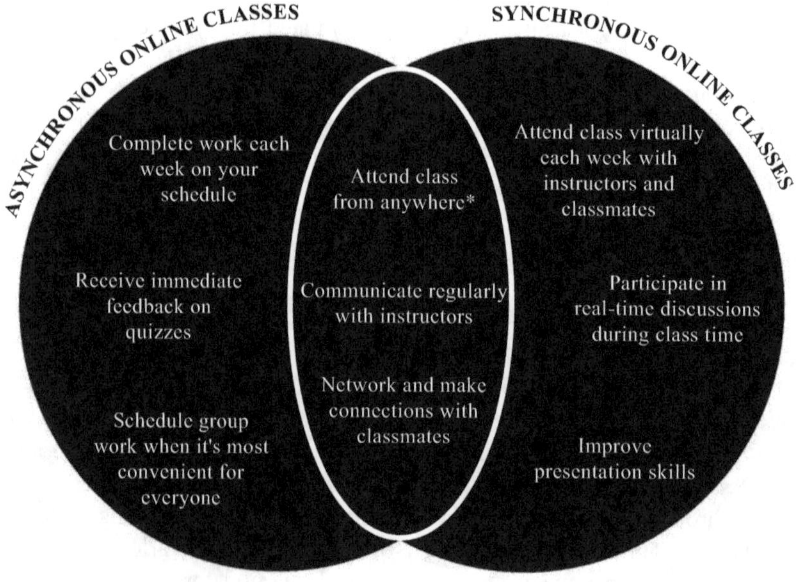

Figure 15.2 Synchronous and asynchronous online classes

15.3.4 Hybrid learning

This type of online education combines both online and in-person instruction, typically with some portion of the class taking place in a traditional classroom setting and some taking place online.

Hybrid learning, also known as blended learning, is a mode of learning that combines both face-to-face and online instruction. In other words, it is a mix of traditional classroom-based instruction and online learning. Hybrid learning provides learners with the benefits of both in-person and online learning [15].

In hybrid learning, students attend some classes in-person, while others are conducted online. The online portion of the course is typically delivered through a learning management system or other online platforms, which can include pre-recorded video lectures, interactive modules, online discussions, and other digital resources (Figure 15.3). The face-to-face portion of the course may include lectures, discussions, group activities, and other in-person learning experiences.

15.3.5 Massive open online courses

These are online courses that are open to anyone, anywhere and often provided by top universities and organizations for free or a small fee.

A massive open online course (MOOC) is an online course that is designed to be open to anyone with an Internet connection. MOOCs typically offer free access to educational resources, including video lectures, interactive modules, discussion forums, and other digital materials. MOOCs are often developed and delivered by universities, colleges, and other educational institutions, as well as by private companies and other organizations [16].

MOOCs can cover a wide range of subjects and topics, from computer science and engineering to business and the humanities. They are typically designed to be self-paced, allowing students to work through the materials on their own schedule. MOOCs can also be customized to suit the needs and interests of individual learners.

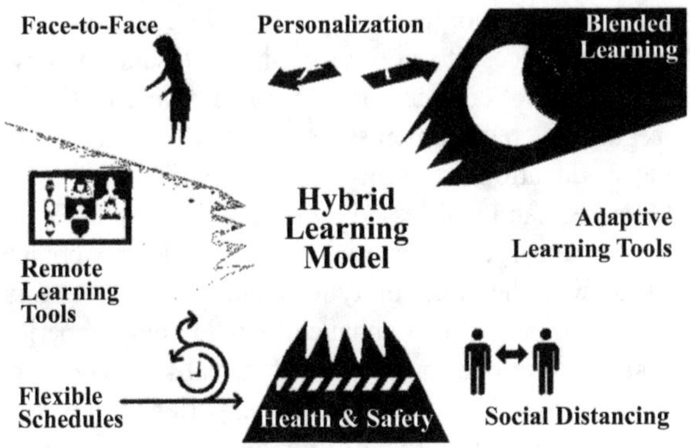

Figure 15.3 Hybrid learning model

15.3.6 Microlearning

This type of online education is characterized by small, targeted content that can be completed in a short period of time.

Microlearning is a form of learning that involves short, focused, and targeted bursts of learning that can be completed in a few minutes or less. It is designed to deliver small, bite-sized pieces of information that can be easily absorbed and retained by learners [17].

Microlearning can take many forms, including videos, interactive modules, quizzes, and other digital resources. It is often used to provide quick and convenient training and support for employees, as well as for personal and professional development.

15.4 Online learning experiences

Online education for physiotherapy students typically includes a combination of synchronous and asynchronous learning, with a focus on interactive and hands-on learning experiences.

Online lectures and video presentations: These provide students with the opportunity to learn the theoretical concepts of physiotherapy at their own pace.

Labs and simulations: These enable students to practice techniques and procedures in a safe and controlled environment.

Case studies and problem-based learning: These help students to apply the knowledge they have learned to real-world scenarios.

Online discussions and peer-to-peer learning: These allow students to share their experiences, ask questions, and receive feedback from their peers and instructors.

Clinical placements: These are essential for physiotherapy students and are typically done in person, but during the pandemic some institutions have offered virtual clinical placements using telerehabilitation for students.

Online assessments and exams: These are used to evaluate students' understanding and mastery of the course material.

It is important to note that online physiotherapy education programs typically require students to have access to certain equipment such as a webcam, microphone, and a reliable Internet connection. Moreover, some institutions might have accreditation or regulatory requirements that need to be met in order to provide online physiotherapy education programs.

Pre-recorded lectures can be accessed by students at any time, allowing them to learn at their own pace and review material as needed. Live webinars, on the other hand, provide students with the opportunity to interact with instructors and other students in real-time, which can help to enhance their learning experience. Interactive activities, such as quizzes, group discussions, and virtual simulations, can also be used to engage students and provide hands-on learning experiences.

Online classes can also include online laboratory sessions and practical sessions, where students can practice skills and procedures in a simulated environment. This can help to prepare students for real-life clinical scenarios. Additionally, online classes can also include remote physiotherapy consultation and telerehabilitation sessions which will enhance the clinical experience of the students [18,19].

15.5 Applications of e-platforms in physiotherapy education

Online learning management systems (LMSs): An LMS is an e-platform that provides access to educational resources, interactive learning activities, quizzes, and tests. LMSs can be used to deliver fully online courses, blended courses, or as a supplement to face-to-face learning. LMSs are particularly useful for physiotherapy students who need to access course content anytime, anywhere.

Video conferencing: Video conferencing allows students to participate in live lectures, tutorials, and group discussions. Video conferencing platform like Zoom, Google Meet, and Skype made it easier for physiotherapy students to interact with instructors and peers in real-time, regardless of their location.

Simulation-based learning: Simulation-based learning is a popular educational tool in physiotherapy education. E-platforms allow students to engage in realistic patient simulations, providing hands-on learning opportunities that may not be possible in a traditional classroom setting.

Virtual reality (VR): VR technology can be used to create immersive physiotherapy learning experiences. VR can be used to simulate patient scenarios, clinical environments, and treatment modalities. This technology provides a safe and controlled environment for students to practice their skills and gain confidence before working with real patients (Figure 15.4).

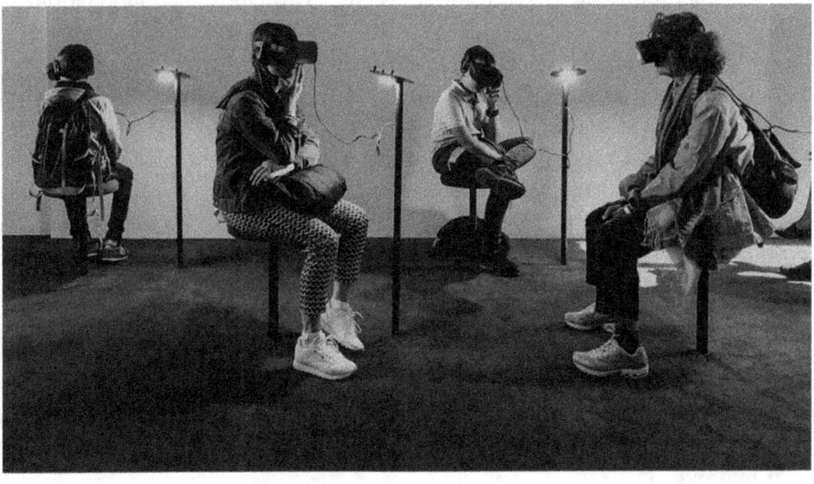

Figure 15.4 Virtual reality

Social media: Social media platforms like Facebook, Twitter, and LinkedIn can be used to create online communities where physiotherapy students can engage in discussions, share resources, and build professional networks. Social media platforms are also useful for sharing news, updates, and research findings relevant to the field of physiotherapy.

15.6 Benefits of online learning/e-platforms in physiotherapy education

E-platforms also offer cost-saving benefits to students and educators. They can reduce the need for students to travel to classrooms or clinics for hands-on learning experiences and can also reduce the need for additional equipment and manpower. This can help to lower the overall cost of education, which is especially important for students who have limited financial resources.

E-platforms in physiotherapy education are becoming increasingly necessary to meet the demand for flexibility and accessibility in learning. Besides, it assists in enhancing hands-on skills and practical learning experiences. However, there are a few challenges in using e-platforms for physiotherapy education, such as ensuring students have access to the technology and are comfortable with it. With the right technological support and orientation to students about e-platforms can be an effective and valuable tool for providing education to students.

Online classes for physiotherapy students can take several forms, including pre-recorded lectures, live webinars, and interactive activities.

E-platforms allow students to access learning materials from anywhere, at any time, making education more accessible and flexible.

Cost-effective: E-platforms can significantly reduce the costs associated with traditional classroom-based education, such as travel, accommodation and materials.

Engaging multimedia: E-platforms can offer interactive and engaging multimedia content, such as videos, animations, and simulations, that enhance learning and retention.

Personalized learning: E-platforms can provide adaptive learning experiences that adjust to each student's pace and learning style.

Increased collaboration: E-platforms can facilitate collaboration and communication between students, instructors, and peers, promoting a sense of community and social learning.

Access to a vast library of resources: E-platforms provide students with access to a vast library of learning resources, including articles, journals, and books, that are easily accessible and searchable.

Automated feedback: E-platforms can provide automated feedback and assessments, allowing students to track their progress and identify areas where they need to improve.

15.7 Demerits of online physiotherapy education

Limited hands-on experience: Online education may lack the hands-on experience that is essential in physiotherapy education, such as practicing clinical skills and procedures.

Technical issues: E-platforms may experience technical problems such as slow Internet connections, software malfunctions, and hardware failures, which can disrupt learning.

Isolation: Online learning can be isolating, with students missing the face-to-face interaction and support of classmates and instructors.

Difficulty in assessing practical skills: Assessing practical skills, such as physical assessment and manual therapy techniques, can be challenging in an online environment.

Quality control: Ensuring the quality and accuracy of online education can be difficult, as there is limited regulation and oversight in this field.

Lack of motivation: Without the structure and accountability of a traditional classroom environment, some students may struggle to stay motivated and engaged in their online studies.

Limited access to equipment and resources: Online students may not have access to the same equipment and resources as those in traditional classroom-based education.

15.8 Conclusion

Overall, online classes can provide physiotherapy students with a flexible and convenient way to learn and practice their skills, while also allowing them to complete their education during times when in-person classes are not possible.

Online education in physiotherapy offers numerous benefits and drawbacks. On the positive side, it provides greater flexibility and convenience for learners as they can attend classes from anywhere and at any time. It also offers a wider range of course options and can be more cost-effective. Additionally, the use of technology allows for interactive learning experiences and the ability to access a wealth of information easily. On the negative side, online education can lack the hands-on experiences and personal interaction found in traditional classroom settings. It also requires a high level of self-motivation and discipline as students are responsible for their own learning. Overall, online education in physiotherapy offers a viable alternative for those seek further their education, but it is important to weigh the advantages and disadvantages to determine if it is the right fit.

In conclusion, e-platforms have revolutionized physiotherapy education, making it more accessible, interactive, and engaging. With the continued evolution of e-platforms, physiotherapy students can expect to benefit from even more innovative and effective learning tools in the future.

References

[1] Hanson C, West J, Neiger B, Thackeray R, Barnes M, and Mcintyre E. Use and acceptance of social media among health educators. *American Journal of Health Education*. 2011;42(4):197–204.

[2] Sandars J and Morrison C. What is the next generation? The challenge for future medical education. *Medical Teacher*. 2007;29(2–3):85–8.

[3] Veletsianos G. Higher education scholars' participation and practices on Twitter. *Journal of Computer Assisted Learning*. 2012;28(4):336–49.

[4] Wells KM. Social media in medical school education. *Surgery*. 2011;150 (1):2–4.

[5] Giordano C and Giordano C. Health professions students' use of social media. *Journal of Allied Health*. 2011;40(2):78–81.

[6] Gardner P, Slater H, Jordan JE, Fary RE, Chua J, and Briggs AM. Physiotherapy students' perspectives of online e-learning for interdisciplinary management of chronic health conditions: a qualitative study. *BMC Medical Education*. 2016;16:1–9.

[7] Soh SE, Morgan PE, Hopmans R, Barker AL, and Ackerman IN. The feasibility and acceptability of a falls prevention e-learning program for physiotherapists. *Physiotherapy Theory and Practice*. 2022;39:1–0.

[8] Salmon G. The future for (second) life and learning. *British Journal of Educational Technology*. 2009;40(3):526–38.

[9] Bastos S, De Oliveira H, Silva M, and Azevedo L. Soft-digital skills in higher education curricula. In *Proceedings of the European Conference on e-Learning* 2019 Nov 1, pp. 70–77.

[10] Ibrahim NK, Al Raddadi R, AlDarmasi M, *et al.* Medical students' acceptance and perceptions of e-learning during the Covid-19 closure time in King Abdulaziz University, Jeddah. *Journal of Infection and Public Health*. 2021;14(1):17–23.

[11] ShahAli S, Shahabi S, Kohan N, Ebrahimi Takamjani I, and Ebrahimi R. Using e-learning methods for physiotherapy students learning – a systematic review and meta-analysis of the impact on knowledge, skills, satisfaction and attitudes. *European Journal of Physiotherapy*. 2022: 1–3.

[12] Divanoglou A, Chance-Larsen K, Fleming J, and Wolfe M. Physiotherapy student perspectives on synchronous dual-campus learning and teaching. *Australasian Journal of Educational Technology*. 2018;34(3).

[13] Ødegaard NB, Myrhaug HT, Dahl-Michelsen T, and Røe Y. Digital learning designs in physiotherapy education: a systematic review and meta-analysis. *BMC Medical Education*. 2021;21:1–8.

[14] İlçin N, Tomruk M, Yeşilyaprak SS, Karadibak D, and Savcı S. The relationship between learning styles and academic performance in TURKISH physiotherapy students. *BMC Medical Education*. 2018;18(1):1–8.

[15] Azahari H. Interactive hybrid learning model for physiotherapy course via knowledge and e-learning integrated platform (KELIP). In *Innovating Education for a Better Tomorrow*.
[16] Hossain MS, Islam MS, Glinsky JV, Lowe R, Lowe T, and Harvey LA. A massive open online course (MOOC) can be used to teach physiotherapy students about spinal cord injuries: a randomised trial. *Journal of Physiotherapy*. 2015;61(1):21–7.
[17] Rickardsson J, Gentili C, Holmström L, *et al.* Internet-delivered acceptance and commitment therapy as microlearning for chronic pain: a randomized controlled trial with 1-year follow-up. *European Journal of Pain*. 2021;25 (5):1012–30.
[18] Chesterton P, Richardson M, and Tears C. Student physiotherapists perceptions of online curriculum delivery during the COVID-19 pandemic. *BMC Medical Education*. 2022;22(1):1–1.
[19] Koleva IB, Yoshinov BR, and Yoshinov RR. Digitalization of educational materials and establishment of electronic archive in the rehabilitation field. *Digital Presentation and Preservation of Cultural and Scientific Heritage*. 2022;12:277–84.

Chapter 16

Challenges and considerations in e-health platforms

Surya Vishnuram[1], Vinodhkumar Ramalingam[1] and Vignesh Srinivasan[1]

Globally healthcare industry has significant advancements. The pandemic's onset further accelerated this process at an unparalleled rate [1]. Technology has found its use in every aspect of healthcare delivery and drug delivery, bringing in the digital health revolution. It is quickly emerging as a solution to the age-old problems of accessibility and affordability by uniting doctors, patients, and other stakeholders on a single platform. With the advancement of technology, e-health has emerged as an innovative solution in various disciplines of healthcare. E-health refers to the use of technology to deliver healthcare services and improve patient outcomes/services.

In recent years, the advent of e-health platforms has revolutionized the healthcare industry, offering new avenues for communication, collaboration, and data management. E-health platforms encompass a wide range of technologies, including electronic health records, telemedicine systems, mobile health applications, and health information exchange networks. While these platforms offer significant benefits, they also bring forth a unique set of challenges and considerations that must be carefully addressed to ensure their successful implementation and use. This chapter delves into some of the key challenges and considerations associated with e-health platforms, exploring issues related to privacy and security, interoperability, user adoption, and regulatory compliance.

E-health initiatives, such as telerehabilitation, provide patients with more opportunities to participate in their own care and stay motivated. In addition, E-health have the potential to improve access, quality, and engagement in patient care [2]. As technology continues to evolve, it is likely that e-health initiatives in physiotherapy will continue to play an increasingly important role in improving patient outcomes and delivering high-quality physiotherapy care.

The foundation of digital health is regarded as being Artificial Intelligence (AI) and Information Technology (IT). AI consciously uses the data produced by digital health systems to enhance diagnosis, choose the best course of therapy,

[1]Saveetha College of Physiotherapy, SIMATS, India

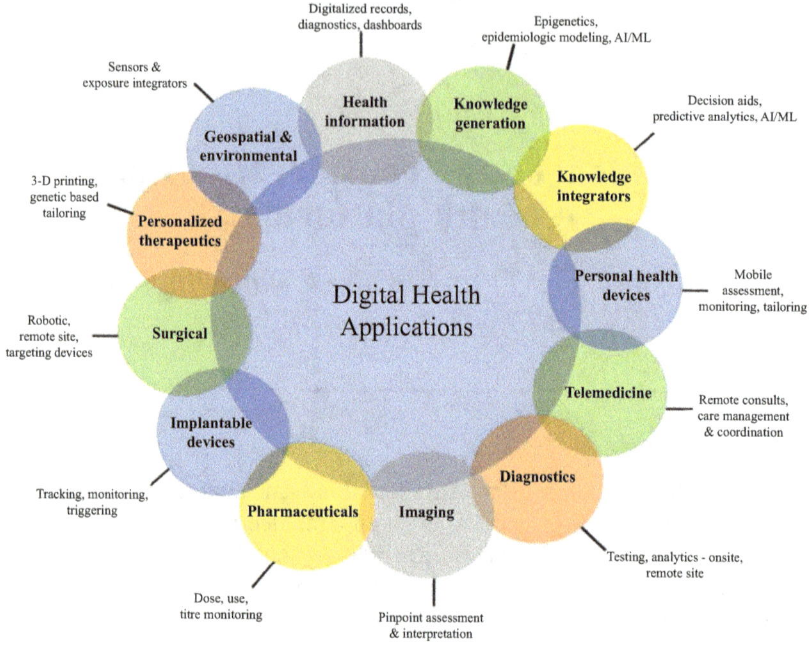

Figure 16.1 Evolving applications of digital technology in health and health care. Source: National Academy of Medicine (2019). Digital Health Action Collaborative, NAM Leadership Consortium: Collaboration for a Value & Science-Driven Health System.

and forecast clinical results in patient care. The effective adoption of digital health is made possible by the established and creative application of such technology [3,4]. Having said that, it is crucial to thoroughly examine the IT and AI system bottlenecks that exacerbate problems with safety, sustainability, and justice.

As shown in Figure 16.1, digital systems equipped with cutting-edge technology are thought to hold greater safety standards than people since AI is seen as the future of technology. Simply said, it is less acceptable for AI systems in digital health to make mistakes. However, little research has been done on how AI systems will affect or pose a risk to human life.

Additionally, the systems' limited training sets on actual data reveal that it is difficult to replicate promising outcomes. Hence, increasing the AI system's overall accuracy can provide clinicians and patients with clear and comprehensible outcomes [5].

However, there are still technical, privacy, and accessibility challenges that must be addressed to ensure that e-health initiatives are accessible and effective for all patients. In this chapter, we will discuss about the challenges and considerations in e-health platforms in detail [6].

16.1 Technical challenges

Technical issues such as unreliable Internet connectivity, hardware malfunctions, and software compatibility can affect the smooth functioning of e-health platforms. Technical issues such as website crashes, slow loading times, and software bugs can cause frustration and negatively impact the user experience [7]. Indeed, the technical issues pose significant challenges to the smooth functioning and user experience of e-health platforms. Here are some considerations to address these technical challenges:

Robust infrastructure: To mitigate issues related to unreliable Internet connectivity, it is essential to have a robust and reliable network infrastructure. This may involve ensuring sufficient bandwidth, redundancy measures, and backup systems to minimize disruptions caused by Internet outages or network congestion. Collaborating with Internet service providers to improve connectivity in underserved areas can also be beneficial.

Hardware and software maintenance: Regular maintenance of hardware and software components is crucial to prevent malfunctions and ensure optimal performance. This includes timely updates, patches, and bug fixes to address software vulnerabilities and compatibility issues. Routine hardware inspections, repairs, and replacements can help in minimizing the risk of hardware failures.

Load testing and scalability: Performing load testing on e-health platforms helps to identify their performance limits and ensures that they can handle increased user traffic without crashing or slowing down. Scalability considerations should be taken into account during the design and development phase of e-health to ensure that the platforms can effectively handle growing user demands.

User support and technical assistance: Establishing a robust user support system is essential to address technical issues promptly. This may involve setting up a dedicated helpdesk or technical support team that can assist users in troubleshooting problems, providing step-by-step guidance and resolving issues efficiently. Offering multiple channels of support, such as phone, email, or live chat, can cater to users with different preferences.

Usability and user experience design: Investing in user experience design can help mitigate frustration caused by technical issues. Designing intuitive and user-friendly interfaces can enhance the overall user experience and minimize errors or confusion. Conducting user testing and gathering feedback during the development process can help identify potential technical issues and improve the usability of the platform.

Continuous monitoring and feedback: Implementing monitoring systems to track the performance of e-health platforms in real-time can help to identify the technical issues as they arise. Proactive monitoring can allow for early detection and resolution of problems, minimizing disruptions. Additionally, encouraging users to provide feedback and report technical issues can help in identifying and addressing recurring or critical issues promptly.

Collaboration with technology providers: Establishing strong partnerships with technology providers, including software vendors and hardware manufacturers, can be beneficial. Collaborating closely with these providers can ensure timely updates, access to technical expertise, and prompt resolution of issues. Regular communication channels and service-level agreements (SLAs) can help maintain a mutually beneficial relationship.

16.2 Privacy and security

Patients' personal and health information must be protected to ensure privacy and security. E-health platforms must comply with regulations such as Health Insurance Portability and Accountability Act (1996) HIPAA and General Data Protection Regulation (2018) GDPR to ensure that sensitive information is not compromised [8]. Confidential health information is at risk of hacking, theft or unauthorized access. One of the primary concerns in e-health platforms is the protection of sensitive patient information. With the digitization of health records and the transfer of data across various platforms, ensuring privacy and security becomes paramount. The challenges in this area include:

Breaches: Unauthorized access or theft of sensitive health information can lead to serious privacy violations. E-health platforms are attractive targets for hackers due to the vast amount of personal health information stored within them. Robust security measures, such as encryption, access controls, and regular security audits, are necessary to mitigate the risk of data breaches.

Hacking: E-health platforms are vulnerable to cyber-attacks and hacking, putting confidential information at risk. It must respect patient autonomy by obtaining informed consent for data sharing and allowing individuals to control their personal health information. Balancing privacy with the need for data exchange and research can be challenging.

Inadequate encryption: Weak encryption methods can leave health information vulnerable to hacking and unauthorized access.

Threats: Employee mistakes or malicious insider activity can result in data breaches and privacy violations.

Data sharing: Sharing health information between healthcare providers and insurance companies can raise privacy concerns and require proper security measures.

Consent: Ensuring patients understand and consent to how their health information is being used and shared is a challenge in e-health platforms.

Limitations: Technical limitations such as limited device compatibility and software bugs can also impact the privacy and security of e-health platforms.

Regulatory compliance: Compliance with privacy and security regulations, such as the Health Insurance Portability and Accountability Act (HIPAA) in the United States, adds an additional layer of complexity to e-health platforms. Ensuring adherence to these regulations is crucial to avoid legal consequences.

16.3 Accessibility

E-health platforms must be accessible to all patients, including those with disabilities or limited access to technology (Figure 16.2). This requires the platform to

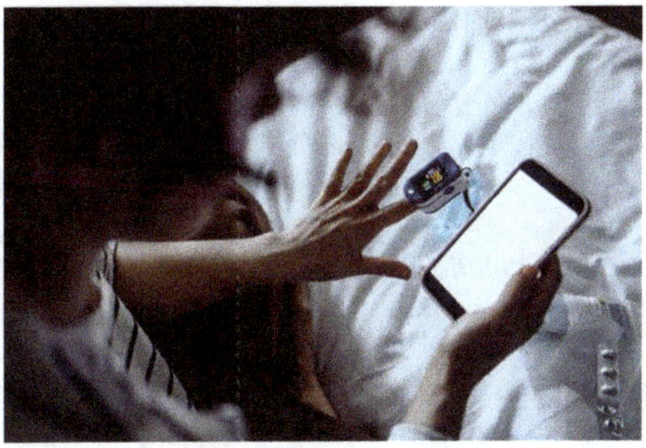

Figure 16.2 Patient data seen in mobile phone

be user-friendly, easy to navigate, and compatible with assistive technologies. Insurance coverage and reimbursement policies for online healthcare services are still evolving, which may vary greatly.

There are several accessibility challenges in online healthcare, including [9] the following:

Internet access: Individuals in rural or remote areas may not have access to reliable or high-speed Internet, making it difficult to use online healthcare services.

Limited literacy: Individuals with limited technical proficiency or digital literacy may have trouble accessing and using online healthcare services.

Language barriers: Online healthcare services may not be available in multiple languages, making it difficult for non-English speaking individuals to access and use the services.

Lack of trust: Some individuals may not trust online healthcare services and prefer in-person interactions with their healthcare provider.

Age: Older adults may have limited experience with technology and may struggle to use online healthcare services.

16.4 Interoperability

E-health platforms must be able to integrate with existing healthcare systems and work seamlessly with other technology solutions, such as electronic health records (EHRs) and telemedicine platforms [10]. Inconsistent data exchange between different e-health systems can lead to errors and duplicated efforts.

Interoperability refers to the ability of different e-health systems to communicate and exchange data seamlessly. Achieving interoperability is critical for the effective coordination of care and the exchange of patient data between healthcare providers. However, several challenges hinder interoperability.

Fragmentation of systems: The healthcare landscape is characterized by a multitude of proprietary systems and legacy technologies that do not communicate with each other effectively. Interoperability standards, such as Fast Healthcare

Interoperability Resources (FHIR), are being developed to address this issue, but adoption remains a challenge.

Data formats and standards: Variations in data formats and standards across different platforms impede the exchange and integration of health information. Agreeing upon common standards is essential to ensure interoperability and enable seamless data sharing.

Governance and coordination: Achieving interoperability requires collaboration and coordination among various stakeholders, including healthcare providers, software vendors, and regulatory bodies. Establishing governance structures and fostering cooperation are crucial to overcome interoperability challenges.

Technical standards: Inconsistent technical standards and protocols across different e-health systems can make data exchange and integration difficult.

Data quality: Ensuring the accuracy, completeness, and consistency of data across different e-health systems can be a challenge.

Vendor lock-in: Dependence on a single vendor or platform can limit the ability of e-health systems to integrate and exchange data with other systems.

Cost and resource constraints: Integrating e-health systems and achieving interoperability can be a complex and resource-intensive process.

Resistance to change: Resistance to change and adoption of new technology can make it difficult to achieve interoperability in online healthcare.

16.5 Data management

E-health platforms must have robust data management systems in place to ensure that patients' health information is accurate, up-to-date, and secure [11].

Data accuracy and completeness: Ensuring all relevant information is collected and recorded correctly.

Data storage and accessibility: Maintaining secure and efficient storage solutions, while ensuring easy accessibility.

Data backup and recovery: Ensuring data is recoverable in the event of a disaster or system failure.

Data analytics and reporting: Extracting meaningful insights from large amounts of data.

Managing health data for remote patients: Ensuring secure and efficient communication of patient information for remote consultations.

16.6 Cost

Implementing and maintaining e-health platforms can be expensive, and it is important to ensure that they provide value for money and deliver positive outcomes for patients and healthcare providers [12].

Some online healthcare services may not be accessible from all devices, such as older smartphones or computers.

Investment in technology: Implementing and maintaining the necessary technology infrastructure can be expensive.

Training and support: Ensuring that healthcare providers and staff are trained on new systems and software.

Data storage and maintenance: The cost of storing and maintaining large amounts of health data.

Cybersecurity measures: Implementing and maintaining security measures to protect sensitive data.

Upgrading technology: Upgrading technology to stay current with the latest advancements in online health care.

16.7 Provider adoption

E-health platforms must be designed to meet the needs of healthcare providers and patients, and providers must be trained and motivated to use the platform effectively [13].

Provider resistance to change: Healthcare providers may be resistant to adapting to new technology and processes.

Technical skill and knowledge gaps: Providers may lack the technical skills and knowledge required to effectively use online healthcare tools.

Workflow integration: Ensuring that online healthcare tools fit seamlessly into existing healthcare provider workflows.

Time and resource constraints: Providers may face time and resource constraints that make it difficult to adopt new technology.

16.8 User experience

The user experience of e-health platforms must be positive, intuitive, and easy to use, to encourage patient engagement and participation in their own care. Encouraging people to adopt e-health technology can be challenging, especially for older adults and those with limited technical proficiency. Users may have trouble accessing e-health services from multiple devices, such as smartphones, tablets, and desktops [14].

User adoption: Ensuring that patients are willing and able to use online health care tools.

User adoption challenges: The success of e-health platforms depends on the willingness of healthcare providers and patients to adopt and utilize these technologies. Traditional healthcare practices often involve paper-based systems and face-to-face interactions. Introducing e-health platforms requires significant changes in workflows and routines, leading to resistance from healthcare professionals who may be hesitant to adopt new technologies.

User education: Educating patients on how to use online health care tools and what to expect from them. E-health platforms should be accessible to all individuals, regardless of their technological literacy or socioeconomic status. Addressing the digital divide and ensuring equitable access to technology is crucial for widespread adoption [15].

Usability: Ensuring that online health care tools are user-friendly and intuitive to use. User-friendly interfaces and intuitive design play a pivotal role in encouraging adoption. Comprehensive training programs and ongoing support are necessary to familiarize users with the features and functionalities of e-health platforms.

Reliable and fast connectivity: Ensuring that online health care tools work effectively and efficiently, even with slow or unreliable internet connections.

Personalized experience: Providing patients with a personalized experience that meets their specific needs and preferences.

16.9 Quality of care

Maintaining quality of care and patient safety is a concern when delivering healthcare services online [16].

Maintaining clinical standards: Ensuring that online healthcare services meet the same clinical standards as in-person care.

Diagnostic accuracy: Ensuring that diagnoses are accurate and made in a timely manner through remote consultations.

Treatment compliance: Ensuring that patients follow through with recommended treatments.

Medication management: Ensuring that patients receive proper medication management, including prescriptions and refill reminders.

Follow-up care: Ensuring that patients receive proper follow-up care, including regular check-ins and monitoring.

Patient–provider communication: Improving patient–provider communication and building trust in remote consultations.

Continuity of care: Maintaining continuity of care for patients who receive care from multiple providers.

Quality monitoring and evaluation: Implementing systems for monitoring and evaluating the quality of online healthcare services.

16.10 Regulation

E-health platforms must comply with local and national regulations and standards, such as data protection and patient safety laws [17]. Online healthcare services are often subject to different laws and regulations, leading to inconsistencies in standards and practices. Regulating the challenges and considerations in e-health platforms is crucial to ensure the safe and effective use of these technologies. The following are some key approaches and strategies that can be employed to regulate e-health platforms:

Legislative frameworks: Governments and regulatory bodies should establish comprehensive legislative frameworks specifically designed for e-health platforms. These frameworks should address privacy, security, interoperability, user consent, and other relevant aspects. Laws and regulations must keep pace with technological advancements and be regularly updated to address emerging challenges.

Privacy and security regulations: Stringent privacy and security regulations should be in place to protect patient data. These regulations should outline strict guidelines for data storage, transmission, access controls, encryption, and data breach reporting. Compliance with existing regulations, such as HIPAA in the United States or the General Data Protection Regulation (GDPR) in the European Union, should be enforced and penalties for non-compliance should be established.

Interoperability standards: Regulatory bodies should encourage the adoption of interoperability standards, such as FHIR, to facilitate seamless data exchange between different e-health platforms. These standards should be widely promoted, and incentives can be provided to healthcare organizations and software vendors that adopt and adhere to them.

Certification and accreditation: Establishing certification and accreditation programs for e-health platforms can ensure that they meet specific quality and safety standards. Independent organizations can evaluate platforms based on criteria related to privacy, security, interoperability, user experience, and regulatory compliance. Platforms that meet the requirements can be certified and accredited, providing assurance to healthcare providers and patients.

Ethical guidelines and codes of conduct: Ethical guidelines and codes of conduct should be developed to govern the use of e-health platforms. These guidelines can address issues such as informed consent, patient autonomy, data sharing, and responsible use of artificial intelligence and machine learning algorithms in healthcare. Professional bodies and industry associations can play a role in establishing and promoting these ethical standards.

Regulatory sandboxes and pilot programs: Regulatory sandboxes or pilot programs can be created to allow for testing and evaluation of new e-health platforms in a controlled environment. This approach enables regulators to assess the risks and benefits of innovative technologies before widespread implementation. Feedback obtained from these programs can inform regulatory decisions and help refine regulations.

International collaboration: Given the global nature of e-health platforms, international collaboration and harmonization of regulations are crucial. Governments and regulatory bodies should engage in partnerships and collaborations to share best practices, exchange information, and work towards harmonizing regulatory frameworks. International standards organizations can play a role in facilitating this collaboration.

Ongoing monitoring and evaluation: Regulatory bodies should establish mechanisms for ongoing monitoring and evaluation of e-health platforms. Regular audits, inspections, and assessments can ensure compliance with regulations and identify any emerging risks or challenges. Continuous evaluation of regulatory frameworks is essential to adapt to changing technology and address new challenges effectively.

16.11 Conclusion

E-health platforms face a number of challenges and considerations, including technical, privacy and security, accessibility, and user experience. To be successful, e-health platforms must be designed and implemented with these challenges in mind and must provide tangible benefits for patients and healthcare providers.

Regulating the challenges and considerations in e-health platforms requires a multi-faceted approach, involving legislative frameworks, privacy and security regulations, interoperability standards, certification programs, ethical guidelines, and international collaboration [18]. By implementing robust regulatory measures, governments and regulatory bodies can foster the safe, secure, and efficient use of e-health platforms, ultimately benefiting healthcare providers, patients, and the healthcare system as a whole.

E-health platforms need to be integrated with existing healthcare systems to ensure that patients receive a seamless and coordinated care experience. However, integrating with existing systems can be challenging, particularly in cases where different systems are used across multiple healthcare providers and institutions.

Overall, addressing these challenges is critical to the successful implementation and adoption of e-health platforms and the delivery of quality, accessible healthcare services.

References

[1] Mbunge E, Batani J, Gaobotse G, and Muchemwa B. Virtual healthcare services and digital health technologies deployed during coronavirus disease 2019 (COVID-19) pandemic in South Africa: a systematic review. *Global Health Journal*. 2022;6:102–113.

[2] Doraiswamy S, Abraham A, Mamtani R, and Cheema S. Use of telehealth during the COVID-19 pandemic: scoping review. *Journal of Medical Internet Research*. 2020;22(12):e24087.

[3] Lupton D. Critical perspectives on digital health technologies. *Sociology Compass*. 2014;8(12):1344–59.

[4] Awad A, Trenfield SJ, Pollard TD, *et al.* Connected healthcare: improving patient care using digital health technologies. *Advanced Drug Delivery Reviews*. 2021;178:113958.

[5] Lupton D. The digitally engaged patient: self-monitoring and self-care in the digital health era. *Social Theory & Health*. 2013;11:256–70.

[6] Ahern DK. Challenges and opportunities of eHealth research. *American Journal of Preventive Medicine*. 2007;32(5):S75–82.

[7] Pagliari C. Design and evaluation in eHealth: challenges and implications for an interdisciplinary field. *Journal of Medical Internet Research*. 2007;9(2):e614.

[8] Kreps GL and Neuhauser L. New directions in eHealth communication: opportunities and challenges. *Patient Education and Counseling*. 2010;78(3):329–36.

[9] Ross J, Stevenson F, Lau R, and Murray E. Exploring the challenges of implementing e-health: a protocol for an update of a systematic review of reviews. *BMJ Open*. 2015;5(4):e006773.

[10] Eng TR. eHealth research and evaluation: challenges and opportunities. *Journal of Health Communication*. 2002;7(4):267–72.

[11] Xiao C, Choi E, and Sun J. Opportunities and challenges in developing deep learning models using electronic health records data: a systematic review. *Journal of the American Medical Informatics Association*. 2018;25(10):1419–28.

[12] Amarasingham R, Patzer RE, Huesch M, Nguyen NQ, and Xie B. Implementing electronic health care predictive analytics: considerations and challenges. *Health Affairs*. 2014;33(7):1148–54.

[13] Beard L, Schein R, Morra D, Wilson K, and Keelan J. The challenges in making electronic health records accessible to patients. *Journal of the American Medical Informatics Association*. 2012;19(1):116–20.

[14] Al-Issa Y, Ottom MA, and Tamrawi A. eHealth cloud security challenges: a survey. *Journal of Healthcare Engineering*. 2019;2019:7516035.

[15] Afzal A, Khan S, Daud S, Ahmad Z, and Butt A. Addressing the digital divide: access and use of technology in education. *Journal of Social Sciences Review*. 2023;3(2):883–95.

[16] El Khaddar MA, Harroud H, Boulmalf M, Elkoutbi M, and Habbani A. Emerging wireless technologies in e-health trends, challenges, and framework design issues. In *2012 International Conference on Multimedia Computing and Systems*, 2012 May 10 (pp. 440–445). IEEE.

[17] Chenthara S, Ahmed K, Wang H, and Whittaker F. Security and privacy-preserving challenges of e-health solutions in cloud computing. *IEEE Access*. 2019;7:74361–82.

[18] Wilkowska W and Ziefle M. Privacy and data security in E-health: Requirements from the user's perspective. *Health Informatics Journal*. 2012;18(3):191–201.

Chapter 17

Telerehabilitation in physiotherapy

Buvanesh Annadurai[1], Preethi Gokulan[1], Jagatheesan Alagesan[1] and Vinodhkumar Ramalingam[1]

Telerehabilitation, also known as telehealth or e-rehabilitation, is the delivery of rehabilitation services remotely through technology. Telerehabilitation can be used to provide physical therapy to patients who are unable to come to a clinic or hospital in person [1]. This can include patients who live in remote areas, have mobility issues, or have been impacted by a pandemic or other event that limits their ability to leave their homes [2].

There are several types of rehabilitation that can be used to deliver rehabilitation services to patients remotely, including: video conferencing, remote monitoring, store-and-forward, asynchronous telerehabilitation, and virtual reality.

These types of telerehabilitation are used in treating musculoskeletal, sports injuries, pulmonary conditions, cardiac conditions, geriatrics, post-natal, parental guidance and drug de-addiction [3].

17.1 Telerehabilitation in musculoskeletal conditions

Telerehabilitation can be used to treat musculoskeletal disorders such as arthritis, low back pain, and musculoskeletal injuries. One-on-one sessions through video conferencing with a trained physiotherapist are the main highlights of telerehabilitation, as they help to specifically design treatment protocol for patients suffering from various musculoskeletal disorders [4].

Telerehabilitation for musculoskeletal disorders can include a variety of interventions, such as exercise prescription, education on pain management and functional assessments [5]. As shown in Figure 17.1, telerehabilitation can be especially beneficial to patients who may not be able to access these services in person due to geographical barriers, mobility limitations, or during the COVID-19 pandemic. Research has shown that telerehabilitation can be as effective as in-person rehabilitation for certain conditions [3].

[1]Saveetha College of Physiotherapy, SIMATS, India

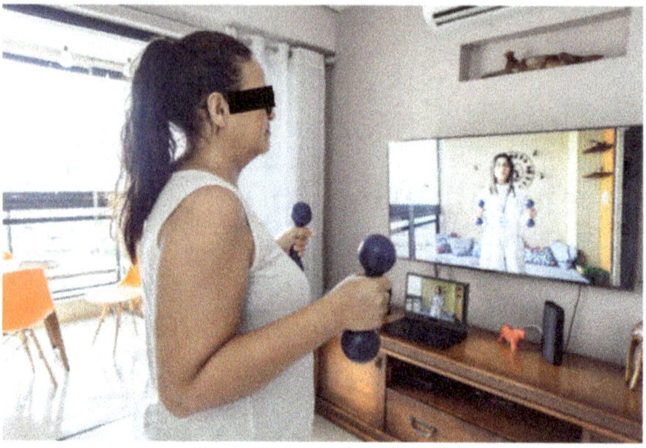

Figure 17.1 Telerehabilitation in musculoskeletal conditions

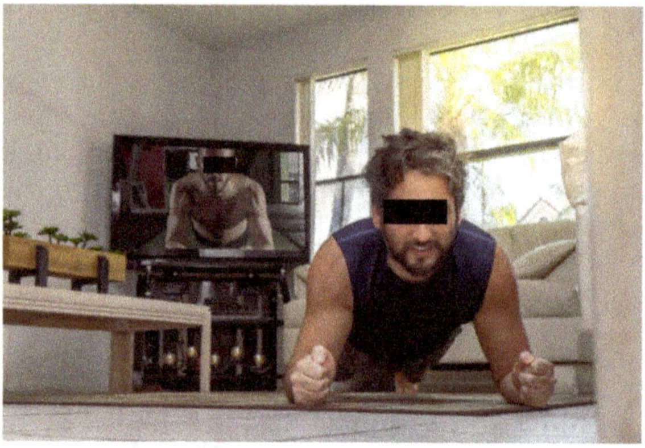

Figure 17.2 Telerehabilitation for sports injuries

17.2 Telerehabilitation for sports injuries

Telerehabilitation in sports injuries can be used to deliver a variety of rehabilitation services remotely, including: virtual consultations with a sports medicine doctor or physical therapist to assess the injury and develop a treatment plan. Remote monitoring of an athlete's recovery progress, including tracking of range of motion, strength, and other functional abilities.

Virtual delivery of physical therapy exercises and other rehabilitation interventions, such as stretching and massage, to help the athlete regain strength, flexibility, and function. Virtual education and training on injury prevention and proper techniques to help reduce the risk of future injuries [6]. Virtual support and communication with the rehabilitation team to provide guidance, encouragement, and feedback throughout the recovery process. As shown in Figure 17.2, telerehabilitation can be particularly beneficial for athletes who live in remote areas or have limited access to in-person rehabilitation services, for athletes who have been injured during the pandemic and have difficulty in visiting physical therapy centers and for elite athletes who want to continue their therapy during the competition travels [3].

However, it is important to note that telerehabilitation should be used as an adjunct to in-person therapy, rather than a replacement, and in some cases, in-person rehabilitation may be necessary [7]. A sports medicine doctor or physical therapist can advise on the most appropriate form of rehabilitation for a specific injury or condition.

17.3 Pulmonary telerehabilitation

Pulmonary telerehabilitation is a type of telehealth service that uses technology such as videoconferencing, remote monitoring, or store-and-forward to provide rehabilitation services to patients with lung conditions, such as chronic obstructive pulmonary disease (COPD), emphysema, or asthma [8].

Pulmonary telerehabilitation includes:

Exercise training: Patients receive instruction and guidance on exercises designed to improve lung function and overall physical fitness as shown in Figure 17.3.

Education: Patients receive education on how to manage their lung condition, including how to use inhalers, how to avoid triggers, and how to maintain overall health [9].

Monitoring: Patients' lung function, symptoms, and overall health are monitored by a healthcare provider remotely, often with the help of wearable devices or smartphone apps [10].

Communication: Patients can communicate with their healthcare provider through videoconferencing, phone calls, or text messaging, to receive feedback and guidance on their treatment plan.

Pulmonary telerehabilitation can be beneficial for patients with lung conditions because it allow them to receive rehabilitation services in the comfort zone in their

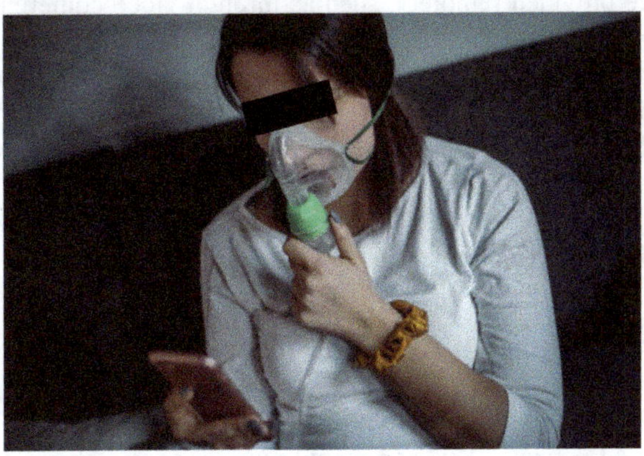

Figure 17.3 Pulmonary telerehabilitation

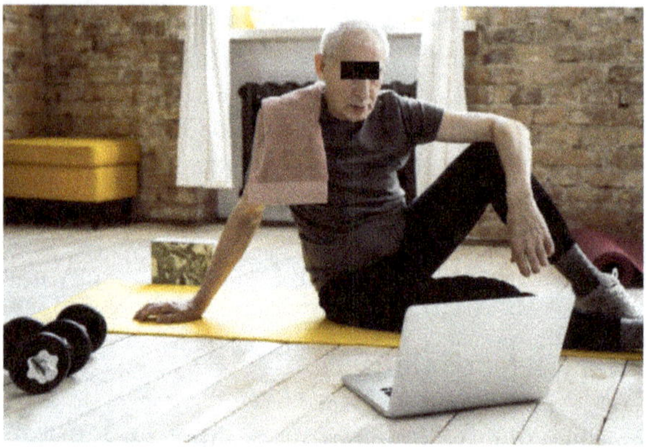

Figure 17.4 Cardiac telerehabilitation

own homes and especially beneficial for those who live in remote areas or have mobility limitations. It also helps to reduce the risk of exposure to COVID-19 or other infections by reducing the need for in-person visits [11]. It is important to note that pulmonary telerehabilitation is not appropriate for all patients and conditions. A healthcare professional should be consulted to determine if this type of telerehabilitation is appropriate for a specific individual [8].

17.4 Cardiac telerehabilitation

Cardiac telerehabilitation is a form of cardiac rehabilitation that uses remote communication technologies, such as teleconferencing, to provide rehabilitation services to patients who are unable to attend in-person sessions. This can include individuals who live in remote or rural areas, those who have mobility limitations, or those who have difficulty attending regular in-person rehabilitation sessions.

Telerehabilitation includes combination of education, exercise, and counseling services that are provided remotely, such as through video conferencing or phone calls as shown in Figure 17.4. The patient may also be provided with equipment, such as a heart rate monitor and pulse oximeter remotely at home during their rehabilitation program [12].

Research has shown that cardiac telerehabilitation can be as effective as in-person rehabilitation in improving patients' physical function and quality of life. It also provides flexibility and accessibility to patients who would otherwise be unable to participate in traditional cardiac rehabilitation programs [13].

17.5 Telerehabilitation in geriatrics

Telerehabilitation can also be used to provide rehabilitation services to older adults, including geriatric patients. This can include virtual consultations with a physical therapist or occupational therapist, remote monitoring of an older adult's recovery

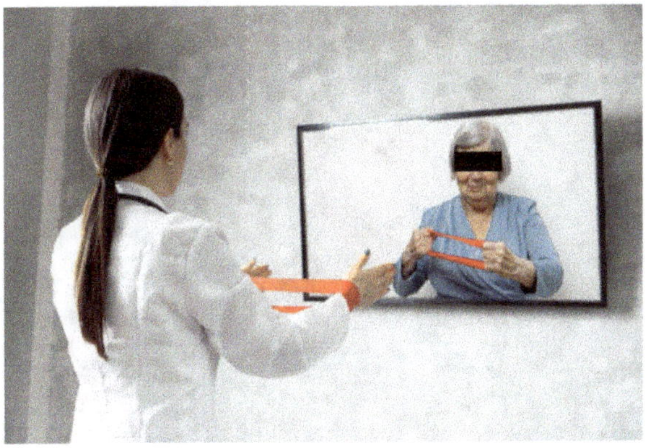

Figure 17.5 Telerehabilitation in geriatrics

progress, and virtual delivery of physical therapy exercises and other rehabilitation interventions.

Telerehabilitation can be particularly beneficial for older adults who live in remote areas or have limited access to in-person rehabilitation services, or for older adults who have difficulty with mobility or transportation. It can also help older adults to avoid the risk of hospitalization, especially during the pandemic as shown in Figure 17.5. Telerehabilitation can be used to help older adults regain strength, flexibility, and function after an injury or illness, and to improve balance and prevent falls. In addition, it can also be used to help older adults manage chronic conditions such as arthritis, diabetes, and heart disease [14].

However, it is important to note that telerehabilitation should be used as an adjunct to in-person therapy, rather than a replacement, and in some cases, in-person rehabilitation may be necessary. A physical therapist can advise on the most appropriate form of rehabilitation for a specific older adult. It is also important to ensure the older adult has access to the right technology and that they are comfortable with it, as well as the safety measures to avoid accidents while performing the exercises at home [15].

17.6 Postnatal telerehabilitation

Postnatal telerehabilitation refers to the use of telehealth technologies to provide rehabilitation services to women after childbirth. This can include virtual consultations with a physical therapist or women's health specialist, remote monitoring of a woman's recovery progress, and virtual delivery of physical therapy exercises and other rehabilitation interventions [16].

Postnatal telerehabilitation can be beneficial for women who have difficulty accessing in-person rehabilitation services due to location, transportation, or other logistical challenges. It can also be beneficial for women who have been discharged from the hospital earlier than expected and have difficulty attending in-person follow-up appointments.

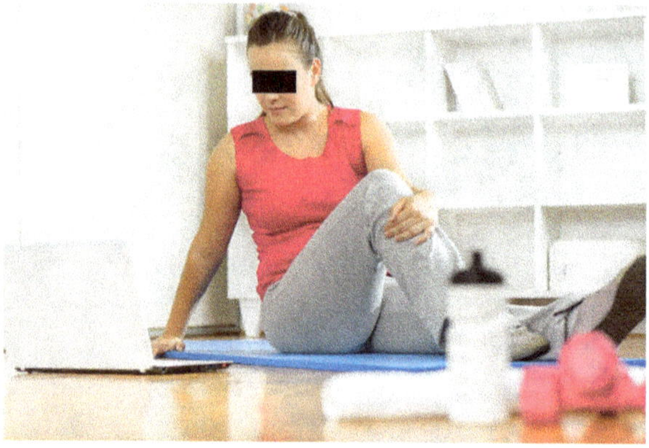

Figure 17.6 Postnatal telerehabilitation

Postnatal telerehabilitation can be used to help women regain strength and function in the pelvic floor and abdominal muscles, which are often weakened during childbirth as shown in Figure 17.6. It can also be used to help women manage conditions such as diastasis recti (abdominal separation), incontinence, and pelvic pain.

It is important to note that telerehabilitation should be used as an adjunct to in-person therapy, rather than a replacement, and in some cases, in-person rehabilitation may be necessary. A physical therapist or women's health specialist can advise on the most appropriate form of rehabilitation for a specific woman, and also ensure the safety of the exercises for postnatal women and new mothers.

17.7 Telerehabilitation on parental guidance

Telerehabilitation can involve parental guidance in order to provide support and assistance to children during the rehabilitation process. Parents or caregivers can play a crucial role in telerehabilitation for children by: assisting with setting up the technology and equipment needed for the therapy sessions. Helping the child understand and follow the therapist's instructions and exercises. Monitoring the child's progress and providing feedback to the therapist. Encouraging and motivating the child to participate in the therapy sessions. Helping the child to apply the exercises and techniques learned in therapy to daily activities. Helping to ensure safety when performing exercises at home [14].

It is important to note that the therapist should also provide guidance and instructions to the parents or caregivers on how to assist the child during the therapy sessions, and also ensure they are informed of the child's progress and any changes in the treatment plan.

Additionally, telerehabilitation can also provide opportunities for parent training and education on the child's condition and how to support the child's development, as well as on injury prevention and proper techniques to help reduce

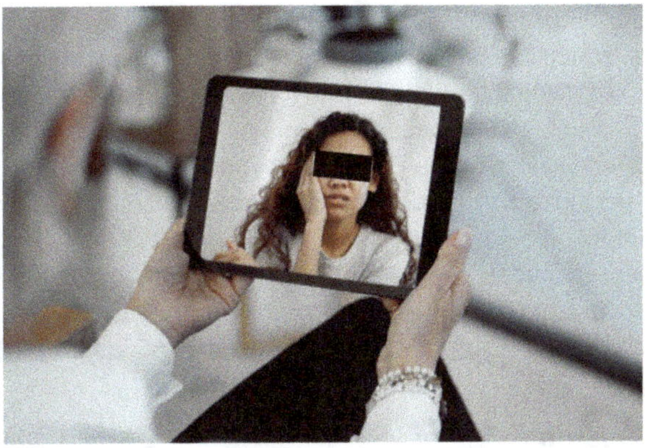

Figure 17.7 Role of telerehabilitation in drug de-addiction

the risk of future injuries. Overall, parent involvement and guidance can play a crucial role in the success of telerehabilitation for children and can help to improve the child's outcomes and overall quality of life.

17.8 Role of telerehabilitation in drug de-addiction

Telerehabilitation can also be used to provide addiction treatment and support to individuals with drug addiction. This can include virtual consultations with a counselor or therapist, remote monitoring of an individual's progress in treatment, and virtual delivery of cognitive-behavioral therapy, motivational interviewing, and other evidence-based therapies.

Telerehabilitation can be an effective way to provide addiction treatment and support to individuals who live in remote areas or have limited access to in-person treatment services as shown in Figure 17.7. It can also be beneficial for individuals who have difficulty engaging in traditional in-person treatment due to transportation issues, childcare responsibilities, or other logistical challenges [17].

However, it is important to note that telerehabilitation is not suitable for all types of addiction treatment, and in some cases, in-person treatment may be necessary. A substance abuse counselor or addiction therapist can advise on the most appropriate form of treatment for a specific individual. Additionally, virtual therapy should be combined with other traditional methods like medication, inpatient or out-patient treatment, peer support groups, and aftercare.

17.9 The benefits of telerehabilitation

Increased accessibility: Telerehabilitation allows patients to receive rehabilitation services regardless of their location, which can be especially beneficial for those who live in remote areas or have mobility limitations.

Convenience: Patients can receive rehabilitation services from the comfort of their own homes, which can be more convenient than traveling to a clinic or hospital.

Reduced costs: Telerehabilitation can reduce the costs associated with transportation and other expenses related to in-person visits.

Improved outcomes: Studies have shown that telerehabilitation can be as effective as in-person rehabilitation in improving outcomes for patients with a variety of conditions, including knee injuries.

It is important to note that telerehabilitation may not be suitable for all patients and conditions. Consultation with a healthcare professional is essential to determine if telerehabilitation is appropriate for a specific individual [18].

17.10 Conclusion

Telerehabilitation, or the use of technology to provide rehabilitation services remotely, has been shown to be effective in a variety of settings. It has the potential to improve access to rehabilitation services for individuals living in rural or remote areas, reduce barriers to care such as transportation and childcare, and increase patient satisfaction. However, there are also potential drawbacks to telerehabilitation, such as the need for reliable internet access and privacy concerns. Overall, telerehabilitation can be a useful addition to traditional rehabilitation services, but further research is needed to fully understand its effectiveness and optimal implementation.

References

[1] Peretti A, Amenta F, Tayebati SK, Nittari G, and Mahdi SS. Telerehabilitation: review of the state-of-the-art and areas of application. *JMIR Rehabil Assist Technol*. 2017;4(2):e7. http://dx.doi.org/10.2196/rehab.7511

[2] Turolla A, Rossettini G, Viceconti A, Palese A, and Geri T. Musculoskeletal physical therapy during the COVID-19 pandemic: Is telerehabilitation the answer? *Phys Ther*. 2020;100(8):1260–4. http://dx.doi.org/10.1093/ptj/pzaa093

[3] Fiani B, Siddiqi I, Lee SC, and Dhillon L. Telerehabilitation: development, application, and need for increased usage in the COVID-19 era for patients with spinal pathology. *Cureus*. 2020;12(9):e10563. http://dx.doi.org/10.7759/cureus.10563

[4] Alsobayel H, Alodaibi F, Albarrati A, Alsalamah N, Alhawas F, and Alhowimel A. Does telerehabilitation help in reducing disability among people with musculoskeletal conditions? A preliminary study. *Int J Environ Res Public Health*. 2021;19(1):72. http://dx.doi.org/10.3390/ijerph19010072

[5] Costa F, Janela D, Molinos M, *et al.* Telerehabilitation of acute musculoskeletal multi-disorders: prospective, single-arm, interventional study. *BMC Musculoskelet Disord*. 2022;23(1):29. http://dx.doi.org/10.1186/s12891-021-04891-5

[6] Dijkstra HP, Ergen E, Holtzhausen L, *et al.* Remote assessment in sport and exercise medicine (SEM): a narrative review and teleSEM solutions for and

beyond the COVID-19 pandemic June 2020. *Journal of Sports Medicine*. 2019;54:2020–2650.

[7] Kim BI, Peairs E, Lander S, Antonelli C, and Lau BC. Telehealth physical therapy for sports medicine rehabilitation: What is its role in the postpandemic era? *Orthop J Sports Med*. 2022;10(10):23259671221127720. http://dx.doi.org/10.1177/23259671221127721

[8] Cox NS, Dal Corso S, Hansen H, *et al.* Telerehabilitation for chronic respiratory disease. *Cochrane Libr.* 2021;2021(1):CD013040. http://dx.doi.org/10.1002/14651858.cd013040.pub2

[9] Tang J, Mandrusiak A, and Russell T. The feasibility and validity of a remote pulse oximetry system for pulmonary rehabilitation: a pilot study. *Int J Telemed Appl*. 2012;2012:798791. http://dx.doi.org/10.1155/2012/798791

[10] Crotty M, Killington M, van den Berg M, *et al.* Telerehabilitation for older people using off-the-shelf applications: acceptability and feasibility. *Journal of Telemedicine and Telecare*. 2014;20:370–6. http://dx.doi.org/10.1177/1357633X14552382. SourcePubMedProject: Telerehabilitation

[11] Sari DM and Wijaya LCG. Cardiac rehabilitation via telerehabilitation in COVID-19 pandemic situation. *Egypt Heart J*. 2021;73(1):31. http://dx.doi.org/10.1186/s43044-021-00156-7

[12] Hwang R, Bruning J, Morris NR, Mandrusiak A, and Russell T. Home-based telerehabilitation is not inferior to a centre-based program in patients with chronic heart failure: a randomised trial. *J Physiother*. 2017;63(2):101–7. http://dx.doi.org/10.1016/j.jphys.2017.02.017

[13] Seron P, Oliveros M-J, Gutierrez-Arias R, *et al.* Effectiveness of telerehabilitation in physical therapy: a rapid overview. *Phys Ther*. 2021;101(6): pzab053. http://dx.doi.org/10.1093/ptj/pzab053

[14] Sarti D, De Salvatore M, Pagliano E, Granocchio E, Traficante D, and Lombardi E. Telerehabilitation and wellbeing experience in children with special needs during the COVID-19 pandemic. *Children (Basel)*. 2021;8(11):988. http://dx.doi.org/10.3390/children8110988

[15] Appleby E, Gill ST, Hayes LK, Walker TL, Walsh M, and Kumar S. Effectiveness of telerehabilitation in the management of adults with stroke: a systematic review. *PLoS One*. 2019;14(11):e0225150. http://dx.doi.org/10.1371/journal.pone.0225150

[16] Zischke C, Simas V, Hing W, Milne N, Spittle A, and Pope R. The utility of physiotherapy assessments delivered by telehealth: a systematic review. *J Glob Health*. 2021;11:04072. http://dx.doi.org/10.7189/jogh.11.04072

[17] Magill M, Ray L, Kiluk B, *et al.* A meta-analysis of cognitive-behavioral therapy for alcohol or other drug use disorders: treatment efficacy by contrast condition. *J Consult Clin Psychol*. 2019;87(12):1093–105. http://dx.doi.org/10.1037/ccp0000447

[18] Pramuka M and Van Roosmalen L. Telerehabilitation technologies: accessibility and usability. *Int J Telerehabil*. 2009;85–98. http://dx.doi.org/10.5195/ijt.2009.6016

Chapter 18

Artificial intelligence in sports

Aravind Ganesh[1]*, Surya Vishnuram*[1] *and Pavithra Aravind*[1]

Artificial intelligence (AI) is rapidly changing the way we think about and interact with technology [1]. In recent years, AI has made its way into a variety of industries, including sports. The integration of AI in sports has the potential to revolutionize the way we train athletes, analyze performance, and even make decisions on the field or court [2].

One of the main ways AI that is being used in sports is through the analysis of performance data. Athlete tracking systems, such as GPS and wearable devices, can collect a vast amount of data on an athlete's movements, heart rate, and other physiological parameters. This data can then be analyzed using machine learning algorithms to gain insights into an athlete's performance and identify areas for improvement [3,4].

Another area where AI is being used in sports is in the realm of decision making. In certain sports, such as baseball and football, coaches and managers must make quick decisions based on a variety of factors. AI algorithms can be used to analyze game data and make predictions about the most likely outcome of a given play. This can assist coaches in making more informed decisions in real-time [5].

AI is also being used in the broadcast of sports events. It can be used to provide real-time statistics, such as player performance, and make predictions about the outcome of the game [6]. This can provide viewers with a more engaging and interactive viewing experience.

In addition to these examples, AI is also being used in sports training and rehabilitation. For example, AI-powered virtual reality systems can be used to simulate game scenarios and provide tailored training programs for athletes. Injuries can be diagnosed and treated with the help of AI-powered medical imaging and analysis [7].

While the use of AI in sports is still in its infancy, it has the potential to greatly enhance the way we train, compete, and watch sports. As technology continues to advance and data becomes more easily accessible, we can expect to see even more innovative uses of AI in the sports industry.

[1]Saveetha College of Physiotherapy, SIMATS, India

In this chapter, we will explore the various ways in which AI is currently being used in sports and discuss the potential benefits and challenges of integrating AI into the sports industry. We will also look at some of the ethical considerations that must be taken into account when using AI in sports, such as data privacy and fairness in competition.

18.1 AI and interactive experience

Sports organizations can better understand their fans' preferences and behavior, and use this information to create more personalized and engaging experiences for them (Figure 18.1).

One example of AI being used in fan engagement is in the analysis of social media data. By analyzing data from social media platforms, such as Twitter and Facebook, AI-powered systems can identify patterns in the way fans engage with teams and players. This can help organizations to understand what content resonates with their fans and what type of engagement is most effective [8].

AI can also be used to create personalized and interactive experiences for fans. For example, an AI-powered chatbot could be used to provide fans with real-time statistics, game predictions, and even personalized recommendations for merchandise or concessions [9].

AI-powered virtual reality systems can also be used to create immersive and engaging fan experiences. For example, a virtual reality system could be used to simulate the experience of sitting courtside at a basketball game or on the sidelines of a football game.

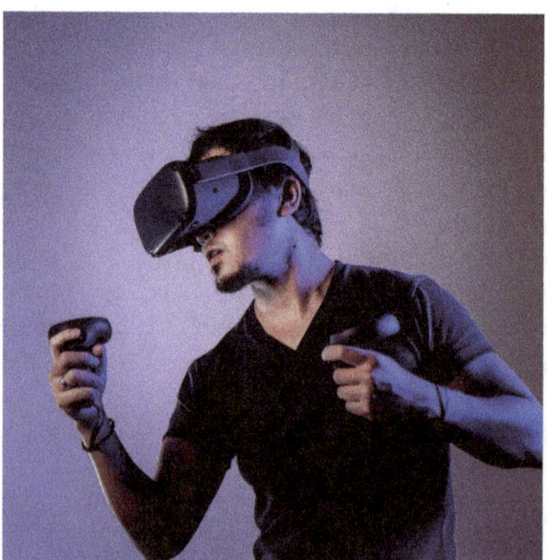

Figure 18.1 Interactive experience through virtual reality

However, while the use of AI in fan engagement has many potential benefits, there are also some challenges that must be addressed. One of the main challenges is the need for high-quality data. In order for AI-powered systems to provide accurate insights and personalized experiences, they must be fed with high-quality data on fan preferences and behavior. Still, there's a need to balance the use of AI with the need for human interaction and engagement. Sports organizations must find the right balance between using AI to provide personalized and engaging experiences for fans and providing opportunities for fans to connect with teams and players in a more traditional, human way [10].

18.2 AI in sports broadcasting

AI is being used in sports broadcasting (Figure 18.2) to enhance the viewing experience for fans. AI-powered systems can analyze live game footage and provide real-time statistics and insights, such as player performance and game predictions. This can make the viewing experience more engaging and interactive for fans, especially for those who enjoy fantasy sports [6,8].

AI is also being used in the field of sports sponsorship and advertising. AI-powered systems can analyze data on fan demographics and behavior, as well as team and player performance, to identify the most effective marketing strategies and target audiences for specific sports teams and events. This can help sports organizations and sponsors to maximize the return on their investment.

AI is making a significant impact in sports is in the field of sports betting. AI algorithms can analyze vast amounts of data on teams and players, including historical performance data, injury reports, and weather conditions, to make predictions on the outcome of games and events. This can give sports bettors a significant advantage in predicting the outcome of games and making informed bet.

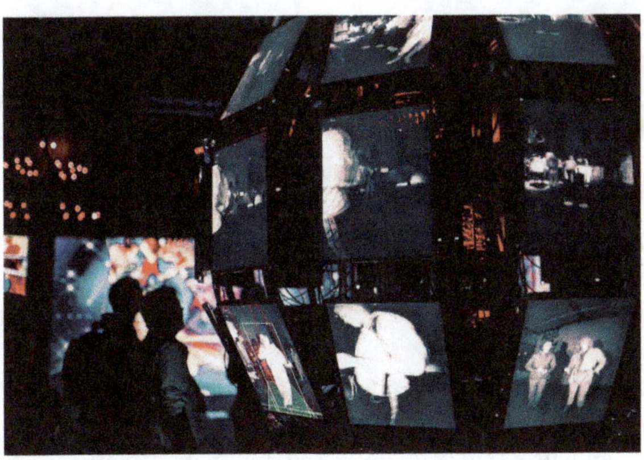

Figure 18.2 Sports broadcasting

18.3 AI as computer vision

One specific application of AI in sports that has gained a lot of attention in recent years is computer vision. Computer vision is a branch of AI that deals with the ability of machines to interpret and understand visual information. In sports, computer vision can be used to track player movements, monitor player performance, and even detect injuries [11].

One example of computer vision being used in sports is in the analysis of a soccer player's movements on the field. By analyzing footage of a player, an AI-powered system can detect patterns in the player's movements and identify areas of improvement. This can help coaches and trainers to tailor training programs to the individual needs of a player.

Computer vision can also be used to monitor player performance in real-time. For example, an AI-powered system could be used to track the movement of a basketball player and provide instant feedback on the player's shooting accuracy. This can help coaches to identify areas of improvement and make adjustments to the player's training program.

Another application of computer vision in sports is in the detection of injuries. By analyzing footage of an athlete, an AI-powered system can detect signs of an injury, such as limping or favoring a specific limb. This can help trainers to quickly identify and treat injuries before they become more serious.

18.4 Athletic tracking systems

Athletic tracking systems are devices or software applications that gather and analyze data related to an athlete's performance and physical activity. This data can include things such as heart rate, speed, distance covered, and calories burned. This information can be used to monitor an athlete's progress, set training goals, and improve overall performance [3]. Some popular examples of athletic tracking systems include Fitbit, Garmin, and Apple Watch.

Athletic tracking systems have revolutionized the way athletes and fitness enthusiasts monitor their performance and physical activity. These systems are designed to gather and analyze data related to an individual's performance, providing valuable insights that can be used to monitor progress, set training goals, and improve overall performance [12].

The primary benefit of athletic tracking systems is their ability to provide real-time feedback and data analysis. For example, a heart rate monitor can track an athlete's heart rate in real-time, allowing them to monitor their level of exertion and adjust their intensity accordingly [13]. Additionally, many athletic tracking systems can provide data on other aspects of performance, such as speed, distance covered, and calories burned.

This data can be used to set realistic training goals and monitor progress over time. For example, an athlete may set a goal to run a certain distance in a certain amount of time and use the data collected by their athletic tracking system to monitor their progress and make adjustments to their training regimen as needed.

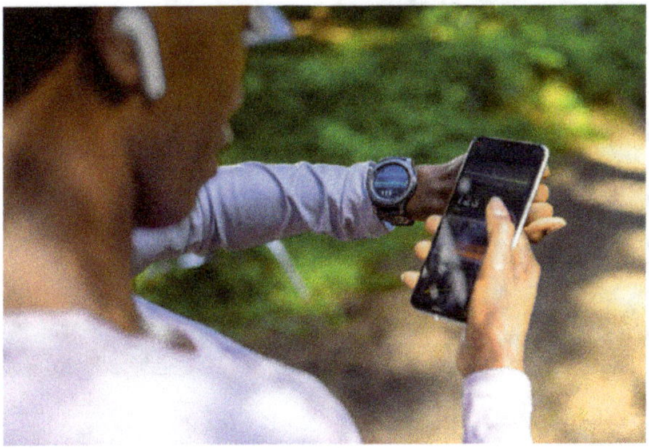

Figure 18.3 Wearable devices and athletic tracking system

Athletic tracking systems (Figure 18.3) can also be used to identify areas of weakness that need improvement. For example, an individual who struggles with stamina may use the data from their athletic tracking system to identify when they are likely to experience fatigue and take steps to improve their endurance [14].

One of the key advantages of athletic tracking systems is their versatility. Many systems are designed to work with a variety of different activities, from running and cycling to weightlifting and swimming. This versatility allows individuals to use the same system for multiple activities, providing a more comprehensive view of their overall fitness level.

Another benefit of athletic tracking systems is their ability to provide a social aspect to fitness. Many systems have online communities where users can connect with others, share their progress, and receive encouragement and support. This social aspect can be especially beneficial for those who struggle with motivation, as it provides a support network that can help keep individuals on track.

Athletic tracking systems have had a profound impact on the way individuals monitor their performance and physical activity. With their ability to provide real-time feedback, data analysis, and social support, these systems have helped individuals set and achieve their fitness goals, leading to improved health and performance.

18.5 AI in sports injury

AI is being increasingly used in the field of sports medicine to help prevent, diagnose, and treat sports injuries (Figure 18.4). The use of AI can help improve the accuracy and speed of injury diagnosis, as well as assist with the development of personalized injury prevention and treatment plans [15].

One of the primary ways AI is being used in sports injury is through the use of machine learning algorithms. These algorithms can analyze large amounts of data related to an athlete's performance and biomechanics, such as movement patterns

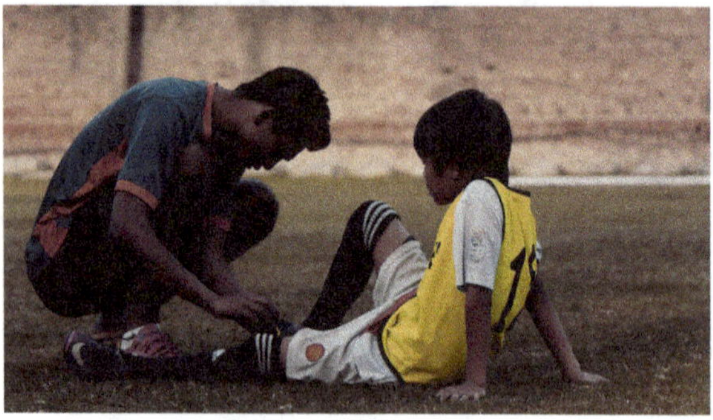

Figure 18.4 Sports injury

and muscle activity, to identify potential injury risks [16]. This information can then be used to develop customized injury prevention programs, helping to reduce the likelihood of injury.

Another application of AI in sports injury is in the diagnosis and treatment of injuries. For example, AI-powered imaging tools can analyze MRI or X-ray images to identify and diagnose injuries more accurately and quickly than traditional methods. This can lead to faster recovery times for athletes, as well as improved outcomes for patients [17].

In addition to helping prevent and diagnose injuries, AI is also being used in the rehabilitation process. For example, AI-powered wearable devices can monitor an athlete's progress during rehabilitation and provide real-time feedback on the effectiveness of their treatments. This information can be used to make adjustments to the treatment plan as needed, leading to improved outcomes and faster recovery times.

Overall, the use of AI in sports injury has the potential to greatly improve the accuracy and speed of injury diagnosis, as well as assist with the development of personalized injury prevention and treatment plans. As technology continues to advance, it is likely that AI will play an increasingly important role in the field of sports medicine.

18.6 Concerns and challenges

However, despite the many potential benefits of AI in sports, there are also some concerns and challenges that must be addressed (Figure 18.5). One of the main concerns is the potential for bias in AI systems, especially when it comes to player evaluation and decision-making. To mitigate this, it is important to ensure that the data used to train AI systems is representative of a diverse population, and that the algorithms are transparent and explainable [18].

Another concern is the potential for AI to be used to gain an unfair advantage in competition. To prevent this, sports organizations may need to establish guidelines and regulations for the use of AI in sports.

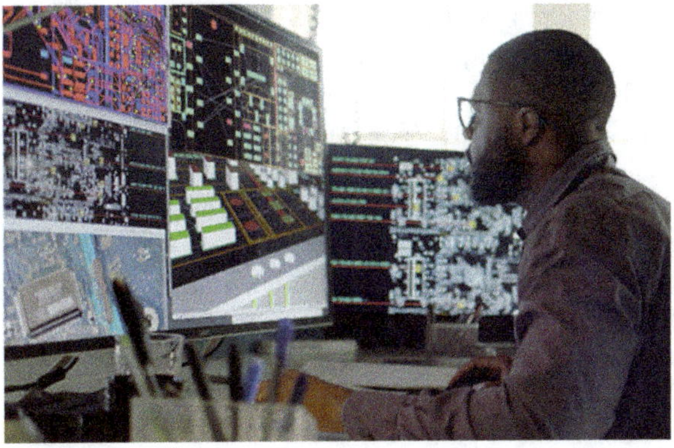

Figure 18.5 Human intelligence versus AI

While computer vision is a powerful tool for sports analysis and training, it also poses some challenges. One of the main challenges is the need for high-quality footage. In order for an AI-powered system to accurately analyze player movements, the footage must be of a high resolution and taken from multiple angles. Additionally, there can be privacy concerns with the use of AI in sports, especially when it comes to player data [19].

18.7 Conclusion

AI has the potential to greatly enhance the way we train, compete, and watch sports. The use of AI in sports is still in its infancy but its application in computer vision, performance analysis, decision-making, and training and rehabilitation can revolutionize the industry. However, we must also consider the ethical implications of using AI in sports, such as data privacy and fairness in competition [20]. As technology continues to advance, we can expect to see even more innovative uses of AI in the sports industry.

In conclusion, AI has the potential to revolutionize the sports industry by enhancing training, analysis, decision-making, and the viewing experience for fans. However, as with any technology, there are also challenges and ethical considerations that must be taken into account. With the continued advancement of AI, it will be important for sports organizations, coaches, and fans to stay informed and stay engaged in the ongoing conversation about the impact of AI in sports [21–34].

References

[1] Pereira SW, Fishman EK, and Rowe SP. The future is now: how technology and entertainment are transforming education in the artificial intelligence era. *Journal of the American College of Radiology*. 2022;19(9):1077–8.

[2] Wei S, Huang P, Li R, Liu Z, and Zou Y. Exploring the application of artificial intelligence in sports training: a case study approach. *Complexity*. 2021;2021:1–8.
[3] Seshadri DR, Drummond C, Craker J, Rowbottom JR, and Voos JE. Wearable devices for sports: new integrated technologies allow coaches, physicians, and trainers to better understand the physical demands of athletes in real time. *IEEE Pulse*. 2017;8(1):38–43.
[4] Cardinale M and Varley MC. Wearable training-monitoring technology: applications, challenges, and opportunities. *International Journal of Sports Physiology and Performance*. 2017;12(s2):S2–55.
[5] García-Aliaga A, Marquina M, Coterón J, Rodríguez-González A, and Luengo-Sánchez S. In-game behaviour analysis of football players using machine learning techniques based on player statistics. *International Journal of Sports Science & Coaching*. 2021;16(1):148–57.
[6] Khan AA and Shao J. Spnet: a deep network for broadcast sports video highlight generation. *Computers and Electrical Engineering*. 2022;99:107779.
[7] Liang F. AI-powered digital media platform and its applications. In *Proceedings of the 2020 Conference on Artificial Intelligence and Healthcare*, 2020 Oct 23, pp. 121–6.
[8] Vale L and Fernandes T. Social media and sports: driving fan engagement with football clubs on Facebook. *Journal of Strategic Marketing*. 2018;26 (1):37–55.
[9] Xiao Z, Zhou MX, Liao QV, *et al.* Tell me about yourself: using an AI-powered chatbot to conduct conversational surveys with open-ended questions. *ACM Transactions on Computer-Human Interaction (TOCHI)*. 2020;27(3):1–37.
[10] Castillo D, Canhoto AI, and Said E. The dark side of AI-powered service interactions: exploring the process of co-destruction from the customer perspective. *The Service Industries Journal*. 2021;41(13–14):900–25.
[11] Naik BT, Hashmi MF, and Bokde ND. A comprehensive review of computer vision in sports: open issues, future trends and research directions. *Applied Sciences*. 2022;12(9):4429.
[12] Li RT, Kling SR, Salata MJ, Cupp SA, Sheehan J, and Voos JE. Wearable performance devices in sports medicine. *Sports Health*. 2016;8(1):74–8.
[13] Waqar A, Ahmad I, Habibi D, Hart N, and Phung QV. Enhancing athlete tracking using data fusion in wearable technologies. *IEEE Transactions on Instrumentation and Measurement*. 2021;70:1–3.
[14] Seshadri DR, Rowbottom JR, Drummond C, Voos JE, and Craker J. A review of wearable technology: moving beyond the hype: from need through sensor implementation. In *2016 8th Cairo International Biomedical Engineering Conference (CIBEC)*, 2016, IEEE, pp. 52–5.
[15] Claudino JG, Capanema DD, de Souza TV, Serrão JC, Machado Pereira AC, and Nassis GP. Current approaches to the use of artificial intelligence for injury risk assessment and performance prediction in team sports: a systematic review. *Sports Medicine-Open*. 2019;5:1–2.

[16] Kakavas G, Malliaropoulos N, Pruna R, and Maffulli N. Artificial intelligence: a tool for sports trauma prediction. *Injury*. 2020;51:S63–5.

[17] Chu WC, Shih C, Chou WY, Ahamed SI, and Hsiung PA. Artificial intelligence of things in sports science: weight training as an example. *Computer*. 2019;52(11):52–61.

[18] Wang S. Trend of competitive sports reform under the background of artificial intelligence. *Journal of Physics: Conference Series*. 2020;1533 (3):032043.

[19] Liu J, Wang L, and Zhou H. The application of human–computer interaction technology fused with artificial intelligence in sports moving target detection education for college athlete. *Frontiers in Psychology*. 2021;12:677590.

[20] Lu H, Li Y, Chen M, Kim H, and Serikawa S. Brain intelligence: go beyond artificial intelligence. *Mobile Networks and Applications*. 2018;23:368–75.

[21] Leong WY. Implementing blind source separation in signal processing and telecommunications. Thesis, The University of Queensland, Australia, 2005.

[22] Palaniswamy M and Leong WY. Mechanical properties of the human vertebrae between normal, post corrective and post operative. In *2014 IEEE International Symposium on Robotics and Manufacturing Automation (ROMA)*, 2014, Kuala Lumpur, Malaysia, pp. 188–93.

[23] Leong WY and Andrew Ng CR. Left-handedness detection. *International Journal on Smart Sensing and Intelligent Systems*. 2022;7(2):442–57.

[24] Leong WY, Chuah JH, and Tuan TB. (eds.) (eds.) . *The Nine Pillars of Technologies for Industry 4.0*. Stevenage, UK: Institution of Engineering and Technology, 2020.

[25] Leong WY. and Ee J. A warehouse management system for 3 dimensional tracking and positioning. *Applied Mechanics and Materials*. 2012;152–154: 1685–90.

[26] Leong WY. *Human Machine Collaboration and Interaction for Smart Manufacturing: Automation, robotics, sensing, artificial intelligence, 5G, IoTs and Blockchain*. Stevenage, UK: Institution of Engineering and Technology.

[27] Leong WY. *Medical Equipment Engineering: Design, manufacture, and applications*. Stevenage, UK: The Institution of Engineering and Technology, 2023.

[28] Leong WY. EEG identification and differentiation for left-handedness. In *2014 IEEE International Symposium on Robotics and Manufacturing Automation (ROMA)*, 2014, Kuala Lumpur, Malaysia, pp. 147–53.

[29] Xiaofan W, Chong PHJ, and Leong WY. Performance comparison of CSMA/CD, CSMA/CA, CSMA/RI, CSMA/PRI and CSMA/PR with BEB. In *2010 5th IEEE Conference on Industrial Electronics and Applications*, 2010, Taichung, pp. 1843–8.

[30] Min HF and Leong WY. Investigating target detection and localization in wireless sensor network. *Procedia Engineering*. 2012;41:75–81.

[31] Mehrotra U and Leong WY. NSEEAR: a energy adaptive routing protocol for heterogeneous wireless sensor networks. In *2009 35th Annual*

Conference of IEEE Industrial Electronics, 2009, Porto, Portugal, pp. 2647–52.

[32] Xiaofan W, Chong PHJ, and Leong WY. Evaluation of performance on random back-off interval and multi-channel CSMA/CA protocols. In *TENCON 2009 - 2009 IEEE Region 10 Conference*, 2009, Singapore, pp. 1–5.

[33] Leong WY, Homer J. EKENS: A learning on nonlinear blindly mixed signals. In Proceedings of IEEE International Conference on Acoustics, Speech, and Signal Processing (ICASSP'05), 2005, pp. iv–81.

[34] Mohankumar P and Leong WY. 3D modelling with CT and MRI images of a scoliotic vertebrae. *Journal of Engineering Science and Technology*, 2016:188–98.

Chapter 19

Case study 1: image processing for medical application of preventing the spread of COVID-19

Suci Dwijayanti[1], *Sukan Agung Perdana*[1], *Zainal Husin*[1] *and Bhakti Yudho Suprapto*[1]

This study presented security system equipped with an ability to detect body temperature to reduce the spread of COVID-19. Generally, temperature screening was done using a thermometer gun. However, its usage was limited and cannot be used together as a security system. Thus, this study developed a smart lock door system with a contactless temperature screening based on Internet of Things (IoT). The built system consists of an ESP32, microcontroller, the MLX90640 sensor as temperature screening, solenoid door lock, the Haar cascade algorithm for face detection, the local binary pattern histogram algorithm for face recognition. The system may send temperature data to the database website, sending an alert if the object has a temperature above 38°C. The results of this study showed that the average temperature difference between thermos gun and the MLX90640 was 0.1°C and 0.09°C at a distance of 10 cm and 12 cm, respectively. Those distances were considered as the effective distance. The proposed face recognition succeeded in recognizing the object with an accuracy of 80% in dark condition and 100% in bright condition. Face recognition and temperature screening were successfully sent to the database with a time difference of sending data was 0.3 s. An alert can be sent to the Telegram in real-time manner when the temperature and face were recognized as a suspect of COVID-19. The security system cannot be opened when the recognized face was not in the database.

19.1 Introduction

During the spread of COVID-19, healthy protocols must be implemented and one of them is to detect body temperature before entering a place [1]. Such body temperature must use a contactless media to prevent the spread of this disease. Usually,

[1]Department of Electrical Engineering, Universitas Sriwijaya, Indonesia

the officer uses a thermometer gun. However, such method may cause an error because it is done manually and depends on the position which part of the body is measured. Thus, a contactless real-time system is needed to replace the role of human in detecting human body temperature.

Some studies have been done to measure a body temperature before accessing a place. The authors of [2] discussed a system to detect heart beat and body temperature based on IoT using firebase database. Meanwhile, the author of [3] studied a monitoring of body temperature and face mask detection. The authors of [4] studied body temperature measurement for infants based on IoT using ESP8266. The authors of [5] designed a wireless monitoring system to measure the human body temperature using an Arduino controller with different sensors and open source Internet connection. However, those studies only focused on body temperature. This study combines both face recognition and body temperature measurement to prevent the spread of COVID-19 based on IoT. The aim of this study is to prevent the spread of COVID-19 bay using the combination of face recognition system and body temperature measurement [6–18].

19.2 Methods

19.2.1 System design

A flowchart of the proposed design can be seen in Figure 19.1. The hardware consists of ESP32 as the controller for temperature detection and internet of things, Arduino uno as a microcontroller for the door lock security system, MLX90640 to detect the body temperature, relay, solenoid door lock, and battery. The prototype can be seen in Figure 19.2.

19.2.2 Face recognition using Haar cascade algorithm and local binary pattern histogram

The proposed system combines the body temperature measurement with the image processing. In this case, the image processing is face recognition as shown in the diagram block in Figure 19.3.

The face recognition system utilizes Haar cascade algorithm and local binary pattern histogram. The Haar cascade algorithm is used to detect the face since face detection is the first process in identifying the face to ensure the possibility of face in an image [19]. Haar cascade algorithm has four stages as follows:

1. Haar feature

   Haar feature consists of one higher interval and one lower interval. In 2D image, they are known as dark and white zones. Some Haar features can be seen in Figure 19.4.

   Each feature produces one value which can be calculated by subtracting pixel values in the bright area to the pixel values in dark area.

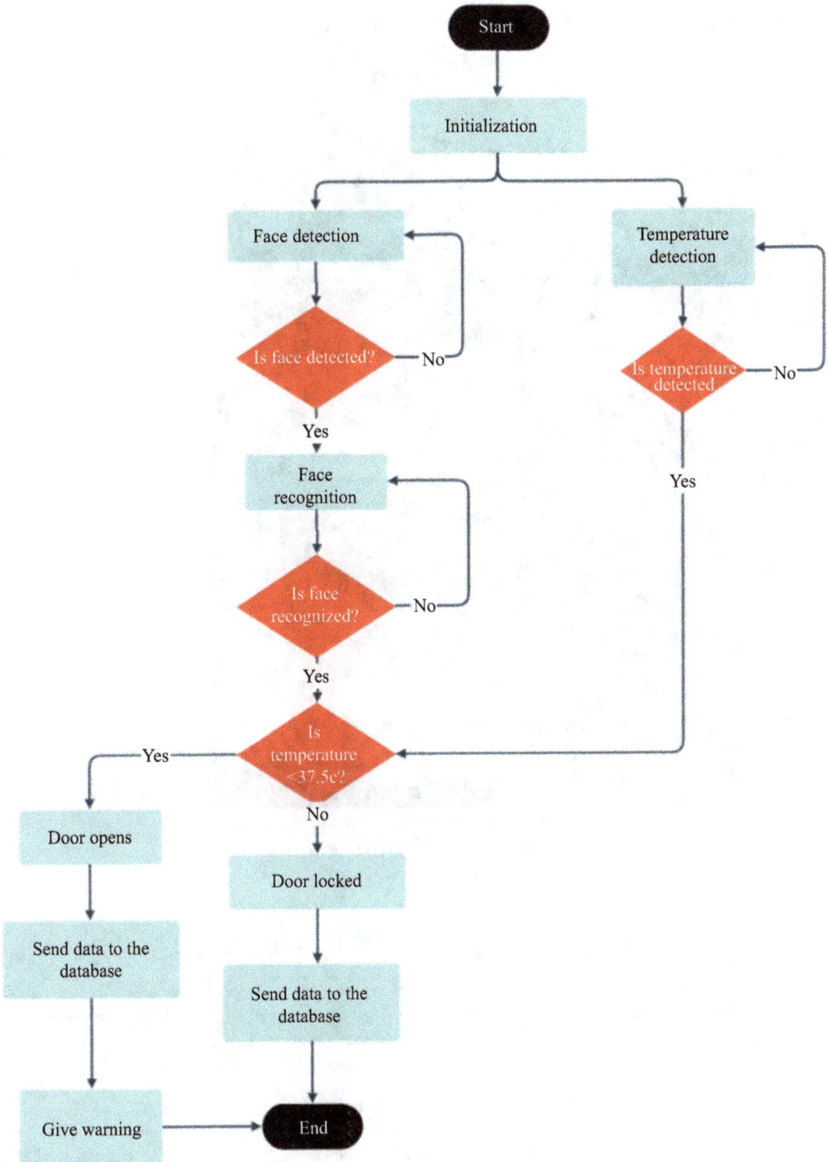

Figure 19.1 Flowchart of the system

2. Integral image

   In this stage, feature value is calculated by changing input image to the integral image which can obtain Haar-like. This integral image is used to calculate the number of pixels in a rectangle by using four values efficiently. Those values are pixels values in integral image on each angle of rectangular. As example as shown in Figure 19.5.

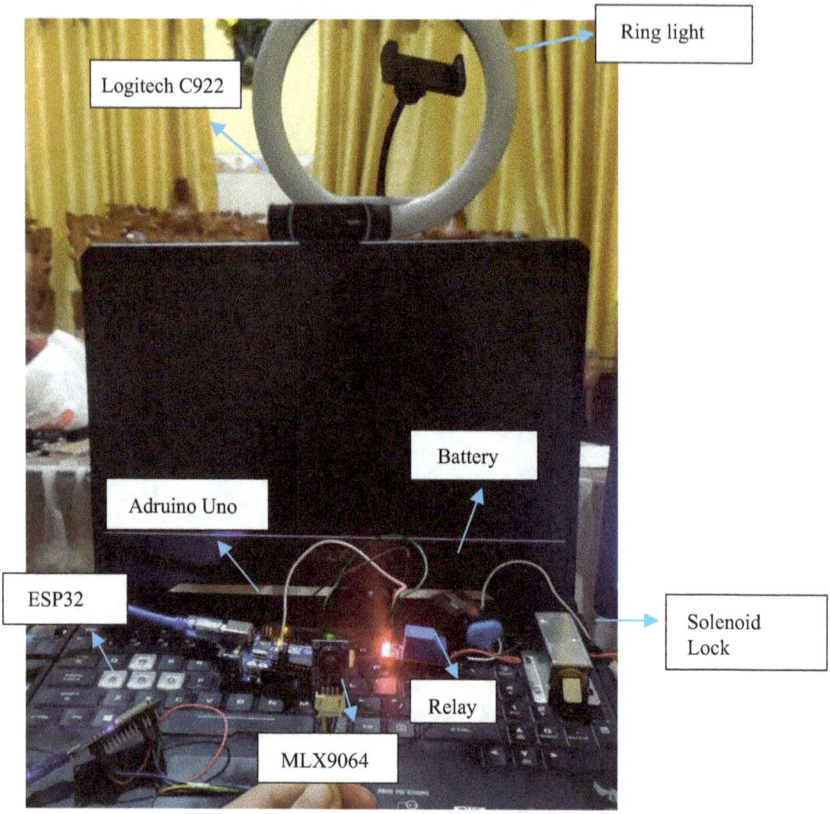

Figure 19.2 Hardware design

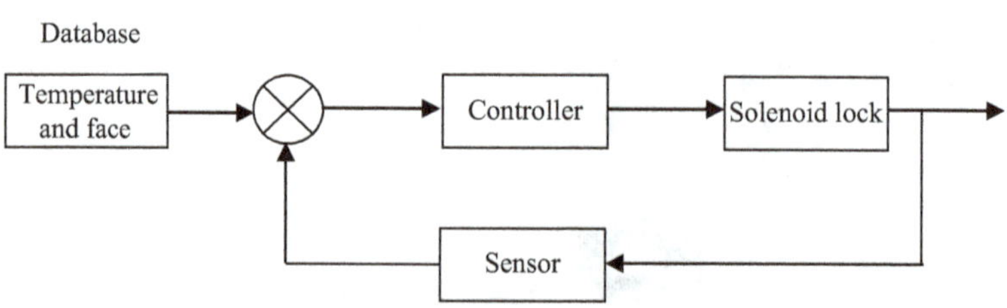

Figure 19.3 Diagram block of system

Number of pixels A in an image can be calculated as follows:

$$A = L_4 - (L_2 + L_3) + L_1$$

After obtaining values of each pixel, the value in integral image must be equal to the numbers of all pixels above and to the next of it as shown in

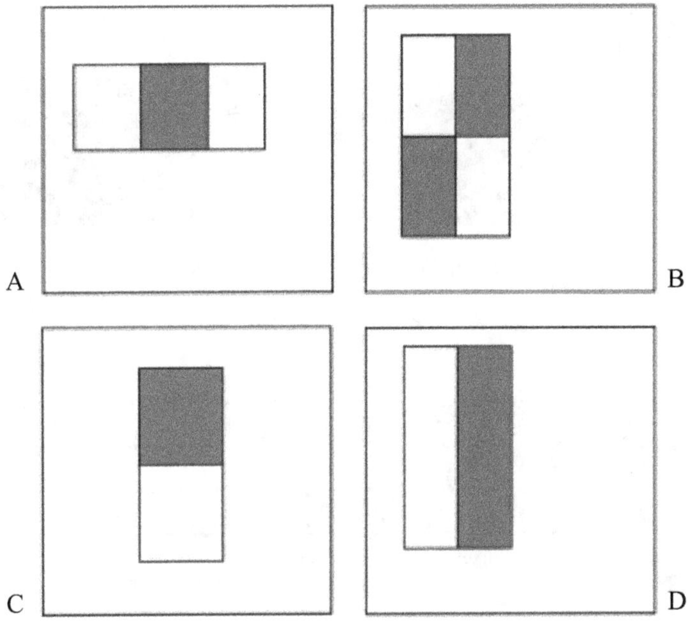

Figure 19.4 Feature Haar [19]

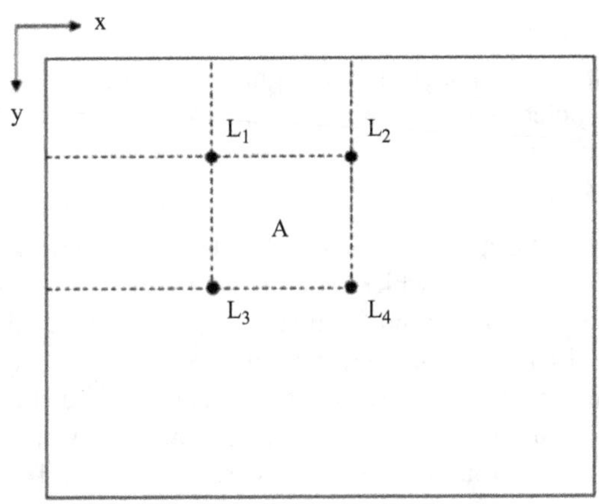

Figure 19.5 Representation of integral image [20]

Figure 19.6. After that, the number of pixels in the bright and dark regions can be determined.

3. AdaBoost

   AdaBoost is a learning algorithm to select the important features and do training to the classifier. AdaBoost has a filter to classify the region of an image.

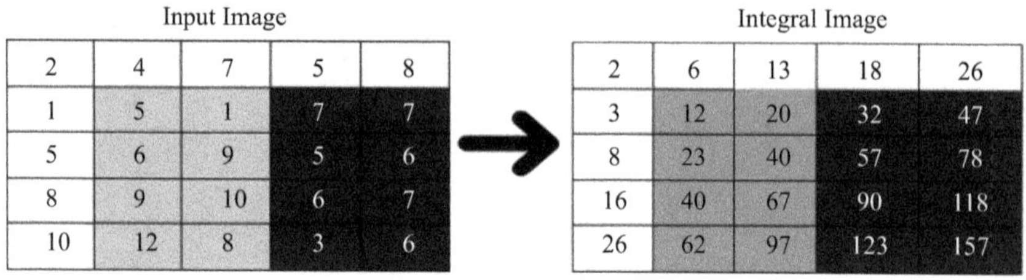

Figure 19.6 Input image to integral image

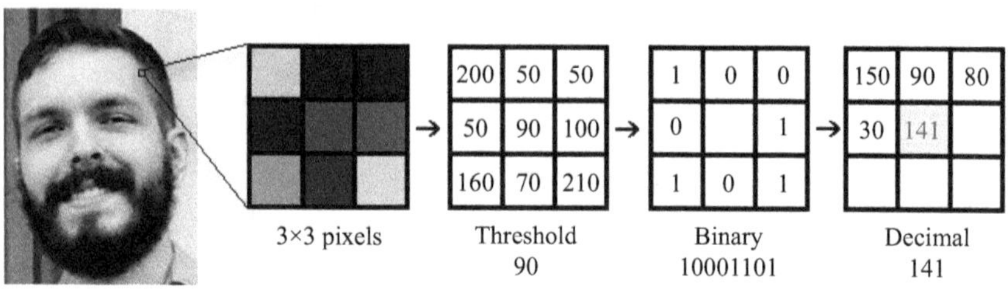

Figure 19.7 Steps to calculate LBP

4. Cascade classifier

   The final stage of Haar Cascade algorithm is the cascade classifier. This classifier will delete non-face images using a strong classifier that has been trained in AdaBoost.

After detecting the face region, the next stage to recognize the face is done using a local binary pattern histogram (LBPH). This algorithm works based on the operator of local binary patter, which label pixels in an image, compare the center pixel with the other 8 pixels around the image, and assume it as the binary number [21]. The stages of LBHP can be seen in Figure 19.7.

As shown in the figure, the grayscale face image is divided into 3 × 3 images. For each of pixel in the image, the binary code is obtained by comparing the center pixel value to the pixels around it. The pixels around become 1 if the value of it is greater or equal to the value of center pixel, and it becomes zero otherwise. Later, the new binary number is arranged to clockwise or counter clockwise with some consistent requirement. These new binary numbers are changed to the decimal and arrange them to center pixel value which is equal to the original image. This image is then extracted to the histogram to determine frequency of binary pattern. The number of bin histogram depends on the pixel number involving in the calculation of LBP. For example, if LBP uses 8 pixels than the histogram bin becomes $2^8 = 256$. Each histogram is added together to obtain new histogram representing the characteristic of original image.

19.2.3 Body temperature measurement with MLX90640

MLX90640 is used to measure the body temperature. In this system, ESP32 is connected to four pins, namely VCC, GND, SCA, and SCL as shown in Figure 19.8. Blue cable connects pin GND MLX90640 to GND ESP32, yellow cable connects VCC MLX90640 to pin 3V3 ESP32, red cable connects SDA MLX90640 to D21 ESP32, and green cable connects SCL to D22 ESP32.

The temperature measurement system is combined with the image processing. If the detected person has higher body temperature which may indicate the high fever, the person is not allowed to access the room to prevent the spread of possibility of COVID-19. This system is connected to the lock door security system as shown in Figure 19.9.

Arduino Uno connecting to relay 5V 1 channel and relay 5V 1 channel connects to solenoid lock and battery. Red cable as shown in the figure connect pin VCC relay to pin 5V Arduino uno. Meanwhile, blue cable connects INT relay to pin 3 Arduino uno and black cable connect GND relay to GND Arduino. Positive cable of solenoid lock connects pin COM relay, positive cable of battery connects pin NO relay, and negative cable connects to negative battery.

19.2.4 Evaluation

Accuracy is used to evaluate the face recognition algorithm. It compares the number of correct recognized face to the whole recognized face, which can be

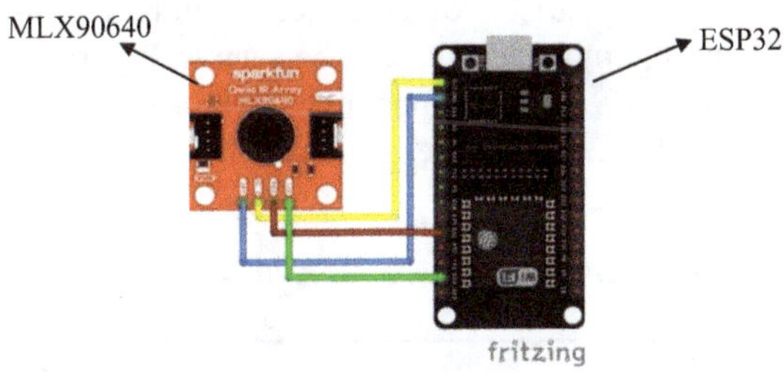

Figure 19.8 Design of temperature sensor MLX90640

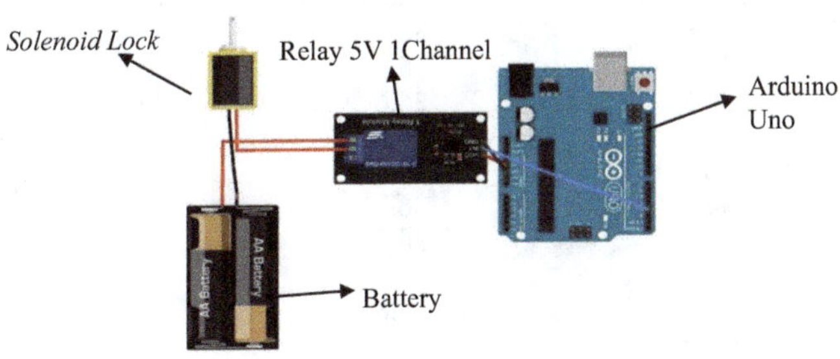

Figure 19.9 Door lock design

calculated as follows:

$$Accuracy = \frac{(\mathrm{TP} + \mathrm{TN})}{(\mathrm{TP} + \mathrm{FP} + \mathrm{TN} + \mathrm{FN})}$$

In this study, the IoT is used to know the time to send the temperature real-time to database website. It is done 10 times, transmitting and receiving time are calculated. The different between transmitting and receiving time is calculated as follows:

$$R = \frac{(WS_1 - W_1) + (WS_2 - W_2) + \ldots + (WS_{10} - W_{10})}{10}$$

where R is the average time of difference between transmitting and receiving time, WS is the received time in database website, and W is the transmitting time to send data to the database.

19.3 Results and discussions

19.3.1 Body temperature measurement

This study uses MLX90640 to measure the body temperature. This sensor has specification of operational temperature range of –40°C to 85°C and an accuracy of ±1°C. To check the accuracy of the body measurement, MLX90640 is compared to thermometer gun with an effective distance of ± 1–3 cm. The results can be seen in Table 19.1 and the comparison of body temperature measurement between sensor MLX90640 and thermometer gun can be seen in Figure 19.10.

As shown in Figure 19.10, the temperature obtained by thermometer gun is between 36.5°C and 36.6°C, meanwhile the sensor MLX90640 is 36.3°C–36.8°C.

Table 19.1 Evaluation of sensor MLX90640

Trial	**Sensor MLX90640 within distance of 2 cm (°C)**	***Thermometer gun* within distance of ± 1–3 cm (°C)**	**Difference (°C)**
1	36,8	36,6	0,2
2	36,5	36,6	0,1
3	36,5	36,6	0,1
4	36,3	36,6	0,3
5	36,5	36,6	0,1
6	36,6	36,7	0,1
7	36,3	36,5	0,2
8	36,5	36,6	0,1
9	36,6	36,6	0
10	36,5	36,6	0,1
The average			0,13

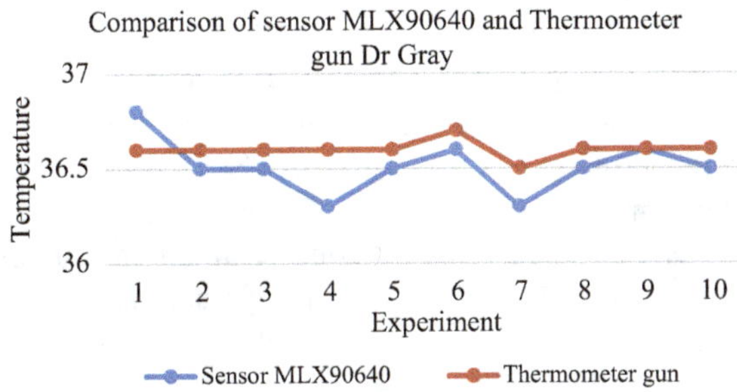

Figure 19.10 Body temperature measurement using sensor MLX90640 and thermometer gun

Table 19.2 Temperature difference for various distance of sensor MLX90640

No.	**Distance of sensor MLX90640 (cm)**	**Average of temperature difference (°C)**
1	2 cm	0.13
2	4 cm	0.29
3	6 cm	0.51
4	8 cm	0.8
5	10 cm	0.1
6	12 cm	0.09
7	14 cm	0.27
8	16 cm	0.72
9	18 cm	0.38
10	20 cm	0.5

The difference is around 0°C–0.3°C with the average difference is 0.13°C. Thus, it indicates that sensor MLX90640 can be used to measure the body temperature contactless. The effective distance to measure the temperature for thermometer gun is ± 1–3 cm. However, sensor MLX90640 does not have any specific distance in measuring the temperature. Thus, this study also performs an experiment to find its effective distance.

Table 19.2 shows the experiment results of average difference of temperature for various distances. As shown in the table, the highest temperature obtained by sensor MLX90640 is 36.9°C with the distance of 6 cm for second trial. The lowest temperature is obtained in the sixth trial with the temperature of 35.5°C and a distance of 8 cm. From the table, the average difference between thermometer gun and sensor MLX90640 is around 0.09°C–0.72°C. The farther the distance between sensor and object may cause the difference becomes bigger, as shown in the trial using the distance of 14–20 cm. Based on the table, the effective distance for MLX90640 is 10 and 12 cm.

19.3.2 Face recognition

The data used for this study was obtained from 10 students, each respondent's face is captured 31 times. Thus, there are 310 images of face. The data is captured using Logitech C922 with resolution of 1080 pixels. The face images are in .JPG and convert to grayscale images.

The images data were then detected using Haar Cascade algorithm to obtain the face area. The example of data detected using Haar cascade algorithm can be seen in Figure 19.11.

The face detected is then preprocessed to grayscale image before recognizing using LBPH. Parameters used for LBPH algorithm consist of four parameters, such as radius to build biner pattern local to circle and represents radius to the center pixel, neighbors are the number of samples to build the biner pattern to local circle, grid X is the number of cells in horizontal, and grid Y is number of cells in vertical.

The training data consist of primary data from 10 respondents and each respondent has 31 images. Totally, the training data is 310 images. The number of classes in this study is labeled to 1–10 representing the identity of face's owner.

After training, the next stage is testing which is performed in the room using Logitech camera C922 in two conditions, namely bright and dim condition. Ring light and lamp are used to obtain the bright condition. Meanwhile, the dim condition is when the door is closed and the lamp in the room turns off. The aim of this evaluation is to get the accuracy of the proposed system in recognizing the face in different conditions. The results can be seen in Tables 19.3 and 19.4, respectively.

The test was done 20 times to recognize the face in two conditions, namely dim and bright conditions. The results show that the accuracy of face recognition in the bright and dim condition is 100% and 80%, respectively. The accuracy of dim condition is lower than the bright ones. It can be caused by the similarity of face between samples 4 and 5 to sample 3. Nevertheless, the system can identify the face well in the bright and dim condition.

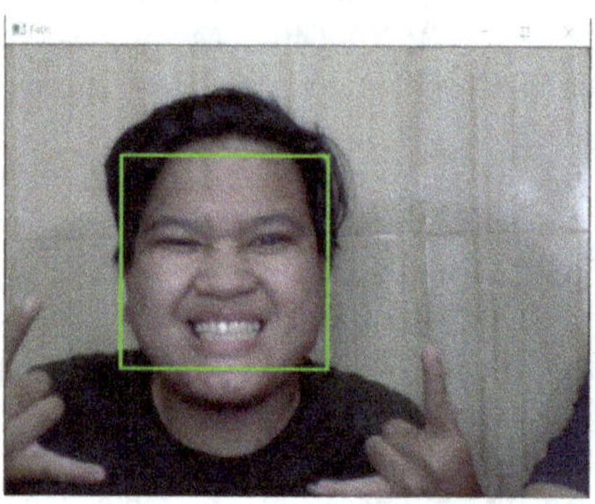

Figure 19.11 Detected face using Haar cascade algorithm

Table 19.3 Result of testing in bright condition

No.	Sample	Result of face recognition	Remark
1	Sample 1	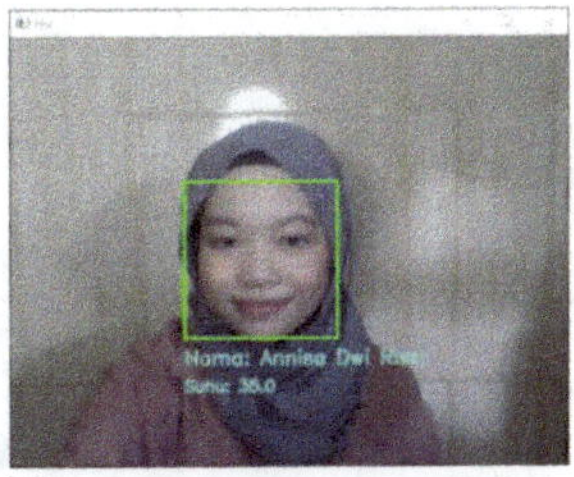	Success
2	Sample 2	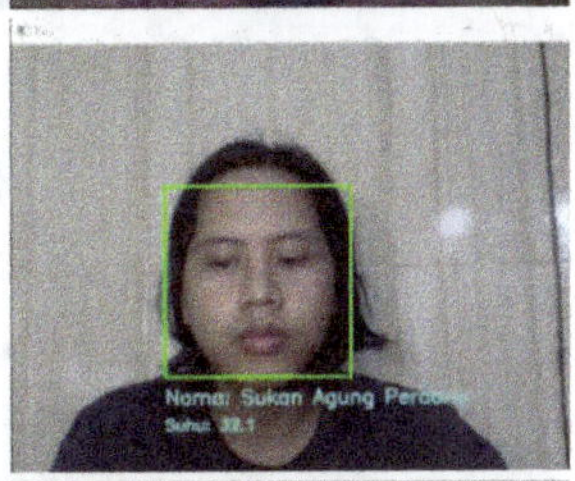	Success
3	Sample 3	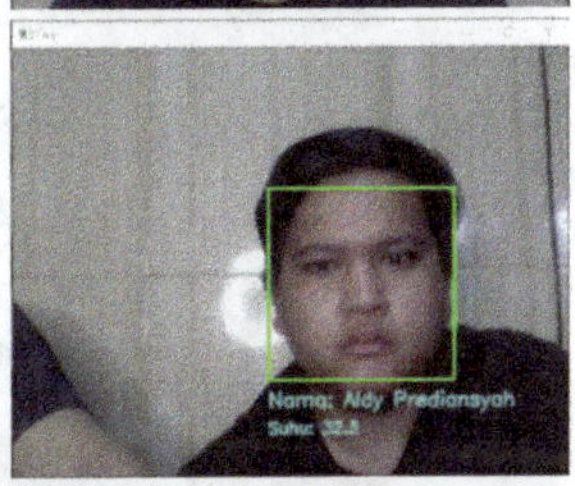	Success
4	Sample 4	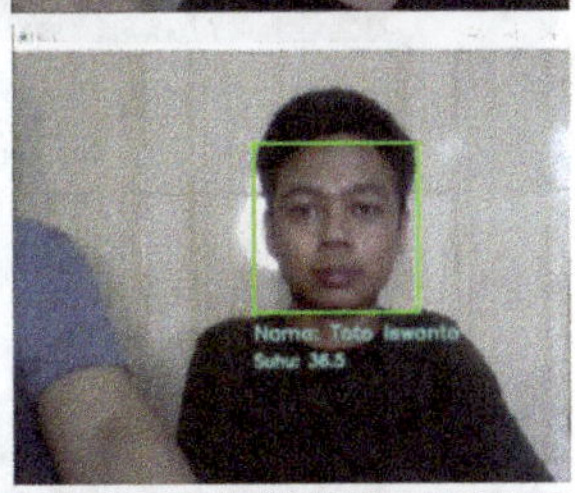	Success
5	Sample 5	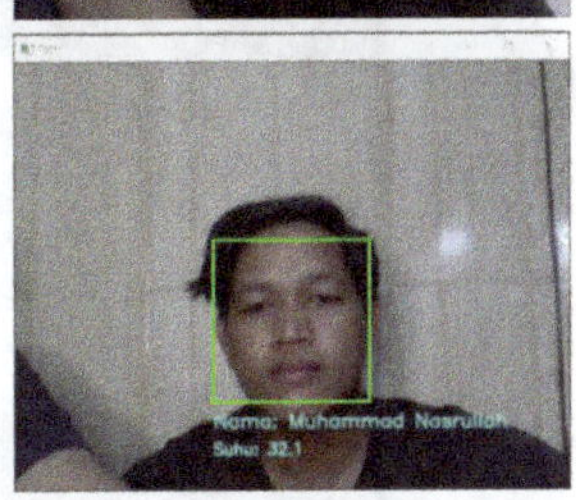	Success

Table 19.4 Result of testing in dim condition

No.	Sample	Result of face recognition	Remark
1	Sample 1	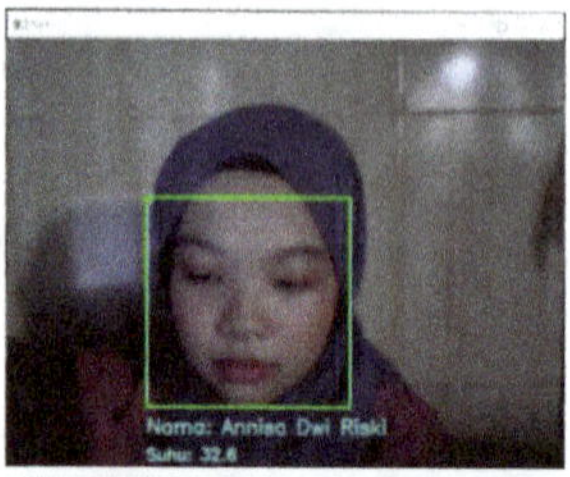	Success
2	Sample 2	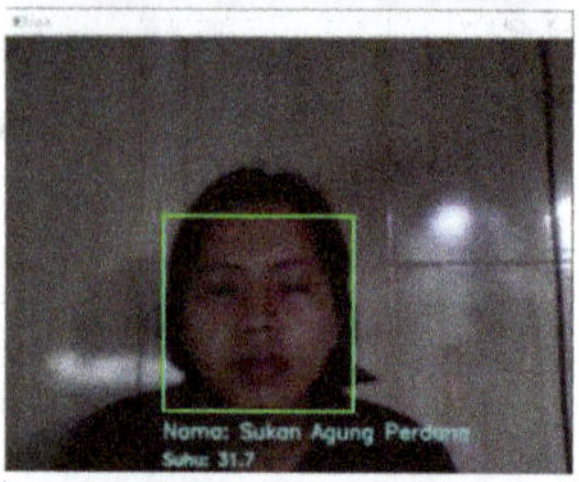	Success
3	Sample 3	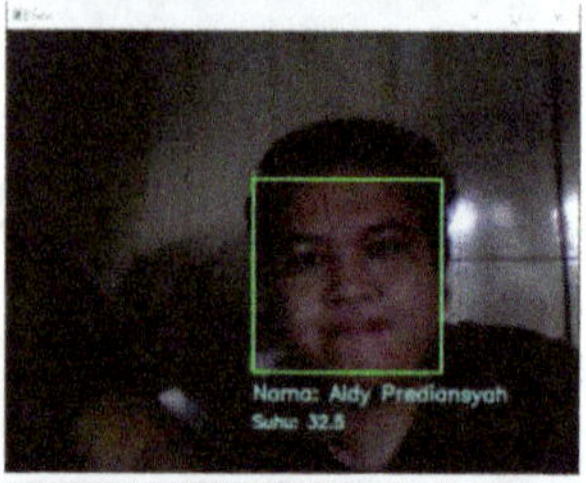	Success
4	Sample 4	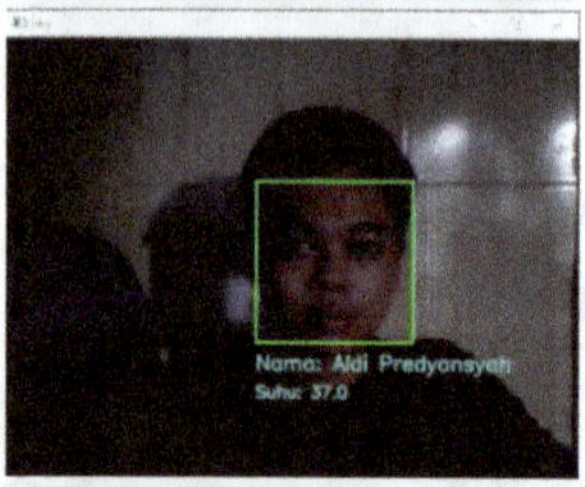	Fail
5	Sample 5	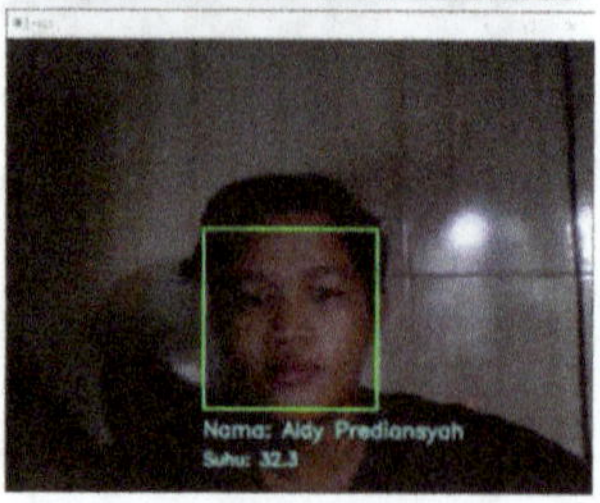	Fail

19.3.3 Security system evaluation

After determining the temperature and recognizing the face, the proposed system in this study is expected to be used for security system. The security system is important to prevent the one with the high body temperature to access the specific location to prevent the spread of COVID-19. This security system works using a solenoid lock. When unknown person accesses the security system, the solenoid lock is locked. Later, the identity of the person which has been recognized using the face recognition system and the body temperature which has been read sent to the database. Figures 19.12 and 19.13 show the example data in database website and website, respectively.

When the person who accesses the room has a temperature above 38°C, *solenoid lock* keeps locked even though the person has been recognized. It aims to prevent the spread of COVID-19 through an interaction between the suspect and the healthy ones. In addition, a warning is sent Telegram at the same time. Figure 19.14 shows the sample of warning sent to Telegram.

19.3.4 Sending the body temperature

This experiment was done to test the time sending the body temperature data to the *database website*. It was done 10 times; the results can be seen in Table 19.5. From the table, sending and receiving time have the difference. The average difference or the delay is 0.3 s from 10 experiments. Thus, it takes 0.3 s to detect the body temperature and face recognition to be shown in the website.

19.3.5 Sending the warning to Telegram

Sending to Telegram is needed to give warning, where the person whose body temperature is above 38°C indicated as a *suspect* of COVID-19.

For this experiment, the limit of body temperature becomes 35°C to test the sending process of data sample indicated as normal temperature. This experiment

id	nama	suhu	waktu
1	Annisa Dwi Rizki	27.5	2021-08-23 11:23:39
2	Sukan Agung Perdana	27.4	2021-08-23 11:31:42
3	Aldi Predyansyah	30.2	2021-08-20 21:45:20
4	Toto Iswanto	34.6	2021-08-19 12:38:14
5	Muhammad Nasrullah	28.1	2021-08-23 11:22:42
6	M. Wildan Muchlisin	30.7	2021-08-23 10:50:59
7	Dicky Pratama Putra	30.9	2021-08-23 11:20:55
8	Rofiqul Abror	27.7	2021-08-23 11:23:46
9	Bayu Dwi Margodigdyo	34.9	2021-08-19 12:38:22
10	Vony Rahma Melista	27.3	2021-08-23 11:30:59
11	Tidak Diketahui	29.6	2021-08-23 11:34:30

Figure 19.12 View in database website (note: nama = name; suhu = temperature; waktu = time)

Nama	ID	Suhu	Waktu
Annisa Dwi Rizki	1	28.6C	2021-08-23 10:51:25
Sukan Agung Perdana	2	28.7C	2021-08-23 10:51:27
Aldi Predyansyah	3	30.2C	2021-08-20 21:45:20
Toto Iswanto	4	34.6C	2021-08-19 12:38:14
Muhammad Nasrullah	5	28.9C	2021-08-23 10:51:21
M. Wildan Muchlisin	6	30.7C	2021-08-23 10:50:59
Dicky Pratama Putra	7	33.6C	2021-08-20 16:02:01
Rofiqul Abror	8	37.4C	2021-08-19 12:37:47
Bayu Dwi Margodigdyo	9	34.9C	2021-08-19 12:38:22
Vony Rahma Melista	10	29.4C	2021-08-23 10:51:06

Figure 19.13 View in website (nama = name; suhu = temperature; waktu = time)

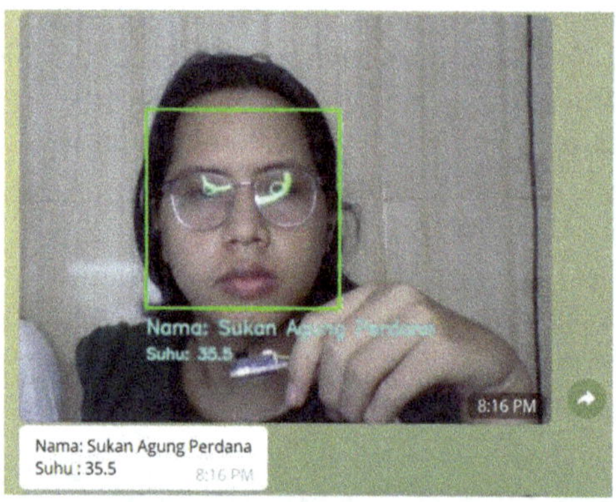

Figure 19.14 Warning in Telegram

Table 19.5 Results of sending temperature data

No.	Sending time	Time shown in website	Difference (s)
1	2021-08-20 16:02:26	2021-08-20 16:02:26	0
2	2021-08-20 16:02:42	2021-08-20 16:02:42	0
3	2021-08-20 16:03:12	2021-08-20 16:03:12	0
4	2021-08-20 16:03:31	2021-08-20 16:03:32	1
5	2021-08-20 16:03:54	2021-08-20 16:03:54	0
6	2021-08-20 16:04:15	2021-08-20 16:04:15	0
7	2021-08-20 16:04:39	2021-08-20 16:04:39	0
8	2021-08-20 16:04:58	2021-08-20 16:04:58	0
9	2021-08-20 16:05:18	2021-08-20 16:05:19	1
10	2021-08-20 16:05:41	2021-08-20 16:05:42	1
Average			0.3

was performed 10 times to determine the difference of sending time. The results can be seen in Table 19.6.

From Table 19.6, it can be seen that there is no time difference between detected time and the time received in Telegram. So, it can be concluded that the system works real-time because no delay time occurs during detection and received time in Telegram.

19.3.6 Unknown face

Another experiment was done to test the system in recognizing unknown person. It aims to ensure that the unknown person cannot access the security system. It compares the face in the database to the face that are not in a database. Besides, it also tests the capability of solenoid door lock to open or close the door. Table 19.7 shows the results of this experiment.

Table 19.6 Result of sending notification to Telegram

No.	Detected time	Time received in Telegram	Difference (s)
1	2021-08-24 20:16:21	2021-08-24 20:16:21	0
2	2021-08-24 20:16:37	2021-08-24 20:16:37	0
3	2021-08-24 20:16:50	2021-08-24 20:16:50	0
4	2021-08-24 20:17:05	2021-08-24 20:17:05	0
5	2021-08-24 20:17:17	2021-08-24 20:17:17	0
6	2021-08-24 20:17:25	2021-08-24 20:17:25	0
7	2021-08-24 20:17:36	2021-08-24 20:17:36	0
8	2021-08-24 20:17:44	2021-08-24 20:17:44	0
9	2021-08-24 20:17:59	2021-08-24 20:17:59	0
10	2021-08-24 20:18:15	2021-08-24 20:18:15	0
Average time			0

Table 19.7 Testing for unknown face

No.	Sample	Face is already in database	System testing	Solenoid lock
1	Sample 2	Yes	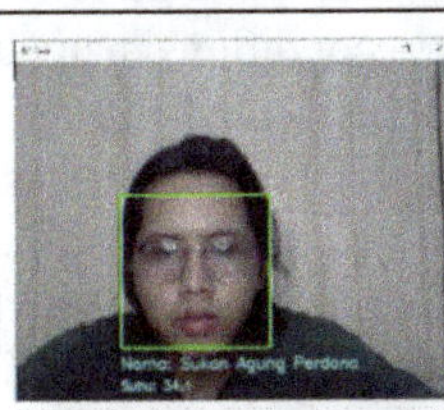	Open
2	Unknown 1	No	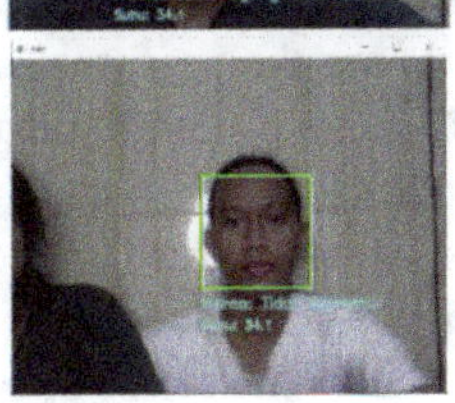	Locked

(Continues)

Table 19.7 (Continued)

No.	Sample	Face is already in database	System testing	Solenoid lock
3	Unknown 2	No	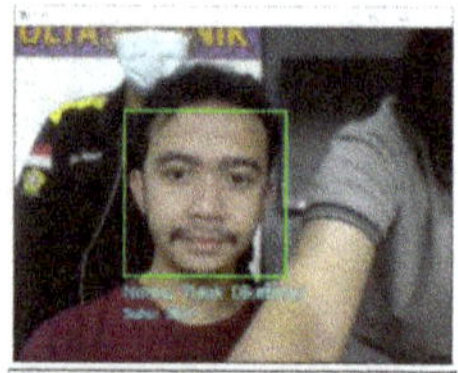	Locked
4	Unknown 3	No	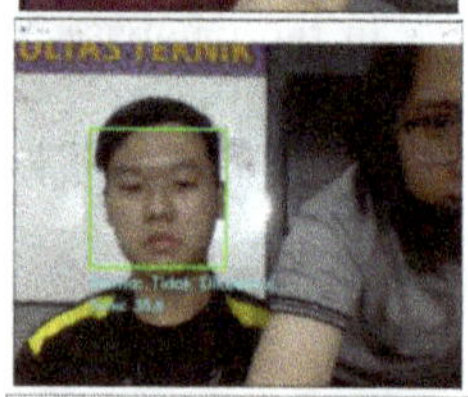	Locked
5	Unknown 4	No	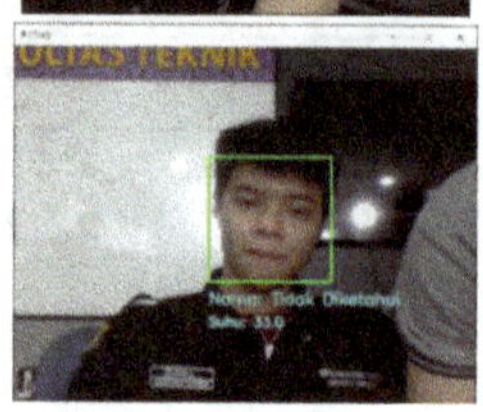	Locked

Table 19.7 shows that the solenoid door lock only opens when the face recognized is a face that is available in the database. On the other hand, the solenoid door lock will not open even though it has detected the face. Thus, it implies the solenoid door lock works well.

19.3.7 Real-time implementation

Real-time implementation is performed in front of laboratory using Logitech C922. It was done in two conditions, namely one object and two objects recognized. The experiments were performed 10 times for the face that has been in database 5 times and not saved in a database 5 times. Then, the experiment for two objects were performed 10 times. It contains of 4 experiments for both of the face available in a database, 2 experiment one is in the database and the other face not, and 4 experiments for both faces not available in a database. The experiment of two objects is done to see the performance of the system in recognizing and detecting the object at the same time. The results can be seen in Tables 19.8 and 19.9.

From Table 19.8, it can be seen that the solenoid door lock opens when the recognized person has been recorded in database and vice versa, it locks for the unknown person. Thus, the accuracy is 100%.

Table 19.9 shows the result of two objects. As shown in the table, the system detects the closest face to the camera. If the face is recognized and the body

Table 19.8 Results using one object

No.	Sample	Face is already in database	Evaluation of system	Temperature	Solenoid lock
1	Sample 2	Yes	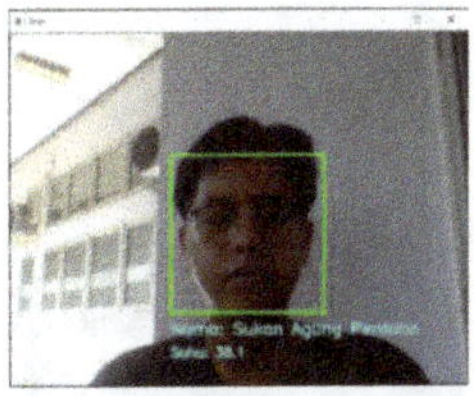	36.1°C	Open
2	Sample 3	Yes	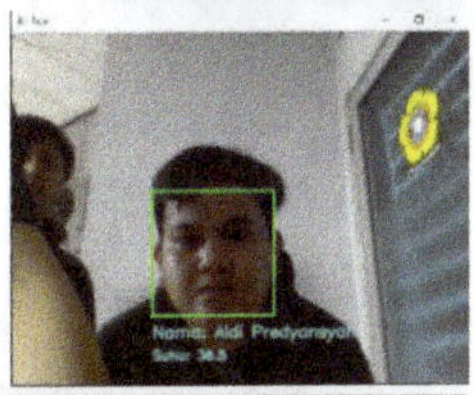	36.5°C	Open
3	Sample 4	Yes	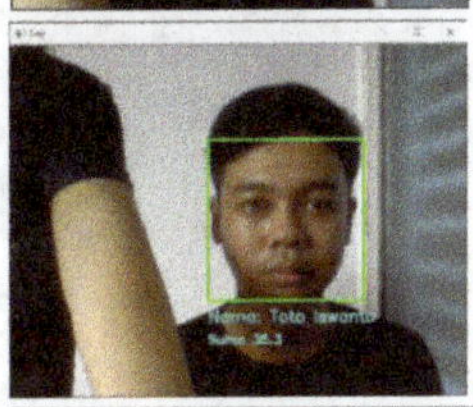	35.3°C	Open
4	Unknown 5	No	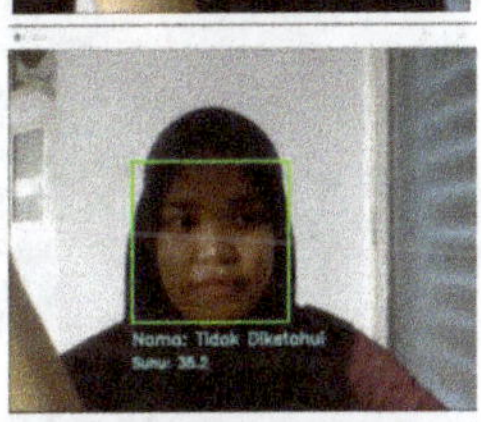	35.2°C	Locked
5	Unknown 6	No	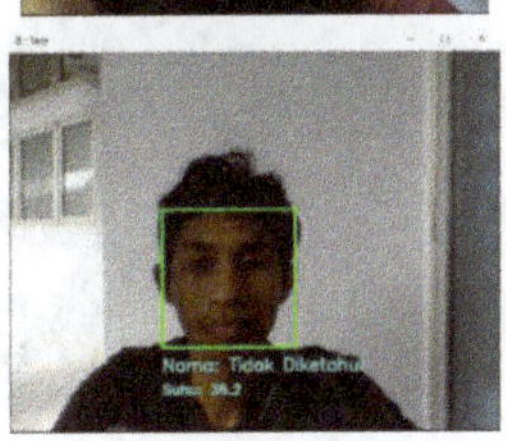	36.2°C	Locked

temperature is below 38°C, but if the face is unrecognized then the door keeps locking. These experiments show that the system is effective for security and prevent the error of the one who has body temperature above 38°C accessing the room.

Table 19.9 Results using two objects

No.	Sample	Face is already in database	Evaluation of system	Temperature	Solenoid lock
1	Sample 2 Sample 5	Yes Yes	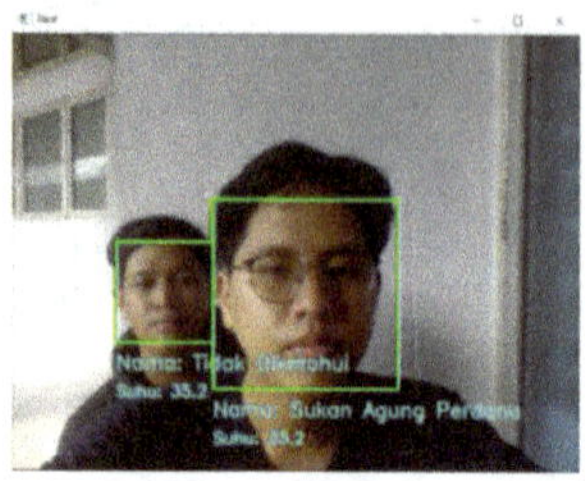	36.1°C 36.1°C	Open
2	Sample 3 Unknown 5	Yes No	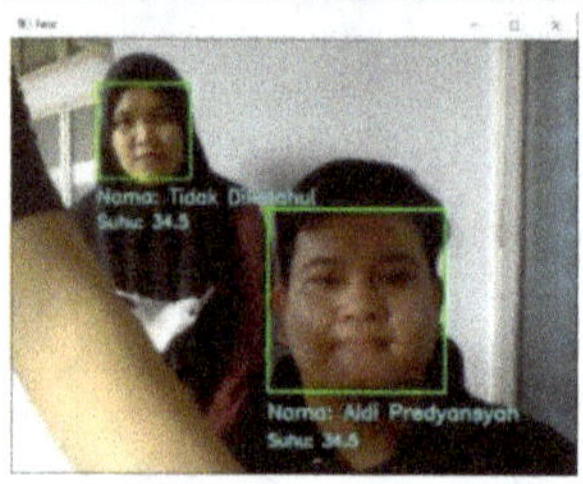	36.1°C 36.1°C	Open
3	Unknown 5 Sample 3	No Yes	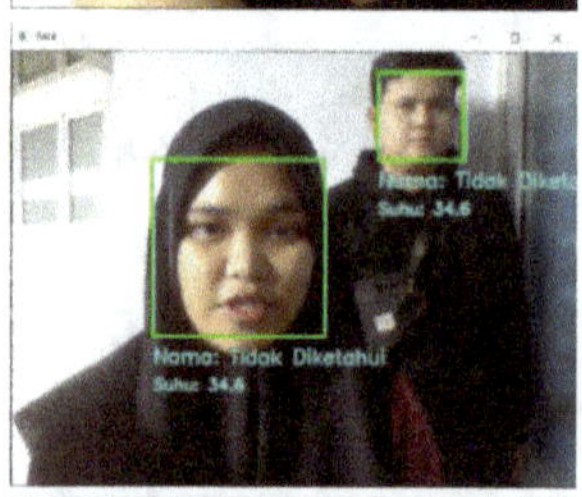	36.1°C 36.1°C	Closed
4	Unknown 6 Unknown 7	No No	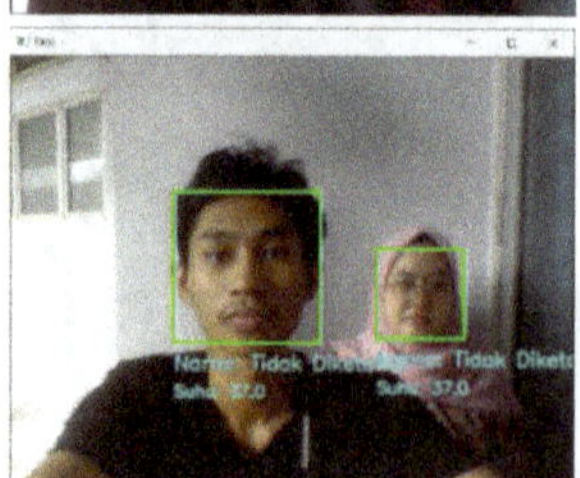	36.1°C 36.1°C	Closed

19.4 Conclusion

This study has shown that sensor MLX90640 can be used as a contactless device for measuring the body temperature. It is shown that the average temperature difference between the thermometer gun and sensor MLX90640 is 0.1°C and 0.09°C the distance of 10 cm and 12 cm, respectively. These distances can be considered as the effective distance to measure the body temperature. The proposed system in this study aims to recognize the face so it can prevent the spread of COVID-19 by ensuring the identity of the one who has high fever. The accuracy of face recognition system for dim and bright conditions are 80% and 100%, respectively. Thus, the light intensity influences the accuracy. Next, the face recognition and temperature measurement can be monitored through IoT with the difference of transmitting and receiving data to the database website is 0.3 s. Warning system which consists of data of body temperature and recognized face suspected as COVID-19 can be sent to Telegram. In addition, this study can also prevent the security system for the unknown person.

References

[1] Lanjar, "Corona Virus Disease," *RistekBrin*, 2020, pp. 1–62.

[2] S. Nookhao, V. Thananant, and T. Khunkhao, "Development of IoT heartbeat and body temperature monitoring system for community health volunteer," in: *2020 Joint International Conference on Digital Arts, Media and Technology with ECTI Northern Section Conference on Electrical, Electronics, Computer and Telecommunications Engineering*, ECTI DAMT NCON 2020, 2020, pp. 106–109.

[3] B. Varshini, H.R. Yogesh, S.D. Pasha, M. Suhail, V. Madhumitha, and A. Sasi. IoT-enabled smart doors for monitoring body temperature and face mask detection. *Global Transitions Proceedings*, 2(2), pp. 246–254, 2021.

[4] N.A. Zakaria, F.B. Mohd Saleh, and M.A.A. Razak, "IoT (Internet of Things) based infant body temperature monitoring," in: *2nd International Conference on BioSignal Analysis, Processing and Systems (ICBAPS)*, ICBAPS 2018, 2018, pp. 148–153.

[5] A.A. Rahimoon, M.N. Abdullah, and I. Taib. "Design of a contactless body temperature measurement system using Arduino," *Indonesian Journal of Electrical Engineering and Computer Science*, 19(3), pp. 1251–1258, 2020.

[6] W.Y. Leong, "Implementing blind source separation in signal processing and telecommunications," Thesis, The University of Queensland, Australia, 2005.

[7] W.Y. Leong and D.P. Mandic, "Towards adaptive blind extraction of post-nonlinearly mixed signals," in: *16th IEEE Signal Processing Society Workshop on Machine Learning for Signal Processing*, 2006, pp. 91–96.

[8] W.Y. Leong, J. Homer, and D.P. Mandic, "An implementation of nonlinear multiuser detection in Rayleigh fading channel," *EURASIP Journal on Wireless Communications and Networking*, pp. 1–9, 2006.

[9] W.Y. Leong, J.H. Chuah, and T.B. Tuan (eds.), *The Nine Pillars of Technologies for Industry 4.0*. Stevenage, UK: Institution of Engineering and Technology, 2020.

[10] W.Y. Leong and J. Ee, "A warehouse management system for 3 dimensional tracking and positioning," in: *Applied Mechanics and Materials* (Vols. 152–154, pp. 1685–1690). Trans Tech Publications, Ltd, 2012.

[11] W.Y. Leong, *Human Machine Collaboration and Interaction for Smart Manufacturing: Automation, robotics, sensing, artificial intelligence, 5G, IoTs and Blockchain*, Stevenage, UK: Institution of Engineering and Technology, 2022.

[12] W.Y. Leong, *Medical Equipment Engineering: Design, manufacture and Applications*, Stevenage, UK: The Institution of Engineering and Technology, 2023.

[13] W.Y. Leong and J. Homer, "Blind multiuser receiver in Rayleigh fading channel," *2005 Australian Communications Theory Workshop*, pp. 155–161, 2005.

[14] W. Xiaofan, P.H.J. Chong, and W.Y. Leong, "Performance comparison of CSMA/CD, CSMA/CA, CSMA/RI, CSMA/PRI and CSMA/PR with BEB," in: *5th IEEE Conference on Industrial Electronics and Applications*, Taichung, pp. 1843–1848, 2010.

[15] H.F. Min, W.Y. Leong, "Investigating target detection and localization in wireless sensor network," *Procedia Engineering*, 41, pp. 75–81, 2012.

[16] U. Mehrotra and W.Y. Leong, "NSEEAR: A energy adaptive routing protocol for heterogeneous wireless sensor networks," in: *35th Annual Conference of IEEE Industrial Electronics*, Porto, Portugal, pp. 2647–2652, 2009.

[17] W. Xiaofan, P.H.J. Chong, and W.Y. Leong, "Evaluation of performance on random back-off interval and multi-channel CSMA/CA protocols," in: *2009 IEEE Region 10 Conference (TENCON 2009)*, Singapore, pp. 1–5, 2009.

[18] W.Y. Leong and J. Homer, "EKENS: A learning on nonlinear blindly mixed signals," in: *2005 IEEE International Conference on Acoustics, Speech and Signal Processing (ICASSP 2005)*. Philadelphia, PA, USA, pp. iv–81, 2005.

[19] Y.Q. Wang, "An analysis of the Viola–Jones face detection algorithm," *Image Processing on Line*, 4, pp. 128–148, 2014.

[20] O.H. Jensen, *Implementing the Viola-Jones Face Detection Algorithm,* Technical University of Denmark, 2008.

[21] F. Deeba, H. Memon, F.A. Dharejo, A. Ahmed, and A. Ghaffar, "LBPH-based enhanced real-time face recognition," *International Journal of Advanced Computer Science and Applications*, 10(5), 0100535, 2019.

Chapter 20

Nanotechnology in biomedical application: pH-responsive starch nanoparticles

Ain Nadirah binti Romainor[1]

20.1 Introduction

Starch is a natural polysaccharide and commonly found in storage parts of the plant such as roots, rhizomes, tubers, and stems. Starch is well known for its biodegradability, bioavailability, and abundance in nature. Starch has been used in commercial applications other than being as a source of carbohydrates in human diet [1]. Starch is a carbohydrate polymer with hydrophilic properties due to an abundance of hydroxyl groups. Therefore, with a necessary modification ensure that the starch exhibits an optimum performance for the desired applications. The physicochemical properties in starch induced by desired modifications allow the optimization and functionalization of various industrial and biomedical applications. A brilliant scientist named Norio Taniguchi had introduced the term nanotechnology in 1974 and he defined that nanotechnology is the process of separation, consolidation, and deformation of materials by one atom or one molecule [2]. Nowadays, nanotechnology has arisen to become one of the most promising technologies for industrial and biomedical applications.

In recent years, the utilization of nanoparticles into potential biomedical applications has grown exponentially due to its good biocompatibility and drug release rates [3]. Other than that, recent studies showed that nanoparticles can be utilized in other applications such as energy storage system [4] and cosmetics [5]. Nanotechnology is one of the innovative strategies that able to comprehend the limitations of native starch such as poor solubility, retrogradation and viscosity. The nanometric size effect has the improved physical and chemical properties of starch. It is found that the nanoparticles had increased the shelf–life and thermal properties of resistant starch [6]. Starch nanoparticles became one of the popular topics in biomedical applications due to their availability in nature, economical, and can be modified through physical and chemical methods. These material had been used in various research such as in nanoencapsulation of catechins for *in vitro* digestion [7], pH-sensitive release carrier [8], and nano-vehicle for ß-carotene

[1]Perdana University, Malaysia

delivery [9]. It was proven that through these research starch nanoparticles are suggested to be one of the promising materials with prospects for novel utilization in industrial and biomedical applications. The starch nanoparticles can be prepared by applying chemical and physical treatments such as nanoprecipitation, acid hydrolysis, high-pressure homogenization, and ultrasonication.

Starch nanoparticles have recently received great attention in drug delivery system as a carrier due to its physicochemical properties. Previous research had integrated starch nanoparticles as a nanocarrier for β-carotene delivery [9], paracetamol [10], and piperine [11]. These materials are excellent for the applications owing to their non-toxic, biodegradability, biocompatibility, and high volume to surface ratio. These properties had certainly improved the drug encapsulation, release kinetic, and allow the drug particles to congregate inside the human organ. Indeed, the outcome of the research had found that it could increase the drug bioavailability and solubility, targeted delivery mechanism, and inconsistency issues of drugs. In other research, the usage of modified starch nanoparticles as a carrier have improved the dissolution of the poorly soluble anti-inflammatory drug, naproxen with good release kinetics [12]. Thus, starch nanoparticles demonstrated a significant effect as a nanocarrier that enhance the drug release of poorly soluble drugs.

The starch nanoparticles have influenced the encapsulation efficiency and release rate of drugs. The modifications of starch nanoparticles had decreasing the water solubilizing group, –OH and its nanoscale formation might enhance the encapsulation efficiency and drug release rate. Hence, starch-based nanoparticles could provide new strategies in the biomedical applications especially in encapsulation of drugs, antioxidants, and vitamins in utilizing target delivery system according to their sizes. Furthermore, the alteration of the parameter and conditions on starch nanoparticles could affect the mechanism and kinetic release of drug loaded starch nanoparticles. Although modified starch nanoparticles are generally regarded as promising effective nanocarriers in biomedical applications, more research is needed to improve the mechanism and kinetic release.

20.2 Starch nanoparticles

Nanoparticle is an ultrafine material that deals with nanometer-size objects, ranging from 1 to 1,000 nm. There are various nanoparticles adapted in nanotechnology application including metal and polymeric nanoparticles. Among them, polymeric nanoparticles made from natural polymers like alginate, chitosan, and starch have aroused great interest for use as potential particulate carriers in biomedical treatment due to their low toxicity and biodegradability [13]. In fact, those polymers can be degraded using microorganism under aerobic conditions by primarily decomposing the polymers into carbon dioxide and water [14].

Starch nanoparticle represents a great source of natural polymeric-based material since the starch material has similar desired characteristics of a versatile polymer as its properties can be tailored for desirable application, as well as having low cost and available abundantly in nature [15]. It is worth to note that at nanoscale, starch offers different properties from its bulk material because of the high surface area to volume ratio of the nanoparticles. Figure 20.1 shows the starch polymeric structure with abundant available of hydroxyl group. The nanoparticles of starch possess highly reactive surfaces covered by hydroxyl group, –OH which commonly contribute to the possible extensive chemical reactions for modification reactions as shown in Figure 20.1 [16]. Thus, it could either enhance or provide new characteristic to the nanoparticulate materials compared to macroparticles of native starch granules [13].

For instance, starch nanoparticles exhibit an emulsifier property which enables them to act as a stabilizer in oil and water emulsion. Due to this reason, starch nanoparticles have gained considerable attention for application in the food industry [17]. Despite that, owing to the fact that starch nanoparticles possess strong reinforcing effects to improve the mechanical properties as well as reducing water vapor barrier of the composite films, starch nanoparticles can be effectively used as bio-filler in composite materials. Therefore, it can increase the shelf-life duration of the product by protecting it from oxidation and humidity [18]. Furthermore, the reduced size of starch from macro to nanoscale leads to greater interaction between the larger surface area of starch drug carrier and solvent system. Thus, starch nanoparticles can increase the solubility of drugs in aqueous solution and make it a promising drug carrier candidate. Figure 20.2 represents the macro size of starch granules and starch nanoparticles respectively.

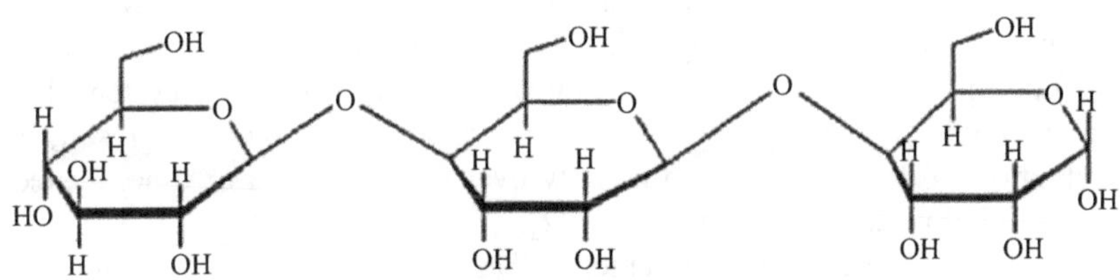

Figure 20.1 Starch polymeric structure

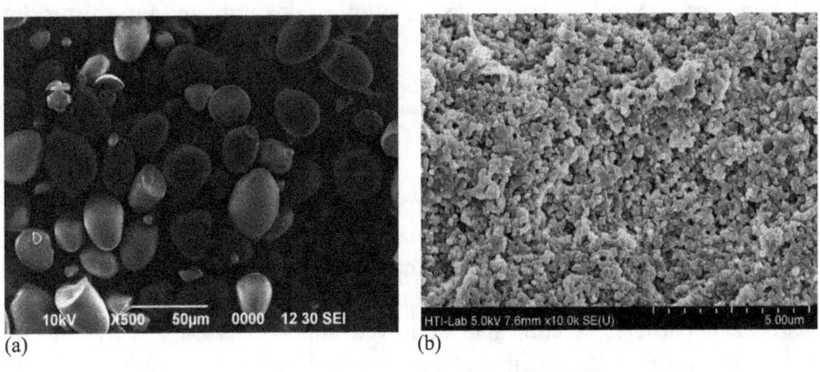

(a) (b)

Figure 20.2 (a) SEM image of starch granules and (b) FESEM image of starch nanoparticles

Nevertheless, it is important to control the size of starch nanoparticles since the applications of nanoparticles primarily depend on the size distribution of the particles [19]. For example, the administration of drugs in a drug delivery system required nanoparticles with sizes ranging between 10 and 240 nm to effectively spread the drugs through the circulatory system (enhance the distribution of the drug since the average size of blood capillaries are 5–10 μM) [20]. In contrast, nanoparticles with smaller size particles are practically providing a larger surface area for the and more intensive studies on controlling the sizes of starch nanoparticles have been conducted widely [15].

20.3 Starch nanoparticles in biomedical application

The use of starch nanoparticles in biomedical application has increased exponentially over the years due to unique properties such as chemical stability, non-toxicity, biocompatible, and can be naturally eliminated from the body [21]. Starch nanoparticles have gained considerable interest as drug carriers in drug release system to prevent major factors limiting the bioavailability of administrated drug including poor drug solubility and initial burst release effect of the drug in drug release system [22]. Most of the drugs showing poor water solubility indicate poor aqueous solubility and poor dissolution in gastrointestinal fluid. Ultimately, these reasons restricted the drug absorption and reduced patient compliance. Meanwhile, initial burst drug release is the rapid diffusion of the drug molecules from the drug carrier during initial contact with the biological fluid in the body system due to lesser retention of the drug carrier in the gastrointestinal tract. As a result, high concentration of drug releases in the body over a short period of time. Hence, it may raise the drug toxicity in the body [22].

Less effective drug–carrier interaction has been recognized as an important factor attributing to low drug bioavailability. Hence, a different mechanism has been modulated and fabricated to enhance drug–carrier interaction by modifying the drug solubility and nanocarrier structure. In a like manner, it was proven that starch nanoparticles had enhanced the solubility of doxorubicin (anti-cancer drug) drug in aqueous medium and delivered a sustainable drug release performance of doxorubicin-loaded starch nanoparticles within 5–7 days in phosphate buffer solution (PBS) compared to fast release of doxorubicin-loaded starch molecules (80% of doxorubicin release within 27 h) [23]. This is because starch nanoparticles carriers possess large specific surface area. Thus, incorporation of the starch nanoparticles substance in drug delivery formulation is undoubtedly able to increase the drug solubility as starch nanoparticles carrier can convert poorly soluble drug and lower drug absorption into efficient deliverable drugs [24].

Besides that, a recent study had demonstrated that dispersion of curcumin drug in starch nanoparticles solution had improved almost 83.70% of curcumin drug stability than in PBS [25]. Their finding was consistent with the other researcher, which found that curcumin drug has poor solubility in aqueous media due to its hydrophobicity but completely dispersible in starch nanoparticles media [10]. In the other report, the functionalization of maleate group onto starch nanoparticles to obtain starch–maleate nanoparticles had successfully increased the curcumin solubility in aqueous by 300 times as compared to starch nanoparticles alone [26]. The presence of carbonyl (C=O) group in starch maleate nanoparticles would interact readily with the OH group of curcumin molecules through hydrogen bonding in an aqueous medium to boost the drug solubility. Due to this reason, the result showed curcumin-loaded starch maleate nanoparticles displaying a constant dose of drug release pattern and eventually recognized as a suitable candidate for controlled drug delivery carrier system [26].

Although starch nanoparticles improved the drug solubility, their particles lack of physiological retention resulted in initial burst release of drugs [27,28]. The physiological retention of the drug carrier could be achieved through functionalization of stimuli-responsive material on the starch nanoparticles structure which could avoid unspecific interactions with the physiological environment and rapid degradation of the drug carrier [27]. Various stimuli-responsive starch nanoparticles drug carriers such as temperature-responsive, light-responsive, and pH-responsive have been employed to address this challenge [28]. In this particular reaction, the entrapped drugs could release the drugs at the appropriate site of action in a controllable manner in response to specific physiological triggers arising from the corresponding stimuli functionalized on the starch nanoparticles carrier. Thus, excessive drug release can be prevented before it reaches the targeted lesion [28].

20.4 pH-responsive starch nanoparticles

Among the responsive stimuli system, pH-responsive drug delivery carrier has drawn much attention in drug delivery system, considering that the pH range of fluids in human bodies varies greatly in various segments which may provide environmental stimuli for responsive drug release. It is well documented that pH in GIT medium between stomach is acidic (pH 1.2–3.5) while intestine is rather neutral to alkaline (pH 6.6–7.5) and colon is acidic to neutral (pH 4.0–7.0) [29]. Apart from that, specific pH gradient also differed in abnormal tissue and normal tissue. For example, tumor tissue cells possess mildly acidic environment (pH 5.5–6.8) whereas normal tissue cells have been found to be at pH 7.4 [30].

pH-responsive drug carriers use various triggers to release drug molecules at the specific targeted site including acidic cleavable linker and ionization of the functional group of the corresponding polymer [31]. Acidic cleavable linkers like hydrazone, acetal, and amine are designed to respond to the acidic physiological pH environment [27]. In contrast, ionization of the functional group for pH-responsive drug carrier involves polyelectrolyte polymers with a functional acidic group (polyanions) or functional basic group (polycations). In response to the pH changes, functional groups on polyelectrolyte polymers are able to go through ionization This ionization reaction causes an abrupt change in the swelling and solubility properties of the polymer to control the drug release in response to their pH-sensitivity [32]. Due to this reason, pH-sensitive polymers play an important role in the development of pH-responsive starch nanoparticles carriers for drug delivery application since starch nanoparticles alone do not employ an electrolyte property because they are considered as neutral polymeric materials [27].

Various pH-sensitive materials have been used to functionalize starch nanoparticles in order to develop an efficient drug delivery system. Previous research had successfully conjugated hydrazine onto starch-coated magnetite nanoparticles to deliver doxorubicin (anticancer drug) through chemical conjugation method [33]. They found that more than 78% of the doxorubicin was released into the buffer solution at pH 5.5 (simulation of tumor tissue environment) and slow drug releases (11%) into neutral buffer solution at pH 7.4 (simulation of normal tissue environment). The plausible mechanism of this drug delivery system is due to the labile hydrazone linkage (hydrazine forms a hydrozone linkage with the drug carrier) observed under acidic condition. Therefore, an adequate amount of drug has been delivered to the targeted lesion to reduce initial burst drug release and systemic toxicity effect [27].

The starch nanoparticles drug carrier was found to be conjugated with polyamidoamin (PAMAM) cationic dendrimer during the release of doxorubicin onto tumor tissue [34]. The *in vitro* drug release profiles showed that hydrolysis of amide linkage (formed between drug carrier and doxorubicin) was observed to release 97% of the drug at pH 5.5 solutions and turned to slow release of 33% at pH 7.4 solutions. Although hydrazine and PAMAM are efficient as pH-sensitive material for drug delivery, however, it should be avoided since hydrazine is carcinogenic and PAMAM is toxic to cell and can cause cell lysis [35].

One of the alternatives to improve this drawback is the use of polyelectrolyte pH-sensitive polymer incorporated onto the starch nanoparticles. In this regard, polyelectrolyte polymer is modified onto starch nanoparticles either through grafting or crosslinking to impart pH-responding on the starch nanoparticles drug carrier [36]. The reason why the polyelectrolyte polymers are sensitive to even slightly changes on gradient pH is greatly associated with the ionization of the polymer's functional group such as COOH and NH_2 [37]. A previous study showed that insulin release from pH-responsive starch nanoparticles grafted poly(L-glutamic acid) (PGA) was much slower (10% of the drug releases) at pH 1.2 solution (simulation of stomach physiological condition) as compared to gradual drug release (70% of the drug releases) at pH 6.8 solution (simulation of intestinal physiological condition) [38]. The result obtained was attributed to the protonation of COOH on PGA chains, which tend to form a compact α-helical structure and made the chain become hydrophobic and aggregated. Consequently, it prevents insulin from degrading in gastric juice. While in an artificial intestinal fluid physiological condition (at pH 6.8), COOH on PGA structure were ionized (deprotonated) and exhibited a hydrophilic and random coil structure in nature. Hence, the insulin was diffused out gradually from the drug carrier and this increased the drug absorption in the intestine.

The effect of swelling behavior of poly(acrylic) acid grafted onto starch composite nanoparticles was investigated and the result obtained was in concomitant with the previous report [39]. This indicated that the protonation of

COOH from poly(acrylic) acid occurred at acidic pH and led to a decrease in swelling ratio of the polymers to slow the drug release rate. In contrast, at neutral to alkaline condition, COOH deprotonated and created the electrostatic repulsion between the carboxylate ion (COO^-) to increase the swelling capacity and induce drug release. Therefore, it was noted that the changes in the physical property of the grafted polymer onto starch composite nanoparticles in response to changes in corresponding pH solution could be used for controlled drug delivery system applications [40].

Most of the pH-sensitive polyelectrolyte polymers used to display tunable pH-responsive property on the starch nanoparticles drug delivery system are derived from synthetic polymers which in turn lead to non-biodegradability concerns [41]. Chitosan is a natural polycationic polymer found in the exoskeleton of crustaceans (shrimp and crabs). Like other pH-sensitive polymers, chitosan has a primary NH_2 group on its structure which main function is to react to changes in pH [42]. In the recent research, the incorporation of chitosan onto starch nanoparticles had enhanced the release of quercetin under the gastrointestinal conditions [43]. The simulated medium consisted of gastric fluid condition (pH 1.6) and intestinal fluid (pH 6.5). The obtained results showed that the quercetin release was nearly 80% after 3 h in the simulated the gastric fluid condition while with intestinal conditions, total quercetin released was about 85% of after four hours.

This finding was probably due to the lack of charge interaction between anionic chitosan with starch nanoparticles and proton in acidic medium at low pH which led to no ionization reaction. In addition, the modified chitosan starch nanoparticles drug carrier is poorly hydrophilic in nature and can withstand acidic environments. Therefore, the matrix showed high resistance in the stomach and decreased the drug release process. On the other hand, this drug carrier is highly hydrophilic in basic medium because of the matrix hydration and dissolves to release drug at higher pH value [44]. In particular, limited studies reported about the utilization of pH-sensitive material from natural resources incorporated onto starch nanoparticles vehicles. There is still room for other natural polyelectrolyte polymers such as alginate, carrageenan, and polycarboxylic acid polymers (such as citric acid and succinic acid) to be considered as pH-responsive agents for the starch nanoparticles drug delivery system [45].

20.5 pH-responsive starch-citrate nanoparticles as controlled drug release

In line with the previous studies, there was another study reported that the preparation of starch-citrate nanoparticles as pH-responsive drug carriers have a potential to release drug in a controllable manner to pH-specific organs [46]. Citric acid was attached to starch molecules to confer pH-responsiveness because it is nontoxic, safe for consumption, and highly water-soluble. The resulting starch-citrate is water soluble and hence, there is no need to use harsh solvents for the dissolution of starch. The potential utility of starch-citrate nanoparticles as drug carriers was evaluated by loading paracetamol as the model drug. The release kinetic profiles were determined in a simulated human gastrointestinal tract (GIT) with the pH of the release media being 1.2 (stomach), 7.4 (venous blood), and 8.6 (intestinal fluid). Cytotoxicity effect of the starch-citrate nanoparticles was investigated using HaCaT cell lines (human skin cells) as *in vitro* model.

20.5.1 Fabrication of pH-starch-citrate nanoparticles

Citric acid was attached to starch molecule backbones by esterification. Hydroxyl (OH) groups of starch molecules were made to react with the carboxylic (COOH) group of citric acid to form the ester bonds of starch-citrate molecules [47]. After esterification, an absorption peak belonging to carbonyl (C=O) ester bonds was observed in the FTIR spectrum of starch-citrate molecules at 1,724 cm^{-1} and the C–O–C stretching of the ester group was present at 1,156 cm^{-1} as shown in Figure 20.3 [48,49]. These peaks were absent in the FTIR spectrum of native starch molecules as in Figure 20.3(a). In addition, the absorption peak of C–O–C glycosidic bonds of anhydroglucose unit (AGU) of starch molecules at 850–854 cm^{-1} was observed to remain intact, suggesting that the aforementioned molecules were not degraded after esterification [48]. It was revealed that peaks in the region 1,648–1,635 cm^{-1} were made up of OH group – 1,648 cm^{-1} (O–H from moisture

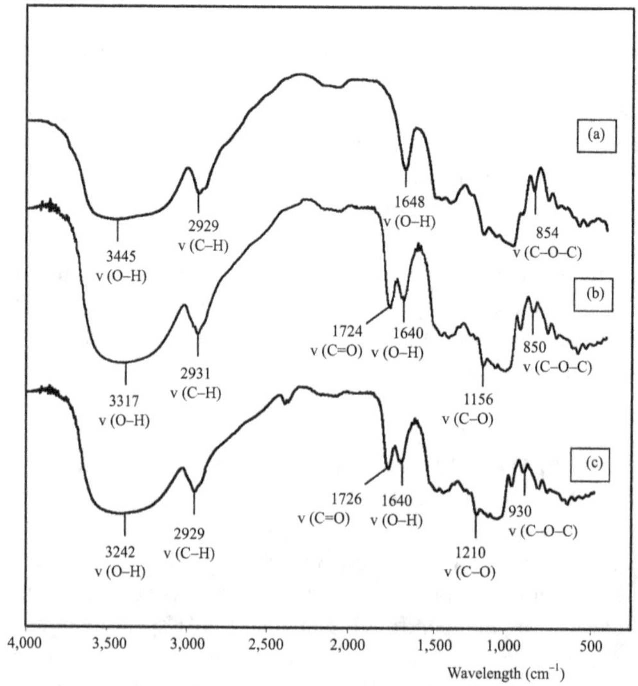

Figure 20.3 FTIR spectra of (a) native starch, (b) starch-citrate molecule, and (c) starch-citrate nanoparticles

absorbency in starch [49] and 1,640 and 1,635 cm^{-1} (O–H from COOH of citric acid substituted onto starch molecules). The characteristic peaks at 2,931–2,929 cm^{-1} indicated the presence of C–H stretching and 3,445–3,242 cm^{-1} was assigned to the OH groups of starch and starch-citrate molecules [50]. As shown in Figure 20.3(b) and (c), FTIR spectra for both starch-citrate molecules and starch-citrate nanoparticles were identical, indicating that the chemical composition of starch-citrate was intact after nanoprecipitation.

Starch–citrate nanoparticles, which were obtained after nanoprecipitation, were spherical with a mean particle diameter of 105 nm as shown in the TEM micrographs in Figure 20.4.

20.5.2 Drug-loading capacity of starch-citrate nanoparticles

Figure 20.5 shows that the loading capacity of paracetamol onto starch nanoparticles increased almost linearly from 1.00 to 5.00 mg mg^{-1} as the concentration

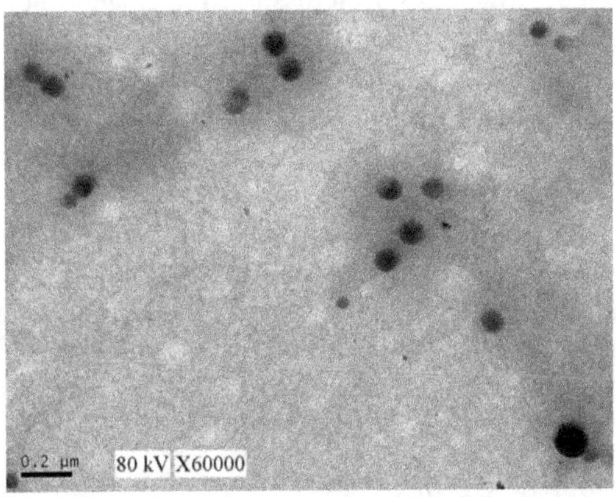

Figure 20.4 TEM images of starch-citrate nanoparticles

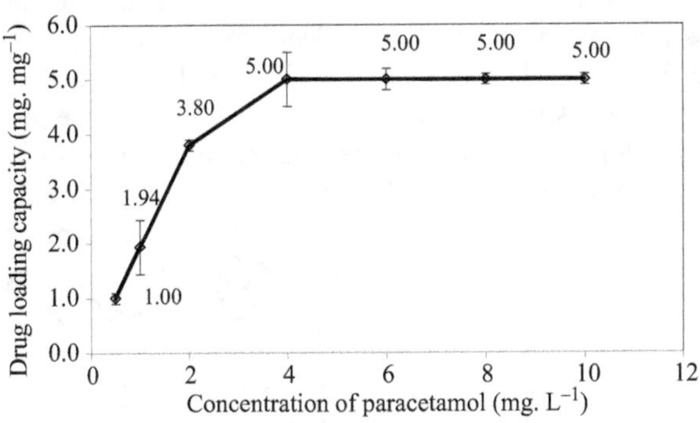

Figure 20.5 Paracetamol-loading capacity of starch-citrate nanoparticles

of paracetamol was increased from 0.5 to 4 mg L^{-1}. When the concentration of paracetamol was 4 mg L^{-1}, a maximum loading capacity of 5.00 mg mg^{-1} was attained, and the latter remained constant even though the former was further increased to 10 mg L^{-1}. The drug-loading capacity plateau can be attributed to the saturation of the adsorption sites of starch-citrate [51].

Previous studies on the possibility of drug loading onto nanoparticles suggested that these particles had relatively lower drug-holding capacities due to conventional absorption loading technique [52]. The previous research found that the paracetamol-loading capacity nanoparticles mesoporous carbon was about 1.5×10^{-1} mg mg^{-1} [53]. Meanwhile, other research showed that showed that the paracetamol-loading capacity of monthmorillonite/N(carboxyacyl) chitosan-coated magnetite nanoparticles was 9.6×10^{-4} mg mg^{-1} [54]. It is noteworthy that starch-citrate nanoparticles displayed a much higher loading capacity of 5.00 mg mg^{-1} for paracetamol encapsulation.

The *in situ* nanoprecipitation drug-loading technique demonstrated a higher drug-loading capacity compared to conventional methods [10]. In the former technique, paracetamol, which has been dissolved in ethanol (non-solvent system), was entrapped in the starch-citrate matrix during the formation of starch-citrate nanoparticles. This process occurred through precipitation and fast diffusion between the solvent and non-solvent systems [55]. Hence, the drug could be easily incorporated into nanoparticle carriers, hence enhancing their drug-loading capacity. Besides, intermolecular interactions between drug molecules and carriers also influenced the drug-loading capacity of the latter [56]. The electrostatic interactions between COO^- groups of starch-citrate nanoparticles and $-OH_2^+$ (leaving group of paracetamol due to protonation of OH of paracetamol occur when in contact with starch-citrate solution) during nanoprecipitation explained the high paracetamol-loading capacity of starch-citrate nanoparticles [54].

20.5.3 Drug release studies

Figure 20.6(a) shows the swelling behavior of the starch-citrate nanoparticles at pH 1.2, 7.4, and 8.6 while Figure 20.6(b) shows the release profiles of paracetamol from starch-citrate nanoparticles at the aforementioned pH values. Paracetamol release profiles were observed to be dependent on the swelling behavior of starch-citrate nanoparticles, which was in turn controlled by the pH of the releasing medium. The pH-responsiveness was due to the difference in the protonation states of starch-citrate nanoparticles. For comparison, the release behavior of tablet forms of paracetamol was investigated at different physiological pH (1.2, 7.4, and 8.6), as shown in Figure 20.6(b). At pH 1.2, paracetamol in tablet form released almost 100% of the drug within the first 4 h (Figure 20.6(b) (ii)). In contrast, at pH 7.4 and 8.6, the tablets disintegrated and abruptly released 100% of the drug within 1 h (Figure 20.6(b) (iv) and (vi)). This implies that paracetamol tablets underwent a brisk drug release (which led to an initial burst release effect of the drug) instead of the controllable release pattern seen when the drug was loaded onto starch-citrate nanoparticles (Figure 20.6(b) (i), (iii) and (v)).

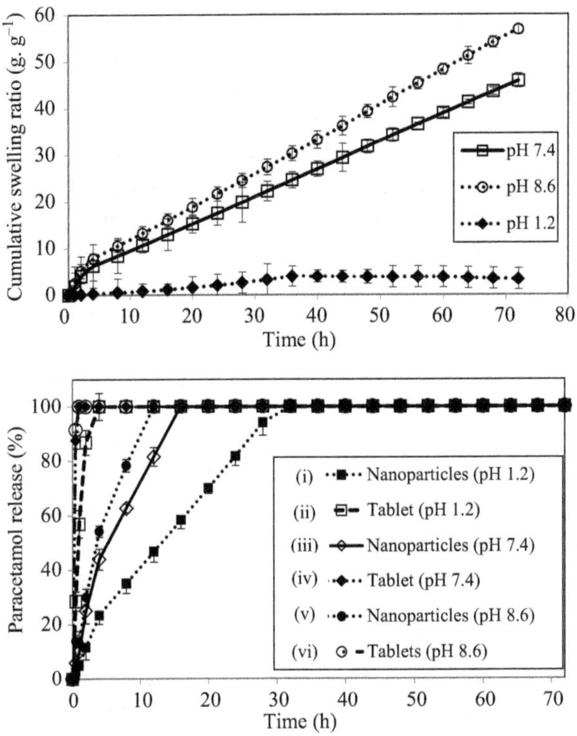

Figure 20.6 *(a) Swelling ratios of starch-citrate nanoparticles in different pH media as a function of time. (b) Percentage of paracetamol released from starch-citrate nanoparticles and tablets in media of various pHs.*

At pH 1.2, paracetamol was completely released from starch-citrate nanoparticles in a slow and sustained manner within 32 h; the initial burst release was not observed. The slower rate of drug release here could be due to the smaller swelling ratio (3.2 g g^{-1}) of starch-citrate nanoparticles in acidic medium (Figure 20.6(a)), which in turn was attributable to the stronger interaction of hydrogen bonds among COOH functional groups of the said nanoparticles [57]. Paracetamol release rates were observed to be more rapid at pH 7.4 (0.38 mg h^{-1}) and 8.6 (0.50 mg h^{-1}) as compared to pH 1.2 (0.18 mg h^{-1}) (Figure 20.6(b) (i), (iii) and (v)). The drug release rates were faster at pH 7.4 and 8.6, whereby 100% of paracetamol were released from starch-citrate nanoparticles within 16 h and 12 h, respectively. However, at pH 1.2, only 58.4% of paracetamol was released. The faster drug release rate was due to the deprotonation of COOH groups of the starch-citrate nanoparticles to form COO^-, leading to electrostatic repulsion and in turn, higher swelling ratios of 45.9 g g^{-1} and 56.8 g g^{-1} at pH 7.4 and 8.6, respectively (Figure 20.6(a)).

20.5.4 Drug-release mechanism

The drug-release data was fitted into various kinetic models as shown in Table 20.1. The correlation coefficients (R^2) of paracetamol released from starch-citrate nanoparticles in all three simulated GIT pH media were nearly equal to 1, which indicated that the release profiles strongly correlated with the zero-order kinetic model. As shown in Table 20.1, the aforementioned release profiles were dominated by simultaneous swelling and erosion of the polymer to enable diffusion of the drug out from the starch-citrate nanoparticles in light of the higher regression line (R^2) (0.9043–0.9987) fitted in both Hixson–Crowell and Higuchi models [58]. The Korsmeyer–Peppas model was applied to further confirm the paracetamol release mechanism from starch-citrate nanoparticles [59]. The R^2 values of the Korsmeyer–Peppas equation were 0.9889, 0.9687, and 0.9717 for pH 1.2, 7.4, and 8.6, respectively. This showed that the drug release was driven by the diffusion of paracetamol molecules out of the starch-citrate nanoparticles matrix. The release mechanism was determined from the slope value (n) of Korsmeyer–Peppas equation. The n values of the releasing media (pH 1.2, 7.4, and 8.6) fell within the range of 0.5–1.0, indicating that the release of paracetamol from starch-citrate nanoparticles was governed by non-Fickian release behavior as well as induced by diffusion through the swelling of the said nanoparticles.

20.5.5 In vitro *cytotoxicity assay*

The starch-citrate nanoparticles were screened for cytotoxic effect *via* MTS [3-(4,5-dimethylthiazol-2-yl)-5-(3-carboxymethoxyphenyl)-2-(4-sulfophenyl)-2*H*-tetrazolium]-

Table 20.1 Kinetics modeling of drug release studies of paracetamol-loaded starch-citrate nanoparticles

pH	Kinetic models	R^2	Features
1.2	Zero-order	0.9905	Drug release rate is concentration independent
7.4		0.9701	
8.6		0.9587	
1.2	First-order	0.8222	Drug release rate is concentration dependent
7.4		0.8359	
8.6		0.8920	
1.2	Hixson–Crowell	0.9043	Drug release mechanism: surface erosion and swelling
7.4		0.9256	
8.6		0.9263	
1.2	Higuchi	0.9887	Drug release mechanism: diffusion
7.4		0.9962	
8.6		0.9957	
1.2	Korsmeyer–Peppas	0.9889, $n = 0.8434$	Drug release mechanism: diffusion and swelling
7.4		0.9687, $n = 0.8800$	
8.6		0.9717, $n = 0.8533$	

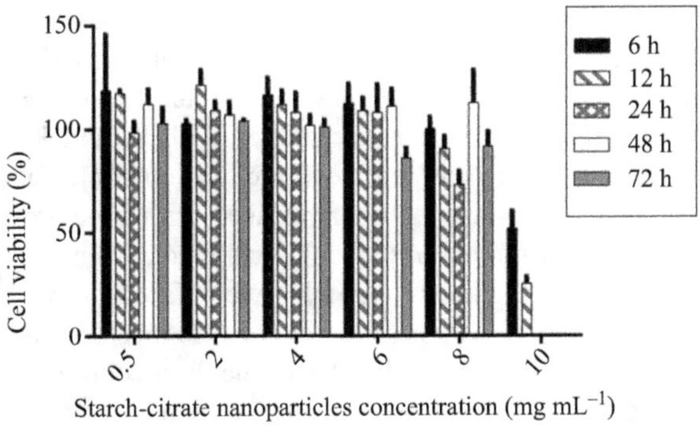

Figure 20.7 Cell viability of HaCaT cells cultured with various starch-citrate nanoparticles concentration from 6 to72 h

based colorimetric assay using HaCaT cells at various concentrations and time points. Pursuant to ISO 10993-5 (practical guidelines for cytotoxicity), percentage of cells viability above 80% are considered as non-cytotoxicity. As seen in Figure 20.7, nanoparticles at low concentrations from 0.5 to 6 mg mL^{-1} showed no cytotoxicity on HaCaT cells until 48 h of incubation time due to the percentage of cells viability were above 100% [60]. There was slight cytotoxic effect with the percentage of cells viability range was within 70–100% at 6 and 8 mg mL^{-1} of nanoparticles at 72 h and various incubation times, respectively. However, the percentage of cells viable was below than 50% at the highest concentration of 10 mg mL^{-1} as shown in Figure 20.7. According to ISO 10993-5 cytotoxicity guidelines, the nanoparticles were cytotoxic towards HaCaT cells [61].

The possible factor that causes cell death at 10 mg mL^{-1} was most likely due to the nature of the nanoparticles whereby the pH value for the nanoparticles was low at around pH 4.0–5.0. In cell culture, pH regulation is crucial as most cells grow well or cellular metabolic activities occur at optimal pH in between 7.0 and 8.0 as cells are usually grown in medium at pH 7.4 that employs a buffering system with probable increasing and reduction at both ends of the optimal pH range [62]. The cells were therefore not able to sustain growth at low pH of the nanoparticles as the cellular activities were disrupted caused by the drastic changed of pH level. The lower concentrations of nanoparticles have pH level at around 7.0–8.0 which was the optimal condition for cell growing hence no cytotoxic effect was observed. The nanoparticles did not exhibit cytotoxic effect towards HaCaT cells at various low concentrations, thus indicate the potential of starch-citrate nanoparticles in biomedical application [62].

20.6 Conclusion

This chapter was devoted to prove the capability of starch nanoparticles as a potential nanocarrier in biomedical applications especially for the drug delivery system. Numerous authors had been introduced starch nanoparticles through physically or chemically modifications and their experiments were designed to investigate the morphological study, pH responsiveness studies, *in vitro* drug release, and kinetic release study of starch nanoparticles with a modeled drug. Further analysis was carried out on the drug releases starch nanoparticles which provided a general statement that percentage of drug released with time from starch nanoparticles was influenced by the pH of physiological media. The obtained data from the release of drug from starch nanoparticles were fitted with different kinetic release equations to determine whether the drug release mechanism was a swelling, diffusion, or surface-erosion controlled system. The drug could release from starch nanoparticles through swelling, surface erosion, or diffusion of the nanoparticles. Thus, the starch nanoparticles were practically a viable solution as a nanocarrier in biomedical applications, with the *in vitro* release data showing the combination of impressive drug release behavior and sensitivity to the pH of the surrounding medium.

This work provides results that suggest the potential of starch nanoparticles as controlled release nanocarriers for drug delivery systems in biomedical applications. The data from the previous experiments can be used as a foundation for future research. More detailed work needs to be carried out to find accurate information on physical and chemical behavior can be obtained to improve the material performance. Future recommended research can involve the *in vivo* drug release from starch nanoparticles and clinical trials. This is crucial because such data could be used as a future guideline to produced starch nanocarrier with better clinical response, tolerability, and lower side effects towards human. Other future extension can be the study of synthesis conditions of starch nanoparticles, the biocompatibility of the material with a different type of drug and other relevant parameters.

References

[1] Dankar, I., Haddarah, A., Omar, F. E., Pujolà, M., and Sepulcre, F., "Characterization of food additive-potato starch complexes by FTIR and X-ray diffraction," *Food Chemistry*, vol. 260, pp. 7–12, 2018.

[2] Bayda, S., Adeel, M., Tuccinardi, T., Cordani, M., and Rizzolio, F. "The history of nanoscience and nanotechnology: from chemical–physical applications to nanomedicine," *Molecules*, vol. 25, no. 1, p. 112, 2019.

[3] Sztandera, K., Gorzkiewicz, M., and Klajnert-Maculewicz, B., "Gold nanoparticles in cancer treatment," *Molecular Pharmaceutics*, vol. 16, pp. 1–23, 2019.

[4] Sheikholeslami, M., and Mahian, O., "Enhancement of PCM solidification using inorganic nanoparticles and an external magnetic field with application in energy storage systems," *Journal of Cleaner Production*, vol. 215, pp. 963–977, 2019.

[5] Jose, J., and Netto, G., "Role of solid lipid nanoparticles as photoprotective agents in cosmetics," *Journal of Cosmetic Dermatology*, vol. 18, no. 1, pp. 315–321, 2018.

[6] Shabana, S., Prasansha, R., Kalinina, I., Potoroko, I., Bagale, U., and Shirish, S. H., "Ultrasound assisted acid hydrolyzed structure modification and loading of antioxidants on potato starch nanoparticles," *Ultrasonics Sonochemistry*, vol. 51, pp. 444–500, 2019.

[7] Ahmad, M., Mudgil, P., Gani, A., Hamed, F., Masoodi, F. A., and Maqsood, S., "Nano-encapsulation of catechin in starch nanoparticles: characterization, release behavior and bioactivity retention during simulated in-vitro digestion," *Food Chemistry*, vol. 270, pp. 95–104, 2019.

[8] Sufi-Maragheh, P., Nikfarjam, N., Deng, Y., and Taheri-Qazvini, N., "Pickering emulsion stabilized by amphiphilic pH-sensitive starch nanoparticles as therapeutic containers," *Colloids and Surfaces B:Biointerface*, vol. 181, pp. 244–251, 2019.

[9] Santoyo-Aleman, D., Sanchez, L. T., and Villa, C. C., "Citric-acid modified banana starch nanoparticles as a novel vehicle for β-carotene delivery," *Science of Food and Agriculture*, vol. 99, no. 14, pp. 6392–6399, 2019.

[10] Troncoso, O. P., and Torres, F. G., 'Non-conventional starch nanoparticles for drug delivery applications'. *Medical Devices & Sensors*. 2020; 3(6), 1–16.

[11] Chong, W. H., Chin, S. F., Pang, S. C., and Kok, K. Y., "Synthesis and characterisation of piperine-loaded starch nanoparticles," *Journal of Physical Science*, vol. 31, no. 1, pp. 57–68, 2020.

[12] Odeniyi, M. A., Adepoju, A. O., and Jaiyeoba, K. T., "Native and modified digitaria exilis starch nanoparticles as a carrier system for the controlled release of naproxen," *Starch-Stärke*, vol. 71, nos. 9–10, p. 1900067, 2019.

[13] Ogunjimi, A. T., Melo, S. M., Vargas-Rechia, C. G., Emery, F. S., and Lopez, R. F., "Hydrophilic polymeric nanoparticles prepared from Delonix galactomannan with low cytotoxicity for ocular drug delivery," *Carbohydrate Polymers*, vol. 157, pp. 1065–1075, 2017.

[14] Harding, K. G., Gounden, T., and Pretorius, S., "Biodegradable plastics: a myth of marketing?," *Procedia Manufacturing*, vol. 7, pp. 106–110, 2017.

[15] Ge, S., Xiong, L., Li, M., Liu, J., *et al.*, "Characterizations of pickering emulsions stabilized by starch nanoparticles: influence of starch variety and particle size," *Food Chemistry*, vol. 234, pp. 339–347, 2017.

[16] Masina, N., Choonara, Y. E., Kumar, P., *et al.*, "A review of the chemical modification techniques of starch," *Carbohydrate Polymers*, vol. 157, pp. 1226–1236, 2017.

[17] Chang, Y., Yan, X., Wang, Q., Ren, L., Tong, J., and Zhou, J., "High efficiency and low cost preparation of size controlled starch nanoparticles through ultrasonic treatment and precipitation," *Food Chemistry*, vol. 227, pp. 369–375, 2017.

[18] Kong, J., Yu, Y., Pei, X., Han, C., Tan, Y., and Dong, L., "Polycaprolactone nanocomposite reinforced by bioresource starch-based nanoparticles,"

International Journal of Biological Macromolecules, vol. 102, pp. 1304–1311, 2017.

[19] Crucho, C. I., and Barros, M. T., "Polymeric nanoparticles: a study on the preparation variables and characterization methods," *Materials Science and Engineering: C*, vol. 80, pp. 771–784, 2017.

[20] Lowe, J.S and Anderson, P.G. (eds.). *Stevens & Lowe's Human Histology*. China: Mosby, 2015, p. 143.

[21] McNamara, K., and Tofail, S. A., "Nanoparticles in biomedical applications," *Advances in Physics: X*, vol. 2, no. 1, pp. 54–88, 2017.

[22] Di Martino, A., Kucharczyk, P., Capakova, Z., Humpolicek, P., and Sedlarik, V., "Chitosan-based nanocomplexes for simultaneous loading, burst reduction and controlled release of doxorubicin and 5-fluorouracil," *International Journal of Biological Macromolecules*, vol. 102, pp. 613–624, 2017.

[23] Raveendran, S. S., Subramani, N., Rahman, S. A., and Palsamy, S., "Formulation and characterization of starch nanoparticles for con-trolled release of doxorubicin," *Nano Science and Technology an Indian Journal*, vol. 10, no. 1, pp. 30–35, 2016.

[24] El-Sheikh, M. A., "New technique in starch nanoparticles synthesis," *Carbohydrate Polymers*, vol. 176, pp. 214–219, 2017.

[25] Sadeghi, R., Daniella, Z., Uzun, S., and Kokini, J., "Effects of starch composition and type of non-solvent on the formation of starch nanoparticles and improvement of curcumin stability in aqueous media," *Journal of Cereal Science*, vol. 76, pp. 122–130, 2017.

[26] Pang, S. C., Chin, S. F., Nadirah, A., Tay, S. H., and Yazid, S. N. A. M., "Fabrication of polysaccharide-based nanoparticles as drug delivery nanocarrier," *The Electrochemical Society Transactions*, vol. 66, no. 37, pp. 15–32, 2015.

[27] Sonawane, S. J., Kalhapure, R. S., and Govender, T., "Hydrazone linkages in pH responsive drug delivery systems," *European Journal of Pharmaceutical Sciences*, vol. 99, pp. 45–65, 2017.

[28] Jong, K., Ju, B., and Zhang, S., "Synthesis of pH-responsive *N*-acetyl-cysteine modified starch derivatives for oral delivery," *Journal of Biomaterials Science, Polymer Edition*, vol. 14, pp. 1525–1537, 2017.

[29] Zhang, L., Sang, Y., Feng, J., Li, Z., and Zhao, A., "Polysaccharide-based micro/nanocarriers for oral colon-targeted drug delivery," *Journal of Drug Targeting*, vol. 24, no. 7, pp. 579–589, 2016.

[30] Pérez-Herrero, E., and Fernández-Medarde, A., "The reversed intra- and extracellular pH in tumors as a unified strategy to chemotherapeutic delivery using targeted nanocarriers," *Acta Pharmaceutica Sinica B*, vol. 11, no. 8, pp. 2243–2264, 2021.

[31] Wu, M., Cao, Z., Zhao, Y., Zeng, R., Tu, M., and Zhao, J., "Novel self-assembled pH-responsive biomimetic nanocarriers for drug delivery," *Materials Science and Engineering: C*, vol. 64, pp. 346–353, 2016.

[32] Rizwan, M., Yahya, R., Hassan, A., *et al.*, "pH Sensitive hydrogels in drug delivery: brief history, properties, swelling, and release mechanism, material selection and application," *Polymers*, vol. 9, no. 4, p. 37, 2017.

[33] Zohreh, N., Hosseini, S. H., and Pourjavadi, A., "Hydrazine-modified starch coated magnetic nanoparticles as an effective pH-responsive nanocarrier for doxorubicin delivery," *Journal of Industrial and Engineering Chemistry*, vol. 39, pp. 203–209, 2016.

[34] Pourjavadi, A., Tehrani, Z. M., and Hosseini, S. H., "Dendritic magnetite decorated by pH-responsive PEGylated starch: a smart multifunctional nanocarrier for the triggered release of anti-cancer drugs," *Royal Society of Chemistry Advances*, vol. 5, no. 60, p. 4858, 2015.

[35] Gomes, J. F., Garcia, A. C., Ferreira, E. B., *et al.*, "New insights into the formation mechanism of Ag, Au and AgAu nanoparticles in aqueous alkaline media: alkoxides from alcohols, aldehydes and ketones as universal reducing agents," *Physical Chemistry Chemical Physics*, vol. 17, no. 33, pp. 21683–21693, 2015.

[36] Li, L., Srivastava, S., Meng, S., Ting, J. M., and Tirrell, M. V., "Effects of non-electrostatic intermolecular interactions on the phase behavior of pH-sensitive polyelectrolyte complexes," *Macromolecules*, vol. 53, no. 18, pp. 7835–7844, 2020.

[37] Gierszewska, M., Ostrowska-Czubenko, J., and Chrzanowska, E., "pH-responsive chitosan/alginate polyelectrolyte complex membranes reinforced by tripolyphosphate," *European Polymer Journal*, vol. 101, pp. 282–290, 2018.

[38] Zhang, Z., Shan, H., Chen, L., He, C., Zhuang, X., and Chen, X., "Synthesis of pH-responsive starch nanoparticles grafted poly(L-glutamic acid) for insulin controlled release," *European Polymer Journal*, vol. 49, no. 8, pp. 2082–2091, 2013.

[39] Hosseinzadeh, H., and Ramin, S., "Magnetic and pH-responsive starch-g-poly (acrylic acid-coacrylamide)/graphene oxide superabsorbent nanocomposites: one-pot synthesis, characterization, and swelling behavior," *Starch*, vol. 68, nos. 3–4, pp. 200–212, 2016.

[40] Liu, L., Yao, W., Rao, Y., Lu, X., and Gao, J., "pH-responsive carriers for oral drug delivery: challenges and opportunities of current platforms," *Drug Delivery*, vol. 24, no. 1, pp. 569–581, 2017.

[41] Shadrack, D. M., Mubofu, E. B., and Nyandoro, S. S., "Synthesis of polyamidoamine dendrimer for encapsulating tetramethylscutellarein for potential bioactivity enhancement I 16(11)," *International Journal of Molecular Sciences*, vol. 16, pp. 26363–26377, 2015.

[42] Kuroiwa, T., Takada, H., Shogen, A., *et al.*, "Cross-linkable chitosan-based hydrogel microbeads with pH-responsive adsorption properties for organic dyes prepared using size-tunable microchannel emulsiemulsification technique," *Colloids and Surfaces A: Physicochemical and Engineering Aspects*, vol. 514, p. 69, 2017.

[43] Barbosa, A. I., Costa Lima, S. A., and Reis, S., "Application of pH-responsive fucoidan/chitosan nanoparticles to improve oral quercetin delivery," *Molecules*, vol. 24, no. 2, p. 346, 2019.

[44] Ahmed, T. A., and Aljaeid, B. M., "Preparation, characterization, and potential application of chitosan, chitosan derivatives, and chitosan metal

nanoparticles in pharmaceutical drug delivery," *Drug Design, Development and Therapy*, vol. 10, pp. 483–507, 2016.

[45] Liu, M., Du, H., Zhang, W., and Zhai, G., "Internal stimuli-responsive nanocarriers for drug delivery: design strategies and applications," *Materials Science and Engineering: C*, vol. 71, pp. 1267–1280, 2017.

[46] Chin, S. F., Romainor, A. N. B., Pang, S. C., Lee, B. K., and Hwang, S. S., "pH-responsive starch-citrate nanoparticles for controlled release of paracetamol," *Starch – Stärke*, vol. 71, nos. 9–10, p. 1800336, 2019.

[47] Ye, J., Luo, S., Huang, A., Chen, J., Liu, C., and McClements, D. J., "Synthesis and characterization of citric acid esterified rice starch by reactive by reactive extrusion: a new method of producing resistant starch," *Food Hydrocolloids*, vol. 92, pp. 135–142, 2019.

[48] Sukhija, S., Singh, S., and Riar, C. S., "Effect of oxidation, crosslinking and dual modification on physicochemical crystallinity, morphological, pasting and thermal characteristic of elephant food yam (*Amorphophallus paeoniifolius*) starch," *Food Hydrocolloids*, vol. 55, pp. 56–64, 2016.

[49] Menzel, C., Seisenbaeva, G., Agback, P., Gällstedt, M., Boldizar, A., and Koch, K., "Wheat starch carbamate: production, molecular characterization, and film forming properties," *Carbohydrate Polymers*, vol. 172, pp. 365–373, 2017.

[50] Awadhiya, A., Kumar, D., and Verma, V., "Crosslinking of agarose bioplastic using citric acid," *Carbohydrate Polymers*, vol. 151, pp. 60–67, 2016.

[51] Parent, M., Baradari, H., Champion, E., Damia, C., and Viana-Trecant, M., "Design of calcium phosphate ceramics for drug delivery applications in bone diseases: a review of the parameters affecting the loading and release of the therapeutic substance," *Journal of Controlled Release*, vol. 252, pp. 1–17, 2017.

[52] Sun, X., Dong, S., Li, X., *et al.*, "Delivery of siRNA using folate receptor-targeted pH-sensitive polymeric nanoparticles for rheumatoid arthritis therapy," *Biology and Medicine*, vol. 2, p. 102017, 2019.

[53] Goscianska, J., Ejsmont, A., Olejnik, A., Ludowicz, D., Stasiłowicz, A., and Cielecka-Piontek, J., "Design of paracetamol delivery systems based on mesoporous carbon," *Materials*, vol. 13, no. 8, p. 4151, 2020.

[54] Anirudhan, T. S., Gopal, S. S., and Sandeep, S., "Synthesis and characterization of montmorillonite/N-(carboxyacyl) chitosan coated magnetic particle nanocomposites for controlled delivery of paracetamol," *Applied Clay Science*, vol. 88, pp. 151–158, 2014.

[55] Gouda, R., Baishya, H., and Qing, Z., "Application of mathematical models in drug release kinetics of carbidopa and levodopa ER tablets," *Journal of Developing Drugs*, vol. 6, no. 2, p. 100071, 2017.

[56] Li, Y., and Yang, L., "Driving forces for drug loading in drug carriers. Journal of microencapsulation," vol. 32, no. 3, pp. 255–272, 2015.

[57] Badakhshanian, E., Hemmati, K., and Ghaemy, M., "Enhancement of mechanical properties of nanohydrogels based on natural gum with

functionalized multiwall carbon nanotube: study of swelling and drug release," *Polymer*, vol. 90, pp. 282–289, 2016.
[58] Wang, H., Poya, Y., Chen, X., Jia, T., Wang, X., and Shi, J., "Hydrogen peroxide as an oxidant in starch oxidation using molybdovanadophosphate for producing a high carboxylic content," *Royal Society of Chemistry Advances*, vol. 5, no. 57, pp. 45725–45730, 2015.
[59] Fan, J., Liu, F., and Wang, Z., "Shear rheology and in-vitro release kinetic study of apigenin from lyotropic liquid crystal," *International Journal of Pharmaceutics*, vol. 49, no. 1, pp. 248–254, 2016.
[60] Jiang, Q., Wang, J., Tang, R., Zhang, D., and Wang, X., "Hypromellose succinate-crosslinked chitosan hydrogel films for potential wound dressing," *International Journal of Biological Macromolecules*, vol. 91, p. 85091, 2016.
[61] Li, Y., and Wang, W. X., "Uptake, intracellular dissolution, and cytotoxicity of silver nanowires in cell models," *Chemosphere*, vol. 281, p. 30762, 2021.
[62] Dubey, A. K., Lavanya, L., Sadananda, D., Gouthami, K., Elfansu, K., and Singh, A., "Inferences of carbon dioxide in present-day cell culture systems: an unacknowledged problem and perspectives," *Austin Therapeutics*, vol. 1033, no. 10, p. 26420, 2021.

Chapter 21

E-Health on ankle rehabilitation

Andrew Anbarason[1], Buvanesh Annadurai[1] and Vinodhkumar Ramalingam[1]

Technology applications in health care provide extensive support for patient management, such as managing patients remotely via telerehabilitation, wearable devices, and mobile health applications. The reality of e-health in physiotherapy practice in a clinical setting is that it is steadily improving people's quality of life by enabling them to have healthier and more satisfying lives. Furthermore, e-health applications will aid in the monitoring of patients' progress by tracking their records in real time and motivating individuals during their rehabilitation. Lateral ankle sprains are a common condition reported in clinical settings among the elderly and sporting population that affect the mobility of an individual. Implementing e-health in ankle rehabilitation would provide patients with better support while they were undergoing rehabilitation [1].

21.1 Anatomy of ankle joint

The articulation of the talus, tibia, and fibula bones results in the hinged synovial joint that makes up the ankle. The ankle mortise is created by the three boundaries.

The lateral boundary of the ankle joint is formed by the articular facet of the lateral malleolus, a bony protrusion on the lower fibula.

The medial border of the joint is formed by the articular facet of the medial malleolus, a bony protrusion on the lower tibia.

The inferior articular surface of the tibia and the superior talar edge combine to form the upper part of the ankle joint.

The ankle joint plays a crucial role in ambulation because it adjusts to the surface one is walking on. The ankle joint provides movements in four directions: plantarflexion, dorsiflexion, inversion, and eversion, anterior, posterior, and lateral compartments make up the leg muscles.

The ankle joint is stabilized by these main supporting ligaments medially deltoid ligament, anterior & posterior talofibular, and laterally calcaneofibular ligament (Figure 21.1) [2].

[1]Saveetha College of Physiotherapy, SIMATS, India

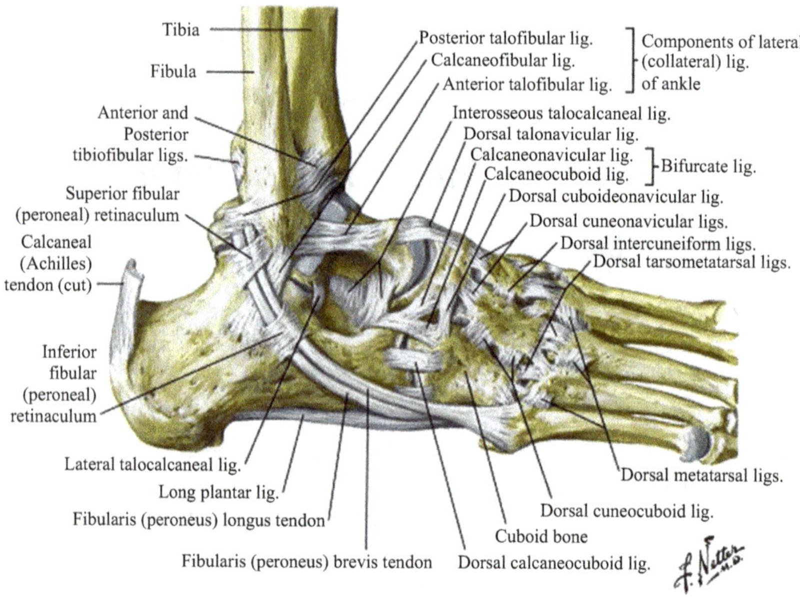

Figure 21.1 The lateral view of ankle joint anatomical structures

21.2 Biomechanics

The motion of the foot and ankle: plantarflexion and dorsiflexion, which occur in the sagittal plane, abduction and adduction, which occur in the transverse plane and inversion–eversion, which occur in the frontal plane, are the main movements of the ankle joint. Supination and pronation are three-dimensional movements produced when these motions are combined across the subtalar and tibiotalar joints as shown in Figure 21.2. The sole faces medially during supination as a result of a combination of plantarflexion, inversion, and adduction. Dorsiflexion, eversion, and abduction help to place the sole facing laterally during pronation.

The axis of rotation of the ankle: many believe the tibiotalar joint to be a straightforward hinge joint; some may say that it may really be multi-axial because of the internal rotation that occurs during dorsiflexion and the outward rotation that occurs during plantarflexion. The tibiotalar joint may be uniaxial, but there is evidence to suggest that its oblique axis is what causes the simultaneous motion that is observed. In the sagittal plane, the line connecting the medial and lateral malleoli serves as the axis of rotation for the ankle joint complex as shown in Figure 21.3. The intersection of the malleoli and the long axis of the tibia in the frontal plane serves as the axis of rotation for the coronal plane.

The long axis of the tibia intersects the midline of the foot to form the transverse plane axis of rotation as shown in Figure 21.4. The medial and lateral parts of the talus exhibit different radial curvatures, which have been highlighted in studies

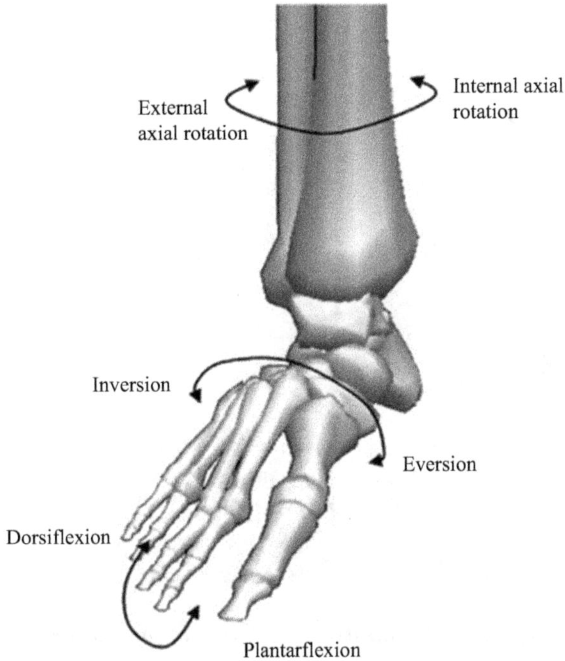

Figure 21.2 The ankle joint actions

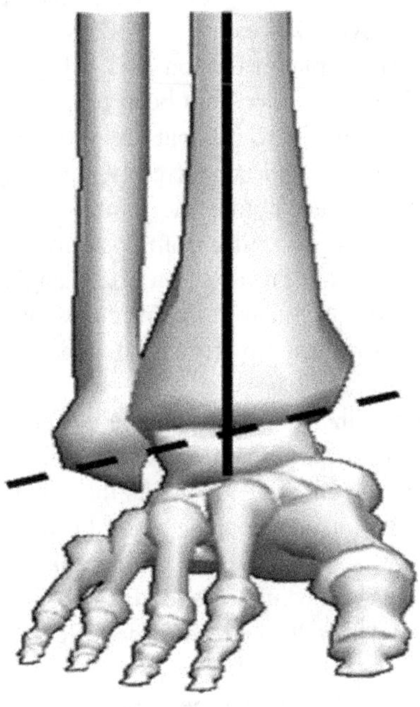

Figure 21.3 Sagittal and frontal plane axis of rotation for the ankle

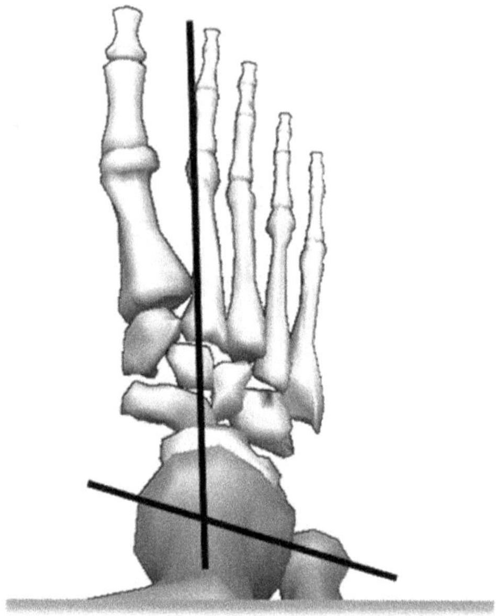

Figure 21.4 Ankle joint axis of rotation in the transverse plane

of the talar anatomy and suggests that the ankle joint's axis of rotation will shift as motion varies. This has led authors to suggest that the ankle joint can move in different directions during everyday exercise. A dorsiflexion axis, which is tilted downward and laterally, and a plantarflexion axis, which points upwards towards the lateral side of the ankle joint, have both been proposed since the 1950s. In the coronal plane, they can vary by up to 30° but are parallel in the transverse plane. These axes cannot be moved around concurrently, and it is thought that the transition between them happens just before the joint is in its neutral position. The subtalar joint's axis is also oblique, going from posterior to anterior and generating an angle of around 40° in the sagittal plane and a 23° angle in the transverse plane with the foot's midline. The subtalar joint produces numerous motions during plantar and dorsiflexion, resulting in pronation and supination, similar to the tibiotalar joint.

Range of motion: according to studies, people's everyday activities and differences in geography and culture can greatly affect the ankle range of motion (ROM).

The ankle ROM during locomotion involves the subtalar joint to complete the dorsiflexion and plantar flexion in the ankle joint. Further, the tibiotalar joint largely participates in plantar- and dorsiflexion during ankle motion, which primarily occurs in the sagittal plane. According to several studies, the range of motion in the sagittal plane ranges from 10 to 20 degrees of dorsiflexion to 40 to 55 degrees of plantarflexion.

A total of 35 degrees of motion can be made in the frontal plane (23° inversions and 12° eversions). However, the ROM needed for daily tasks is significantly less, with a maximum of 30° for walking and 37° for standing and 56° for stair climbing and stair lowering, respectively.

Gait analysis can be used to objectively measure the mobility of lower limb joints and forces acting on those joints, but it cannot measure upper limb joints. Due to the significant difficulty in precisely measuring talus motion with skin-mounted markers, the talocalcaneal (subtalar), tibiotalar (talocrural), and transverse-tarsal (talocalcaneonavicular) joints were separated. Gait analysis is nevertheless often employed, despite this drawback, to quantify the complicated kinematics and kinetics of the ankle joint [3].

21.3 Pathomechanics

With a lateral ankle sprain, the ATFL is the first ligament to sustain damage, with the CFL coming in second most frequently. Studies using cadaveric-sectioning have shown that when the ATFL is torn, the rearfoot's transverse-plane motion (internal rotation) significantly increases, placing additional strain on the ligaments that are still intact. When examining laxity patterns in the sprained ankle, it is common to overlook the "rotational instability" phenomenon of the ankle.

Also typical of lateral ankle sprains is a concurrent injury to the talocrural joint capsule and the ligamentous stabilisers of the subtalar joint.

Following total CFL disruption, Martin *et al.* found that the cervical ligament was subjected to noticeably increased tension.

Patients with acute lateral ankle sprains have been shown to have a subtalar joint injury up to 80% of the time. Only severe ankle sprains frequently result in PTFL injury, which is frequently accompanied by fractures, dislocations, or both.

According to a patho-mechanical model, Fuller described an increased supination moment at the subtalar joint is what causes lateral ankle sprains.

The position and strength of the vertically projected ground response force at first foot contact contribute to the enhanced supination moment. Fuller postulated that compared to a foot with a more lateral relationship between the centre of pressure (COP) and the joint axis, one with the COP medial to the subtalar-joint axis would experience a stronger supination moment from the vertical ground reaction force. After an acute injury, the ankle often swells, becomes tender, and hurts to move and bear weight on. Function normally returns over the period of a few days to a few months, depending on the severity of the injury. Recurrent ankle sprains are assumed to be caused by the same mechanism as first acute ankle sprains; however, negative changes that take place after the original injury are likely to predispose people to recurring sprains. Mechanical instability and functional instability have historically been proposed as two possible causes of CAI [4].

21.4 Incidence

Lateral ankle sprains are referred to as inversion ankle sprains or as supination ankle sprains. Men and women are thought to sustain lateral ankle sprains at

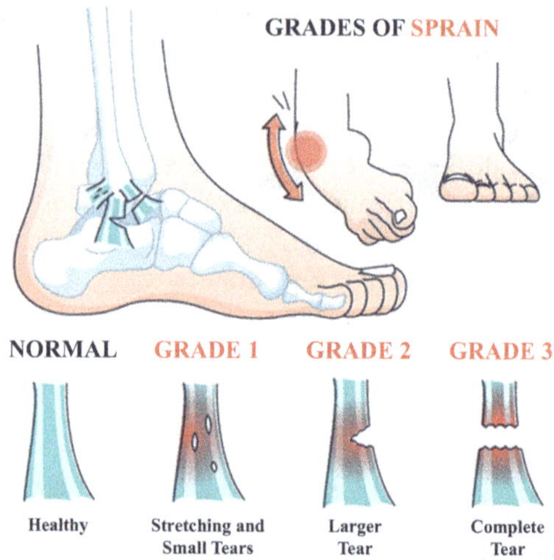

Figure 21.5 Grades of ankle sprain

roughly the same rates, but it has been reported that female interschool and university basketball players are 25% more likely than their male peers to sustain grade I ankle sprains. Despite the generally benign nature of the ankle sprain, 55–72% of patients still experience residual symptoms six weeks to eighteen months following the injury. Numerous recurrent ankle sprains have been linked to functional and mechanical instability, as well as an increased risk of reinjury.

The ligament sprains are graded as shown in Figure 21.5.

- Grade 1 – mild, painful, minimal tearing of the ligament fibers.
- Grade 2 – moderate, painful, significant tearing of the ligament fibers.
- Grade 3 – severe, sometimes not painful, complete rupture of the fibers.

Common problems addressed in rehabilitation were the following:

- Reducing swelling and pain.
- Improving the ankle range of motion.
- Strength training.
- Re-training of proprioception.
- Return to sports or return to functional activity.

21.5 Conventional management

21.5.1 Reducing swelling and pain

Within the first 48–72 h, initial management starts for acute lateral ligament to reduce pain and swelling following *PEACE AND LOVE.*

P – Protect
E – Elevate

A – Avoid anti-inflammatory modalities
C – Compression
E – Educate

PEACE Protocol is applied for the first 3 days and followed by *LOVE* Protocol to manage the acute condition of ankle sprains.

L – Load
O – Optimism
V – Vascularization
E – Exercise

21.5.2 Restoring range of motion

The patient moves with pain free active range of movement exercises such as ankle pumps, ankle inversion/eversion, ankle rotation & toe curls.

21.5.3 Rebuilding strength

Strength training for general population and athletic community. Less Intensity for General Population and Medium to High intense strength training for athletic population such as ankle exercises with resistance bands.

21.5.4 Proprioception

Training proprioception skills such as Tippy Toe Walk and Heel Walk were practiced to improve the patient coordination and overall dynamic stability in physical and sports activities.

The above exercise for patients is the common practice they need to undergo to improve the range of motion, strength, and proprioception in the injured ankle before resuming to full functional activity. On the other hand, if the athlete plans to resume sport, they need to be urged to tape or wear an ankle brace for an additional 6 months to give external support. Besides, they were trained for balance using the Wobble Board activities, Heel Toe Balance and Stork Balance [5].

21.6 E-Rehabilitation for ankle injuries

Electronic (E) rehabilitation involves the use of technology-based devices and tools to aid in the rehabilitation and recovery process for ankle injuries. It may include wearable devices for tracking progress, virtual reality exercises, and gamified therapy sessions to increase engagement and motivation. The goal is to improve outcomes, reduce recovery time, and enhance the overall rehabilitation experience for ankle injury patients [6,8,10].

21.7 E-Assessment for ankle injuries

E-assessment for ankle injuries involves the use of electronic devices and technologies to evaluate the functional status and injury severity of a patient's ankle.

This may include the use of wearable sensors to track range of motion, gait analysis software to assess walking patterns, and virtual reality simulations to evaluate balance and stability. The aim of e-assessment is to provide accurate, objective, and timely information to healthcare providers to inform diagnosis and treatment planning, and to monitor progress during the rehabilitation process [9].

21.8 E-Preventive measures for ankle injuries

E-preventive measures for ankle injuries involve the use of electronic technology and devices to help prevent the occurrence of ankle injuries. This may include wearable devices to monitor and track physical activity, virtual reality games for injury prevention and training, and online education platforms to provide information and guidance on safe exercise and movement practices. The goal of e-preventive measures is to improve awareness and understanding of risk factors, and promote healthy movement habits [7].

21.9 Conclusion

In conclusion, e-health technology plays an important role in the rehabilitation of ankle injuries, and in the present global tech support environment, its use is drastically increasing. By leveraging technology-based tools and devices, patients can receive effective and accessible rehabilitation services, whether it is through telerehabilitation, e-assessment, or e-preventive measures. The use of e-health in ankle rehabilitation has the potential to improve outcomes, increase patient engagement and satisfaction, and reduce recovery time. It also offers a cost-effective and convenient alternative to traditional in-person rehabilitation services. As technology continues to evolve, it is likely that the use of e-health in ankle rehabilitation will become more widespread, transforming the way patients receive care and recover from ankle injuries.

References

[1] Anton D, Berges I, Bermúdez J, Goñi A, and Illarramendi A. A telerehabilitation system for the selection, evaluation and remote management of therapies. *Sensors (Basel)*. 2018;18(5):1459. http://dx.doi.org/10.3390/s18051459

[2] Ankle Joint. *Physiopedia*. [cited 2023 Feb 24]. https://www.physio-pedia.com/Ankle_Joint

[3] Brockett CL and Chapman GJ. Biomechanics of the ankle. *Orthop Trauma*. 2016;30(3):232–8. http://dx.doi.org/10.1016/j.mporth.2016.04.015

[4] Hertel J. Functional anatomy, pathomechanics, and pathophysiology of lateral ankle instability. *J Athl Train*. 2002;37(4):364–75.

[5] Lateral Ligament Injury of the Ankle. *Physiopedia*. [cited 2023 Feb 25]. https://www.physio-pedia.com/Lateral_Ligament_Injury_of_the_Ankle.

[6] Karamians R, Proffitt R, Kline D, and Gauthier LV. Effectiveness of virtual reality- and gaming-based interventions for upper extremity rehabilitation poststroke: a meta-analysis. *Arch Phys Med Rehabil.* 2020;101(5):885–96. http://dx.doi.org/10.1016/j.apmr.2019.10.195

[7] Attia M and Taher MF. A wearable device for monitoring and prevention of repetitive ankle sprain. In: *2015 37th Annual International Conference of the IEEE Engineering in Medicine and Biology Society (EMBC)*. IEEE, 2015.

[8] Dicianno BE, Parmanto B, Fairman AD, *et al.* Perspectives on the evolution of mobile (mHealth) technologies and application to rehabilitation. *Phys Ther*. 2015;95(3):397–405. http://dx.doi.org/10.2522/ptj.20130534

[9] Wikstrom EA, Hubbard-Turner T, and McKeon PO. Understanding and treating lateral ankle sprains and their consequences: a constraints-based approach. *Sports Med.* 2013;43(6):385–93. http://dx.doi.org/10.1007/s40279-013-0043-z

[10] Cottrell MA and Russell TG. Telehealth for musculoskeletal physiotherapy. *Musculoskelet Sci Pract.* 2020;48(102193):102193. http://dx.doi.org/10.1016/j.msksp.2020.102193

Chapter 22

Medical equipment for back pain

Dineshwaran Naidu a/l K. Subramaniam[1] and Wai Yie Leong[1]

Back pain has become a major problem in most of the community, though those symptoms sometimes resolve on their own over time. In some people, the back pain normally resolves as soon as they rest their body by lying down or simply sitting on their favorite chair. Some of them even attend massage centers or physiotherapy to ease their pain that is not resolved with simple sitting and lying down. The pain should be more concerning when none of these methods ease the pain away and make it even worse. In many severe cases, a phenomenon known as sciatica occurs, where the back pain usually radiates to your legs, causing muscle strain and making it harder for you to even walk or sit. On the bright side, some medical equipment has been and is being built in order to help those people with unresolved back pain. Back pain is one of the most prevalent pain disorders, with significant individual and social implications [1]. Back pain or lower back pain, commonly known as LBP, is defined based on the length of the pain symptoms, with acute pain lasting less than 4 weeks, subacute pain lasting between 4 and 12 weeks, and chronic back pain lasting more than 12 weeks [2]. Despite the fact that many patients heal completely with no residual abnormalities, 15–20% of patients continue to experience pain symptoms after 12 weeks [2,3]. Surgery to repair any damage to the spine is rarely the first option unless the damage or injury is pervasive that it is beyond repair. Despite the fact that each major or minor spine injury may be treated surgically, there are several restrictions to spinal surgery. According to Bajwa and Haldar [4], the subject of pain is always brought up when considering back surgery. Most surgeries are performed in the belief that the discomfort would go away. In many circumstances, surgery does not relieve pain, particularly in the long run. Often, the freedom to move and the suffering worsen. Whenever a person's motion is restricted, the regions adjacent to it must make up for the shortfall and work harder. Because of the added tension, the surrounding regions become weary much faster. Moreover, when motion is restricted post-spinal surgery, the patient will have to sit or lie down for a very long period as part of the recovery. When this happens, the patients are at high risk for developing deep vein thrombosis as there

[1]Graduate School of Medicine, Perdana University, Malaysia

will be a blood clot formation in the leg area which will lead to unbearable pain and swelling of the posterior thigh of the leg. The clots will eventually block the blood vessels supplying the leg and prevent them from being properly perfused with blood. In extreme cases, the clots might break into tiny pieces and travel throughout the blood vessels and may eventually end up in the lungs or brain leading to pulmonary embolism, risk of stroke, or even death. Besides surgical repair, many medical equipment that are solely meant for the spine can be widely used to correct and facilitate some minor and non-invasive injuries to the spine.

22.1 Transcutaneous electrical nerve stimulation (TENS)

TENS is a small-scaled device that comprises electrode wires and sticky patches at the end that can be adhesively placed on the desired skin area. According to Gibson *et al.* [5], transcutaneous electrical nerve stimulation (TENS) is a therapeutic application of electrical nerve stimulation through the skin. It primarily treats pain in people suffering from miscellaneous acute and chronic pain problems.

As illustrated by Figure 22.1 below, TENS gadgets usually utilize battery-powered adhesive electrodes placed on the skin's surface to deliver pulsed electrical stimulation that may be adjusted in frequency (stimulation rate), intensity, and endurance [6]. Similarly, Johnson *et al.* [7] have stated that transcutaneous electrical nerve stimulation (TENS) is a conventional pain-relieving non-invasive peripheral stimulation therapy that delivers pulsed electrical currents over the entire skin surface to trigger and activate the underlying nerves to ease the pain. Johnson *et al.* [7] also stated that TENS could be classified into three techniques, which are conventional TENS, acupuncture-like TENS, and intense TENS. TENS

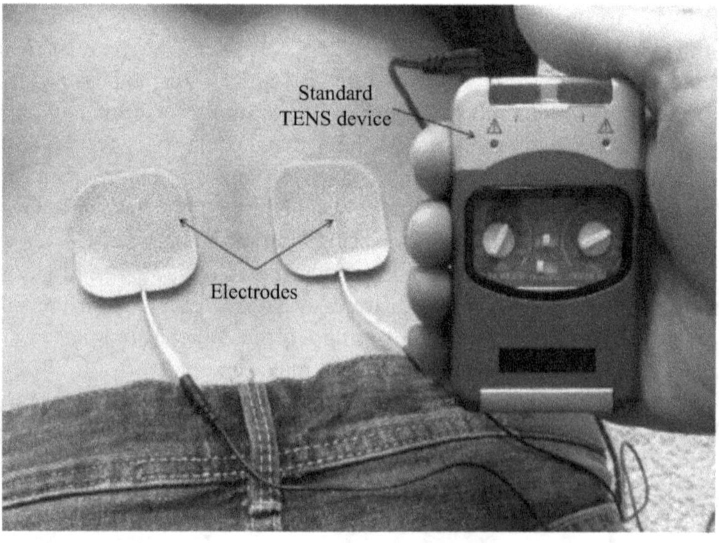

Figure 22.1 A TENS device placed on the lower back [8]

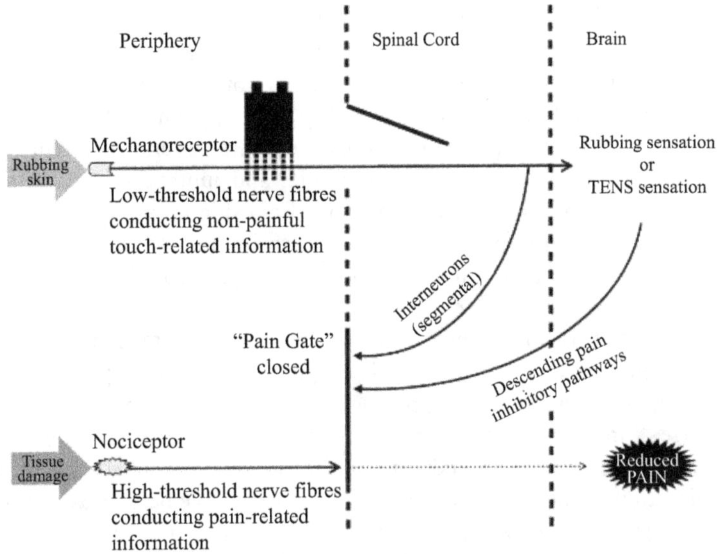

Figure 22.2 TENS generates low-threshold afferent waves that carry non-painful touch-related information to the brain leading to the closing of the pain gate and pain-related fibers are blocked with TENS sensation of low-threshold afferent fibers [8]

produces firm but comfortable TENS paresthesia by eliciting segmental analgesia by preferentially triggering large diaphragms whenever there is pain at a specific site [7].

According to Figure 22.2, TENS is administered in a high-intensity and low-frequency mode that will induce extra segmental analgesia by causing muscle spasms and activating small-diameter motor afferents, whereas the intense TENS is provided in a high-intensity and high-frequency mode that triggers peripheral nerve blocking and extra segmental analgesia by activating small-diameter noxious afferents. Moreover, the TENS device is self-administrable and affordable as the patients or individuals can just follow the instructions given by the physiotherapists or manual so that they can operate it on their own. TENS is a non-invasive method of pain relief. People who get pain relief via TENS may be able to cut back on pain drugs, some of which might be addictive or have adverse side effects. TENS devices are also useful since they are compact, portable, and generally inconspicuous. People can carry a TENS unit in their pocket or clip it to their belts to enjoy instant pain relief throughout the day.

22.2 Spinal orthoses

In Greek, the word orthoses represents "straightening" in lame end terms known as braces. Spinal orthoses, often known as braces, are prostheses used to straighten and support the spine. Cervical orthoses were documented in the fifth Egyptian dynasty, and thoracic bandages were used to cure scoliosis in the mid-eighteenth century [9]. To date, various external spinal orthoses are medically being used as a method of management among those patients with various spinal disorders. According to Agabegi *et al.* [10], there are several different types of braces available to assist the cervical, thoracic, and lumbar spines, along with junctional areas that require unique mechanical consideration. The primary biomechanical purpose of these spinal orthoses is to immobilize a motion segment and relieve pressure on that spine segment and also to provide complete touch, three-point pressure, endpoint control, or heightened pressure as a kinesthetic reminder. As stated by Jones and Uustal [9], most spinal braces require a minimum of three-point pressure control, which in turn requires three points of contact on a certain plane with balanced opposing pressures. A three-point pressure system comprises three forces: one applied via the rotation axis, one applied from underneath the rotation axis, and one applied above the rotation axis in the opposite direction as the other two forces [11]. There have been pressure-tolerant tissues and pressure-intolerant tissues, such as those found around the nerves or bony protrusions. The capacity to endure pressure can be altered by adjusting the length of the lever arm or altering the size of the contact pad. Because the pressure to an area is calculated by multiplying force by distance, the longer the lever arm, the less pressure per square area is necessary to regulate forces around a joint. Hence, expanding pressure points is critical for increasing patient comfort and reducing discomfort. Unfortunately, improper or incorrect spinal orthoses application may lead to therapy failure and contribute to severe trauma with long-standing complications. As reported by Agabegi *et al.* [10], the inability to change one's body posture in reaction to severe external pressure, whether due to cognitive impairment or a lack of protective feeling, is a relative contraindication to using spinal orthoses. Furthermore, extreme pressure will contribute to soft-tissue contractures due to limited movement. Long-term use of spinal orthoses also may lead to osteopenia [9]. Finally, another major and most common contraindication that can be related to spinal orthoses is the entrapment of moisture underneath the braces if they were left for a long period which will lead to loss of skin integrity or in much worse case ulcers.

Types of spinal orthoses

1. Semirigid spinal orthoses (corsets)

According to Weppner and Alfano [12], corsets are commercially available and come in a variety of shapes, sizes, and materials. The design of a corset is determined by the body part that needs to be stabilized, the degree of control required, and the patient's anatomical measurements.

These semirigid spinal orthoses are corsets, which have an inelastic construction made of supple canvas, cotton, or Dacron, and fortification with both hard and flexible supports, which can partially immobilize the spine. These types of spinal orthoses can be used to relieve any lumbosacral muscular strain and eventually manage spinal lordosis. Hence, the corsets can be worn in such a way that the

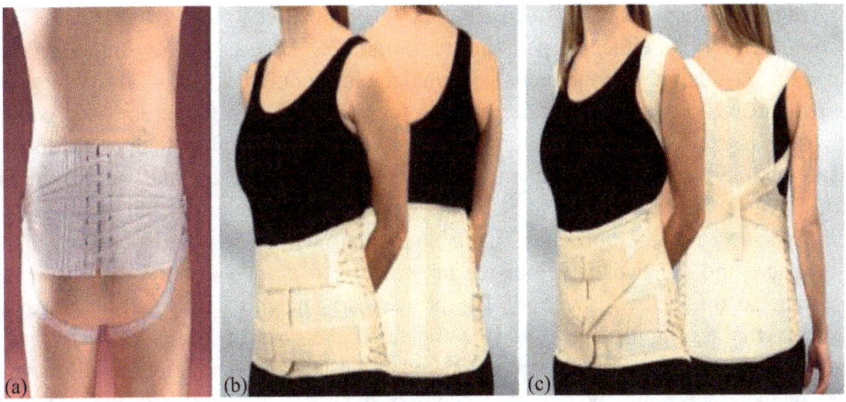

Figure 22.3 The types of semirigid spinal orthoses: (a) Sacroiliac; (b) Lumbosacral; and (c) Thoracolumbosacral (dorsolumbar) [12]

tightness increases the intraabdominal pressure leading to lower axial strain on the vertebral bodies and abdominal support [12]. As shown in Figure 22.3(a), the sacroiliac corset provides support solely to the pelvic region which covers the endpoints that are lower than the waist and higher than the pubis surrounding the pelvis. For minor disorders, sacroiliac corsets are normally used to slightly enhance the abdominal circumferential pressure and support the sacral joint only as these corsets provide very little spinal stabilization. Unlike the sacroiliac corset, the lumbosacral corset from Figure 22.3(b) accounts for a three-point pressure system while raising intracavitary pressure in the abdomen along the inferior angle of the scapula to the sacrococcygeal junction posteriorly, superior to the pubic symphysis and inferior to the xiphoid process' inferior boundary anteriorly [12]. As for the thoracolumbosacral corsets, see from Figure 22.3(c).

For minor disorders, corsets are normally used to slightly enhance belly circumferential pressure. Corsets provide very little spinal support.

1. Rigid spinal orthoses
2. Cervical orthoses
3. Orthoses for spinal deformity

22.3 Spinal decompression table and traction therapy

According to Choi *et al.* [13], around 80% of individuals encounter lumbar pain at least once in their lives, and intervertebral discs are responsible for 80% of lumbar pain structures. Intervertebral disc herniation can be usually treated using both surgical and non-surgical approaches whereas traction treatment is one of the most often utilized procedures. Traction therapy ultimately relieves the pressure imposed by gravity and soft tissues, and enough tension allows spinal separation and the intervertebral disc to be extended. Negative pressure inside the intervertebral disc promotes hydration and relieves nerve root pressure by decreasing the force imparted to the vertebral pulp. The traction therapy can either be periodic relaxation with cycles of a few minutes, sustained for 20–60 min, or continuously maintained for hours to days [14]. It may also be classified based on the principal force's direction, whether axial (superoinferior axis of the spine) or distracting (axial force combined with off-axis forces such as flexion or lateral bending). In short, the patients will be fastened to the table and various props, such as cushions, are utilized to keep the patient comfortable and the spine in the proper position for decompression. The table program will be activated after the patient is in place, and the two halves of the table begin to draw away from one another according to the desired direction. The primary advantage of spinal decompression therapy is that it is highly less invasive compared to the surgical approaches that can be done to decompress a spine. When compared to surgical interventions, spinal decompression therapy is a method that has recently been used as a conservative treatment for intervertebral disc herniation [13]. Another major benefit of this spinal traction therapy is that it will create negative pressure within the intervertebral discs and relieves the pressure that might be compressing the nerves or other spinal cord structures. This eventually will prevent or reduce the risk of permanent damage to the spinal components that might give out unpleasant symptoms to the patients. Furthermore, the negative pressure also will make sure that the spinal cord structures are properly hydrated with the cerebrospinal fluid surrounding it which is rich in oxygen and nutrients required for maintaining a healthy spine.

References

[1] Gore, M., Sadosky, A., Stacey, B. R., Tai, K.-S., and Leslie, D. (2012). The burden of chronic low back pain: clinical comorbidities, treatment patterns, and health care costs in usual care settings. *Spine*, 37(11):E668–E677.

[2] Chou, R. (2010). Low back pain (chronic). *BMJ Clinical Evidence*, 2010:1116.

[3] Chou, R., Gordon, D. B., de Leon-Casasola, O. A., *et al.* (2016). Management of postoperative pain: a clinical practice guideline from the American Pain Society, the American Society of Regional Anesthesia and Pain Medicine, and the American Society of Anesthesiologists' Committee on Regional Anesthesia, Executive Committee, and Administrative Council. *The Journal of Pain*, 17(2):131–157.

[4] Bajwa, S. J. S., and Haldar, R. (2015). Pain management following spinal surgeries: an appraisal of the available options. *Journal of Craniovertebral Junction & Spine*, 6(3):105–110.

[5] Gibson, W., Wand, B. M., Meads, C., Catley, M. J., and O'Connell, N. E. (2019). Transcutaneous electrical nerve stimulation (TENS) for chronic pain – an overview of Cochrane Reviews. *Cochrane Database of Systematic Reviews*. https://doi.org/10.1002/14651858.cd011890.pub3

[6] Johnson, M. I., and Bjordal, J. M. (2011). Transcutaneous electrical nerve stimulation for the management of painful conditions: focus on neuropathic pain. *Expert Review of Neurotherapeutics*, 11(5):735–753.

[7] Johnson, M. (2007). Transcutaneous electrical nerve stimulation: mechanisms, clinical application and evidence. *Reviews in Pain*, 1(1):7–11.

[8] Johnson, M. I. (2014). *Transcutaneous Electrical Nerve Stimulation (TENS): Research to Support Clinical Practice*. Oxford University Press.

[9] Jones, P. S. and Uustal, H. (n.d.). *Spinal Orthoses: Principles, Designs, Indications, and Limitations*. https://medicine.missouri.edu/sites/default/files/pm-r/Jones_Article_CH38SpinalOrthoses3rdEd0037_v1.pdf

[10] Agabegi, S. S., Asghar, F. A., Herkowitz, H. N. (2010). Spinal orthoses. *American Academy of Orthopaedic Surgeon*, 18(11):657–667.

[11] Kadhim, F. M. and Al-Din Tahir, M. S. (2020). Design and analysis of three-point pressure for varus foot deformity. *Journal of Biomimetics, Biomaterials and Biomedical Engineering*, 45:1–11.

[12] Weppner, J. L., and Alfano, A. P. (2019). Principles and components of spinal orthoses. In: *Atlas of Orthoses and Assistive Devices* (pp. 69–89.e2). Philadelphia, PA: Elsevier.

[13] Choi, J., Lee, S., and Hwangbo, G. (2015). Influences of spinal decompression therapy and general traction therapy on the pain, disability, and straight leg raising of patients with intervertebral disc herniation. *Journal of Physical Therapy Science*, 27(2):481–483.

[14] Gay, R. E. and Brault, J. S. (2012). Traction therapy. In *Evidence-Based Management of Low Back Pain*, New York, NY: Elsevier, pp. 205–215. https://doi.org/10.1016/b978-0-323-07293-9.00015-5

Index

www.ingramcontent.com/pod-product-compliance
Lightning Source LLC
LaVergne TN
LVHW011839200926
848484LV00002B/375